Nephrology: Diagnosis and Treatment of Kidney Diseases

Nephrology: Diagnosis and Treatment of Kidney Diseases

Editor: Adriana Jones

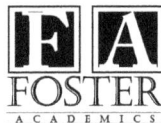

FA FOSTER
ACADEMICS

www.fosteracademics.com

www.fosteracademics.com

FA Foster
ACADEMICS

Cataloging-in-Publication Data

Nephrology : diagnosis and treatment of kidney diseases / edited by Adriana Jones.
   p. cm.
Includes bibliographical references and index.
ISBN 978-1-63242-964-3
1. Nephrology. 2. Kidneys--Diseases. 3. Kidneys--Diseases--Diagnosis.
4. Kidneys--Diseases--Treatment. I. Jones, Adriana.
RC902 .N47 2020

616.61--dc23

Foster Academics,
118-35 Queens Blvd., Suite 400,
Forest Hills, NY 11375, USA

ISBN 978-1-63242-964-3 (Hardback)

Contents

Permissions

List of Contributors

Index

Preface

This book has been an outcome of determined endeavour from a group of educationists in the field. The primary objective was to involve a broad spectrum of professionals from diverse cultural background involved in the field for developing new researches. The book not only targets students but also scholars pursuing higher research for further enhancement of the theoretical and practical applications of the subject.

Nephrology is a field of medicine which is concerned with the evaluation of kidney function, diagnosis and treatment of kidney diseases, and preservation of kidney health. The kidneys can be affected by a host of pathological conditions such as kidney diseases and systemic conditions. Kidney diseases can also cause various systemic diseases, like renal osteodystrophy and hypertension. Kidney diseases include chronic kidney disease, acute kidney injury, nephritic and nephrotic syndromes, and pyelonephritis. The chemical and microscopic analysis of the urine, kidney biopsy and CT scan, and measurement of kidney function through serum creatinine tests are common techniques of diagnosing kidney diseases. Kidney transplantation or dialysis may be required to treat kidney failure, while in cases of renal carcinoma, nephrectomy may be performed. The various studies that are constantly contributing towards advancing technologies and evolution of nephrology are examined in detail in this book. Its objective is to give a general view of the different types of kidney diseases, and their diagnosis and treatment. This book includes contributions of experts and scientists which will provide innovative insights into this field.

It was an honour to edit such a profound book and also a challenging task to compile and examine all the relevant data for accuracy and originality. I wish to acknowledge the efforts of the contributors for submitting such brilliant and diverse chapters in the field and for endlessly working for the completion of the book. Last, but not the least; I thank my family for being a constant source of support in all my research endeavours.

Editor

ANKS1B is a smoking-related molecular alteration in clear cell renal cell carcinoma

Jeanette E Eckel-Passow[1], Daniel J Serie[2], Brian M Bot[3], Richard W Joseph[4], John C Cheville[5] and Alexander S Parker[2*]

Abstract

Background: An association between cigarette smoking and increased risk of clear cell renal cell carcinoma (ccRCC) has been established; however, there are limited data regarding the molecular mechanisms that underlie this association. We used a multi-stage design to identify and validate genes that are associated with smoking-related ccRCC.

Methods: We first conducted a microarray study to compare gene expression patterns in patient-matched ccRCC and normal kidney tissues between patients with (n = 23) and without (n = 42) a history of smoking. Analyses were first stratified on obesity status (the other primary risk factor for ccRCC) and then combined and analyzed together. To identify genes where the fold change in smokers relative to non-smokers was different in tumor tissues in comparison to patient-matched normal kidney tissues, we identified Affymetrix probesets that had a significant tissue type-by-smoking status interaction pvalue. We then performed RT-PCR validation on the top eight candidate genes in an independent sample of 28 smokers and 54 non-smokers.

Results: We identified 15 probesets that mapped to eight genes that had candidate associations with smoking-related ccRCC: ANKS1B, ACOT6, PPWD1, EYS, LIMCH1, CHRNA6, MT1G, and ZNF600. Using RT-PCR, we validated that expression of ANKS1B is preferentially down-regulated in smoking-related ccRCC.

Conclusion: We provide the first evidence that ANKS1B expression is down regulated in ccRCC tumors relative to patient-matched normal kidney tissue in smokers. Thus, ANKS1B should be explored further as a novel avenue for early detection as well as prevention of ccRCC in smokers.

Background

Currently, cigarette smoking is an established risk factor for the development of clear cell renal cell carcinoma (ccRCC) [1]. Indeed, authors of a meta-analysis involving 26 epidemiologic studies spanning 37 years concluded that the risk of ccRCC among ever smokers is approximately 40% higher compared to lifetime never smokers [2]. From a population-based perspective, previous investigators have suggested that cigarette smoking alone accounts for approximately 20-25% of the ccRCCs diagnosed in the U.S. [3,4]. While smoking is an established risk factor for ccRCC, what remain unclear are the specific somatic molecular alterations that underlie this well-reported association. Identification of specific alterations at the cellular level that link smoking to ccRCC development

has the potential to further solidify a causal association, advance our understanding of the etiology of this disease and possibly extend even further into more focused measures of early detection and prevention.

To address the need to better understand the molecular underpinnings of smoking-related ccRCC, we sought to identify candidate genes that are differentially expressed in ccRCC tumors that develop in smokers compared to non-smokers. Thus, we employed the Affymetrix U133 Plus 2.0 platform to compare somatic gene expression profiles between patient-matched ccRCC and normal kidney tissues from patients with and without a history of smoking, controlling for obesity status (the other primary risk factor for ccRCC [4,5]). Although other risk factors have been reported in the literature, smoking and obesity are the only epidemiological risk factors that have been consistently validated as increasing risk of ccRCC. Following our microarray-based discovery efforts, we then validated our top candidate genes by employing RT-PCR on an independent set of ccRCC and patient-matched normal kidney tissue samples from smokers and non-

* Correspondence: parker.alexander@mayo.edu
[2]Department of Health Sciences Research, Mayo Clinic, 4500 San Pablo Road, Jacksonville, FL 32224, USA
Full list of author information is available at the end of the article

smokers. Using this multi-stage design, we report that ANKS1B is a smoking-related alteration in ccRCC.

Methods
Ethics statement
This study was approved by the Mayo Clinic Institutional Review Board. All participants provided written consent to participate in this study.

Overview
For this investigation, we employed a multi-stage design that allowed us to take into account potential confounding effects of obesity, the other consistently-reported risk factor of ccRCC [5], and seek validation of our top candidate genes. Briefly, in stage 1 we only considered non-obese subjects and used the Affymetrix platform on patient-matched ccRCC and normal kidney tissues from smokers and non-smokers to identify candidate smoking-related gene expression changes in ccRCC. In stage 2, we again used the Affymetrix platform on patient-matched ccRCC and normal kidney tissues from smokers and non-smokers; however, this time we included only obese subjects. That is, we aimed to identify smoking-related genes that were not dependent on obesity status. With the list of candidate genes narrowed down, in stage 3 we performed RT-PCR validation on the top candidates in an independent set of patient-matched ccRCC and normal kidney tissues. We provide more detail on the design and selection of the subjects for each stage in the sections below.

Patient selection
Stage 1: Affymetrix microarrays on non-obese ccRCC subjects
The objective of stage 1 was to perform a genome-wide scan and identify candidate genes that are associated with smoking-related ccRCC. To do so, we compared gene expression between patients with and without a history of smoking across patient-matched tumor and normal kidney samples. Upon approval from our Institutional Review Board, we identified patients treated with radical nephrectomy or nephron-sparing surgery for unilateral, sporadic ccRCC between 2000 and 2006 from our Nephrectomy Registry. We then excluded all patients with a body mass index (BMI) > 30 kg/m^2 as well as patients with late stage tumors (pT4) and patients with high-grade tumors (grade 4). The decision to remove patients with a BMI > 30 in stage 1 was based on the fact that obesity represents the only other widely reproducible risk factor for ccRCC development and thus we wanted to match by obesity status. The removal of late-stage and high-grade subjects was based on our desire in stage 1 to identify changes that occur early in ccRCC carcinogenesis. Based on these criteria, we identified 46 non-obese subjects that had both fresh-frozen normal kidney and tumor tissue

available for study; 16 of which had a history of smoking and 30 had no history of smoking. We obtained smoking data from risk factor questionnaires completed at time of surgery and from medical chart review where necessary. Using these data, we defined non-smokers as anyone who reported never smoking cigarettes on the questionnaire or to their physician during a standard patient history taken prior to surgery. For smokers, we required that the subject report greater than 20 pack-years of smoking on either the questionnaire or during the patient history.

Stage 2: Affymetrix microarrays on obese ccRCC subjects
As noted above, because obesity is the other widely acceptable risk factor and we wanted to identify molecular markers that were not dependent on obesity status, we performed a two-stage design stratifying by obesity status. Thus, we repeated our design and analysis from stage 1 but this time we only used obese subjects. Our rationale for this second stage of discovery is that by moving into an obese population we would have the opportunity to further screen the candidates from stage 1 by looking for genes that still have a smoking-related expression signal even among subjects with another primary risk factor for ccRCC. The subjects in stage 2 were similar to stage 1 (i.e. unilateral, sporadic, pT stage 1-3, grade 1-3) with the exception that they all had a BMI > 30 kg/m^2 at time of surgery. As such, stage 2 consisted of 19 obese ccRCC subjects that had both fresh-frozen normal kidney and tumor tissue available for study; 7 of which had a history of smoking and 12 had no history of smoking. We used the same criteria to define smokers and non-smokers as described above for stage 1.

Stage 3: RT-PCR validation on non-obese ccRCC subjects
With our discovery-based steps complete, the objective of stage 3 was to seek independent validation of the candidate genes we identified in stages 1-2. The patients in stage 3 consisted of 82 non-obese patients that had both fresh-frozen normal kidney and tumor tissue available for study; 28 of which had a history of smoking and 54 had no history of smoking. For this important validation step we moved back into the setting of only evaluating non-obese patients to allow for the most robust chance of validation. For this validation stage, we used the same criteria to define smokers and non-smokers as described above for stage 1.

Tissue preparation and laboratory assays
Tissue samples
An experienced urologic pathologist identified fresh-frozen blocks with representative tumor and normal kidney tissue for each patient involved in stages 1-3. For those patients with a ccRCC tumor that showed mixed grade, the study pathologist selected the block with the highest grade

tumor for dissection. After the appropriate blocks were selected, a histotechnologist macrodissected two five-micron sections from each of the fresh-frozen tumor and corresponding normal kidney tissue blocks. The Mayo Biospecimen Accessioning and Processing Core performed RNA extractions using kits and protocols from the Qiagen miRNEasy kit and Qiagen Qiacube instrument. The RNA was DNAse treated on the column prior to elution. We assessed RNA quantity and quality using Nanodrop Spectrophotometer and Agilent.

Affymetrix microarrays
Microarray analysis was conducted according to manufacturer's instructions for the Affymetrix One Cycle Target Labeling and Control Reagents kit (Santa Clara, CA). Briefly, cDNA was generated from five micrograms of total RNA using SuperScript II reverse transcriptase (Invitrogen, Carlsbad, CA) and T7 Oligo(dT) primer. Subsequently, the products were column-purified (Affymetrix) and then *in vitro* transcribed to generate biotin-labeled cRNA. The IVT products were then column-purified, fragmented, and hybridized onto Affymetrix U133 Plus 2.0 GeneChips® at 45°C for 16 h. Subsequent to hybridization, the arrays were washed and stained with streptavidin-phycoerythrin, then scanned in an Affymetrix GeneChip® Scanner 3000 (Santa Clara, CA). All control parameters were confirmed to be within normal ranges before normalization was initiated. The data discussed in this publication have been deposited in NCBI's Gene Expression Omnibus and are accessible through GEO Series accession number GSE46699 (http://www.ncbi.nlm.nih.gov/geo/query/acc.cgi?acc=GSE46699).

Microarray data normalization and statistical methods
The data used herein are comprised of two batches of samples that were processed at two different time periods (see Supplementary Methods in [6]). Base-2 logarithm transformed intensity data from the two batches of samples were normalized within each batch using frozen robust multi-array analysis (frozen RMA) [7]. Frozen RMA was specifically designed to preprocess arrays in batches and subsequently allow the data to be combined for downstream analyses.

The samples used in stage 1 and stage 2 are shown in Figure 1. Stage 1 and stage 2 data were analyzed separately and then combined and analyzed as a whole. Linear mixed models were fit to the normalized intensity data for each probeset. Within the linear mixed model, tissue type (tumor/normal), smoking status (smoker/non-smoker) and a smoking status-by-tissue type interaction were included as fixed effects while a random intercept was fit on a per patient basis to account for the patient-matched tumor and normal samples. The smoking status-by-tissue type interaction was included to identify probesets where

the fold change between smokers versus non-smokers was different in tumor in comparison to normal tissue. Probesets with a smoking status-by-tissue type interaction p-value <0.01 in stage 1 were identified as having a potential association with smoking-specific alterations in ccRCC and therefore were determined to be good candidates for further evaluation in stage 2. We acknowledge that this p-value threshold does not account for multiple testing at the conservative Bonferroni level. However, probesets that are consistently identified in stage 1 at this nominal significance and subsequently in stage 2 with a smoking status-by-tissue type interaction pvalue <0.05 and then maintained a smoking status-by-tissue type interaction p-value <0.01 in the analysis of the combined data were deemed to be good candidates for further validation in stage 3. To determine how the fold change differed across tumor and normal specimens, we also calculated the fold change of normalized expression for smokers versus non-smokers in normal tissue as well as the fold change of smokers versus non-smokers tumor tissue. All statistical tests were performed using a Linux release of R version 2.14. All probeset-to-gene mapping was done using the hgu133plus2.db (version 2.9.0).

Gene expression by fluidigm quantitative PCR
Samples were reverse transcribed according to the manufacturer's instructions for the High Capacity Reverse Transcription kit (Applied Biosystems, Foster City, CA). Briefly, 50 ng of total RNA was reverse transcribed in a 20 μl reaction mixture containing 0.8 μl of 100 nM dNTP, 2.0 μl RT buffer, 1.0 μl of reverse transcriptase (50U/μl), 2 μl of RT primer. The reaction mixture was mixed and incubated as follows; 25°C for 10 min, 37°C for 2 h, and then 85°C for 5 min, followed by a 4°C hold. Pre-amplification of cDNA was initiated by creating a pool of 24 TaqMan mRNA Assays at a final concentration of 0.2X for each assay. The pre-PCR amplification reaction was then performed in a 5 μl reaction mixture containing 2.5 μl TaqMan PreAmp Master Mix (2X), 1.25 μl of 24-pooled TaqMan assay mix (0.2X) and 1.25 μl of cDNA. The pre-amplification PCR was performed according to the following cycling conditions: one cycle 95°C for 10 min, 14 cycles at 95°C for 15 sec and then 60°C for 4 min. After pre-amplification PCR, the product was diluted 1:5 with dH$_2$O and stored at -20°C until needed for amplification.

Quantitative PCR of the mRNA targets was carried out using the 48.48 dynamic array (Fluidigm, South San Francisco, CA) following the manufacturer's protocol. Briefly, a 5 μl sample mixture was prepared for each sample containing 2x TaqMan Universal Master Mix (with UNG), 20X GE Sample Loading Reagent and each of diluted pre-amplified cDNA. Five microliters of Assay mix was prepared with one 20X TaqMan mRNA assay

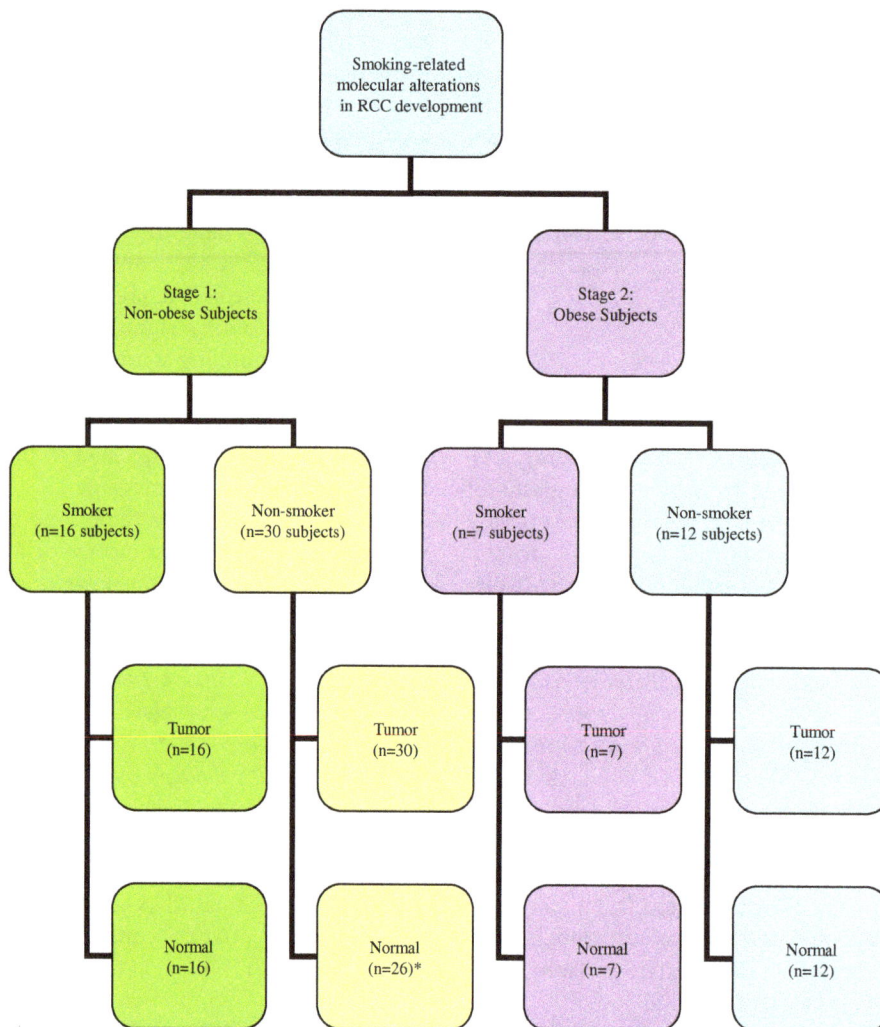

Figure 1 Experimental design for stage 1 and stage 2. *Normal tissue did not pass RNA or microarray quality-control metrics for 4 normal tissue samples.

(final concentration 10x) and 2X Assay Loading Reagent. The dynamic array was primed with control line fluid in the IFC controller and samples and assay mixes was loaded into the appropriate inlets. The chip was then returned to the IFC controller for loading and mixing, and then placed in the BioMark Instrument for PCR at 50°C for 2 min and 95°C for 10 min, followed by 40 cycles at 95°C for 15 sec and 60°C for 1 min. The data were analyzed with the Real-Time PCR Analysis Software (Fluidigm, South San Francisco, CA).

RT-PCR data normalization and statistical methods
Normalization was carried out as discussed previously [8]. In brief, the negative CT (denoted hereafter as -CT) values for the two control genes (POLR2A and ACTB) were averaged on a per sample basis and the average was subtracted from the -CT value for each sample. As was done for the Affymetrix microarray data, linear mixed models were fit

to the normalized −CT data for each gene. Within the linear mixed model, tissue type (tumor/normal), smoking status (smoker/non-smoker) and a smoking status-by-tissue type interaction were included as fixed effects while a random intercept was fit on a per patient basis.

Results
Patient characteristics
We provide a comparison of demographic and clinical characteristics between smokers and non-smokers for the patients in each of the three stages of our study in Table 1. Although in all three stages there was a trend for smokers to more likely be male than the non-smokers, this trend was only statistically significant in stage 3. In contrast, we observed no differences in age categories or in tumor grade between smokers and non-smokers across the three stages. In stage 1, smokers were more likely to have later stage disease compared to non-smokers; however, the

Table 1 Demographic and clinicopathologic characteristics for subjects in each stage of the multi-stage design

| | Affymetrix microarray | | | | | | RT-PCR | | |
| | Stage 1: non-obese subjects | | | Stage 2: obese subjects | | | Stage 3: non-obese subjects | | |
	Non-smokers 30 (65%)	Smokers 16 (35%)	p-value	Non-smokers 12 (63%)	Smokers 7 (37%)	p-value	Non-smokers 54 (66%)	Smokers 28 (34%)	p-value
Gender			0.2170			0.1698			0.0273
Male	14 (47%)	11 (69%)		4 (33%)	5 (71%)		30 (56%)	23 (82%)	
Female	16 (53%)	5 (31%)		8 (67%)	2 (29%)		24 (44%)	5 (18%)	
Age at surgery			0.2537			0.8584			0.4597
<50	3 (10%)	3 (19%)		2 (17%)	1 (14%)		9 (17%)	5 (18%)	
50-79	24 (80%)	13 (81%)		9 (75%)	6 (86%)		41 (76%)	23 (82%)	
≥80	2 (7%)	0		1 (8%)	0		4 (7%)	0	
Unknown	1 (3%)	0		0	0		0	0	
Nuclear grade			0.2032			0.5834			0.2000
1	3 (10%)	1 (6%)		4 (33%)	2 (29%)		5 (9%)	3 (11%)	
2	18 (60%)	7 (44%)		8 (67%)	4 (57%)		17 (32%)	7 (25%)	
3	9 (30%)	8 (50%)		0	1 (14%)		24 (44%)	11 (39%)	
4	0	0		0	0		8 (15%)	7 (25%)	
Pathologic tumor stage			0.0123			0.5926			0.4713
pT1	24 (80%)	7 (44%)		9 (75%)	6 (86%)		31 (57%)	11 (39%)	
pT2	2 (7%)	2 (12%)		2 (17%)	1 (14%)		4 (7%)	4 (14%)	
pT3	4 (13%)	7 (44%)		1 (8%)	0		18 (33%)	13 (46%)	
pT4	0	0		0	0		1 (2%)	0	
Presence of necrosis			0.2829			1.0000			0.4739
Yes	5 (17%)	5 (31%)		1 (8%)	1 (14%)		19 (35%)	13 (46%)	
No	25 (83%)	11 (69%)		11 (92%)	6 (86%)		34 (63%)	15 (54%)	
Unknown	0	0		0	0		1 (2%)	0	

stage distribution was similar between smokers and non-smokers among patients in stages 2-3. Finally, across all three stages, there was no significant difference in presence of necrosis in smokers compared to non-smokers.

Discovery of genes associated with smoking-related ccRCC (stage 1 and stage 2 results)

We identified 305 probesets that had a smoking status-by-tissue type interaction p-value <0.01 in stage 1 (non-obese cohort). Of the 305 probesets we identified in stage 1, 15 also had a smoking status-by-tissue type interaction p-value <0.05 in stage 2 (obese cohort) and maintained a p-value <0.01 in the analysis of the combined data (Table 2). Of these 15 probesets, only nine were mapped to known genes. Due to the fact that the Affymetrix platform contains multiple probesets that map to the same gene, in addition to showing the 15 probesets that met our pre-defined filtering criteria, Additional file 1 provides results for all additional probesets that map to these 9 genes and demonstrates that the fold change estimates are consistent across probesets that map to the same gene. In normal kidney tissue ANKS1B, ACOT6, EYS, CHRNA6, MT1G and UTY were up regulated in smokers in comparison to non-smokers; however, these genes tended to be down regulated in smokers versus non-smokers in ccRCC tumor tissue. Conversely, in normal kidney tissue PPWD1, LUMCH1 and ZNF600 were down regulated in smokers compared to non-smokers; however, these genes were up regulated in smokers versus non-smokers in ccRCC tumor tissue. We selected eight of these nine candidate genes for follow-up validation using RT-PCR in stage 3; we chose not to attempt to validate UTY since it is located on chromosome Y and likely reflects the fact that smokers were more likely to be male than non-smokers.

Independent RT-PCR validation (stage 3 results)

Of the eight genes interrogated via RT-PCR in stage 3, only ANKS1B validated as having an expression pattern that was consistent with what was observed in stages 1 and 2 (Table 3). Specifically, in stage 1 (non-obese cohort) ANKS1B had a tissue type-by-smoking status interaction p-value of 0.0008; the fold change of expression between smokers and non-smokers was 1.08 (p = 0.02) in normal tissues and 0.92 (p = 0.01) in tumor tissues (Table 2). These results were consistent in stage 2 (obese cohort) with an interaction p-value of 0.018 and a fold change of expression between smokers and non-smokers of 1.11 (p = 0.005) in normal tissue and 0.98 (p = 0.64) in tumor tissue (Table 2). Furthermore, the additional 4 probesets that map to ANKS1B showed similar fold change estimates as the proband probeset that met our pre-defined filtering criteria (Additional file 1). Performing RT-PCR on an independent cohort of 82 non-obese

subjects (stage 3), we validated these results with an interaction p-value of 0.0051; the fold change of expression between smokers and non-smokers was 1.35 (p = 0.06) in normal tissues and 0.95 (p = 0.76) in tumor tissues.

Discussion

Based on the current literature, there is little question regarding the role of cigarette smoking in the etiology of ccRCC; however, what remains unclear is exactly how smoking acts within the body (specifically within the kidney itself) to increase a person's risk of developing ccRCC. Related to this, tobacco smoke contains a vast number of chemicals, with about 50 of those chemicals being classified as human carcinogens [9]. Inhaled chemical carcinogens from cigarette smoke, like any other chemical that enters the human body, are subject to extensive metabolism. The majority of this metabolism is directed toward deactivation of the particular chemical and eventual excretion. However, an important fraction of the metabolic process results in the conversion of the ingested compound to highly reactive metabolite(s) that possess the ability to bind to intercellular components (i.e. DNA) and induce changes in their structure; changes that may or may not lead to the transformation of normal cells to tumor cells. Given that the kidney is the main filtration organ of the blood and is known to locally produce enzymes involved in xenobiotic metabolism, it is theorized to be at high exposure to any smoking-related carcinogen. In fact, researchers have reported that the urine of smokers has increased mutagenic activity compared to non-smokers [10]. While this primary theory of how smoking increases the risk of ccRCC does exist, little progress has been made towards illuminating the actual molecular target(s) that are altered by smoking carcinogens in the development of ccRCC.

ANKS1B, Ankyrin repeat and sterile alpha motif domain-containing protein 1B, is a tyrosine kinase signal transduction gene that is primarily expressed in the brain and testis. Here, we demonstrate for the first time that expression of the ANKS1B gene is associated with smoking-related ccRCC development. ANKS1B is involved in apoptosis and thus has the potential to play a key role in cancer development [11]. From our observational data, we show that ANKS1B is up regulated in smokers relative to non-smokers in normal kidney tissue; however, it is down regulated in smokers relative to non-smokers in ccRCC tumor tissue. Thus, ANKS1B expression in smokers is down regulated in the tumor tissue in comparison to the patient-matched normal kidney tissue and this down regulation is potentially a key event that supports ccRCC development. Interestingly, Lin et al. [12] recently evaluated the association of germline SNPs within apoptotic pathway genes with lung cancer risk – in which smoking is also a major risk factor – and identified

Table 2 Results for stage 1, stage 2 and the combined samples from stage 1 and stage 2

| Affymetrix probeset | Gene | Chrom | Smokers vs non-smokers | | | | | | | | |
| | | | Stage 1: non-obese patients | | | Stage 2: obese patients | | | Combined (stage 1 + stage 2) | | |
			Fold change in tumor tissue (p-value)	Fold change in normal tissue (p-value)	Interaction p-value	Fold change in tumor tissue (p-value)	Fold change in normal tissue (p-value)	Interaction p-value	Fold change in tumor tissue (p-value)	Fold change in normal tissue (p-value)	Interaction p-value
240292_x_at	ANKS1B	12	0.92 (0.013)	1.08 (0.02)	0.00082	0.98 (0.64)	1.11 (0.005)	0.018	0.94 (0.014)	1.09 (0.0013)	0.00005
241949_at	ACOT6	14	0.88 (0.0098)	1.07 (0.15)	0.00085	0.89 (0.1)	1.04 (0.56)	0.034	0.88 (0.0019)	1.06 (0.13)	0.00006
236999_at	PPWD1	5	1.13 (0.0062)	0.99 (0.74)	0.0015	1.2 (0.0034)	1.04 (0.5)	0.038	1.14 (0.00023)	1.0 (0.99)	0.00016
233996_x_at	EYS	6	0.94 (0.022)	1.03 (0.27)	0.0022	1.0 (1)	1.06 (0.045)	0.046	0.96 (0.033)	1.04 (0.077)	0.00026
241459_at	LIMCH1	4	1.27 (0.06)	0.89 (0.37)	0.0077	1.9 (0.0032)	1.09 (0.65)	0.02	1.43 (0.0011)	0.95 (0.62)	0.00047
207568_at	CHRNA6	8	0.92 (0.24)	1.15 (0.064)	0.0075	0.95 (0.62)	1.23 (0.034)	0.037	0.93 (0.2)	1.17 (0.0069)	0.00058
210472_at	MT1G	16	1.0 (0.97)	1.47 (0.00013)	0.0045	0.93 (0.62)	1.4 (0.032)	0.018	0.98 (0.82)	1.45 (0.0000099)	0.00061
242463_x_at	ZNF600	19	1.48 (0.0064)	0.98 (0.87)	0.0077	1.78 (0.001)	1.31 (0.083)	0.045	1.56 (0.00013)	1.07 (0.53)	0.0012
210322_x_at	UTY	Y	0.98 (0.76)	1.13 (0.079)	0.0086	0.96 (0.72)	1.22 (0.075)	0.0093	0.98 (0.68)	1.16 (0.012)	0.00029
1557478_at	NA	NA	1.22 (0.03)	0.95 (0.55)	0.00052	1.88 (0.00002)	1.31 (0.022)	0.0011	1.38 (0.00012)	1.04 (0.62)	0.000002
1558410_s_at	NA	NA	1.42 (0.013)	0.93 (0.58)	0.0049	2.49 (0.0000087)	1.63 (0.0038)	0.017	1.66 (0.000044)	1.1 (0.44)	0.0006
210717_at	NA	NA	1.74 (0.00062)	0.89 (0.47)	0.0033	2.12 (0.00026)	1.41 (0.053)	0.027	1.83 (0.000011)	1.03 (0.8)	0.00086
232324_x_at	NA	NA	1.17 (0.004)	0.97 (0.52)	0.0081	1.27 (0.0018)	1.03 (0.61)	0.039	1.2 (0.000058)	0.99 (0.77)	0.0011
232369_at	NA	NA	1.36 (0.021)	0.89 (0.4)	0.0081	2.07 (0.00065)	1.3 (0.15)	0.031	1.53 (0.00016)	1.0 (0.99)	0.00078
244290_at	NA	NA	1.32 (0.0038)	0.99 (0.94)	0.0015	1.66 (0.000041)	1.26 (0.022)	0.033	1.4 (0.000035)	1.06 (0.42)	0.00019

The smoking status-by-tissue type interaction p-value is provided as well as the fold change of expression in smokers relative to non-smokers and corresponding p-values.
Chrom denotes chromosome.
NA denotes that there is no gene annotation available for the corresponding Affymetrix probeset.

Table 3 RT-PCR results for stage 3

Gene	Chrom	Stage 3: non-obese patients		
		Fold change in tumor tissue (p-value)	Fold change in normal tissue (p-value)	Interaction p-value
ANKS1B	12	0.95 (0.76)	1.35 (0.06)	0.0051
ACOT6	14	1.21 (0.53)	1.03 (0.92)	0.56
PPWD1	5	0.97 (0.66)	0.94 (0.44)	0.67
LIMCH1	4	1.04 (0.81)	1.05 (0.76)	0.93
CHRNA6	8	0.92 (0.71)	0.63 (0.038)	0.095
MT1G	16	1.15 (0.72)	1.27 (0.55)	0.80
ZNF600	19	1.05 (0.62)	1.00 (0.99)	0.52

The smoking status-by-tissue type interaction p-value is provided as are the fold change of expression in smokers relative to non-smokers and corresponding p-values.
Chrom denotes chromosome.

2 SNPs in ANKS1B (rs1549102 and rs11110099) that had statistically significant associations. What remains unclear is whether these SNPs are also found in lung cancer tissues and whether they are functionally associated with expression or activity of the ANKS1B protein. That notwithstanding, these results from another smoking-related cancer further suggest a possible role for ANKS1B to be a smoking-related molecular alteration in cancer and underscore the potential for these results to advance the knowledge of ccRCC etiology and prevention. Indeed, in addition to advancing our understanding of the pathways involved in smoking-related ccRCC, alterations in ANKS1B could also potentially be used for early detection and prevention in smokers. That being said, we acknowledge that our findings must first be validated at the protein level. Moreover, there is a need to link alterations in ANKS1B to smoking-related ccRCC in a more robust epidemiologic study design. Particularly, using a larger case–control study or a large prospective-cohort study where it would be feasible to adjust for additional reported risk factors, to study the dose–response relationship of smoking with ANKS1B and lastly, to study the association of smoking with molecularly-defined ccRCC subtypes.

We used a discovery-based approach to identify smoking-specific molecular alterations associated with ccRCC development that can be followed up in more focused investigations. Having said that, the key limitations of our approach include our focus on expression changes at the RNA level (compared to protein expression or alterations at DNA level) and our overall limited generalizability (tertiary referral center, >95% of patients are Caucasian). We acknowledge that our cohort has differences between the ccRCC tumors in the smokers and non-smokers that were studied. First, smokers were more likely to be male than non-smokers. Additionally, smokers in our study were more likely to have later stage disease compared to non-smokers in stage 1; however, the stage distributions were similar between smokers and non-smokers in stages 2-3. Since ANKS1B showed similar results in all 3 stages it is likely not simply a marker associated with later-stage disease. With those limitations in mind, the specific strengths of our design include the use of only clear cell RCC subtype (the most common histologic subtype), exclusion of late stage and high grade tumors in the discovery stages (to focus on events linked to early ccRCC development), use of packyears > 20 years to define smokers (those at theorized high exposure to smoking carcinogens) and access to data on obesity in order to account for the other primary risk factor for ccRCC.

Our study was designed specifically to identify smoking-related molecular alterations that are associated with ccRCC development. As a result, we evaluated patient-matched tumor and normal kidney samples from both smokers and non-smokers. Thus, our potential targets of interest were those that had a statistically significant smoking status-by-tissue type interaction. It is worth noting that if cancer is not of interest and future investigators are interested in simply identifying genes that are associated with only smoking, our publicly available data could be further explored to identify genes with a significant smoking main effect.

Conclusion
In summary, we demonstrated that ANKS1B expression is associated with smoking-related ccRCC. Interestingly, ANKS1B was recently shown to be associated with cancer by Lin et al. [12], where they showed that 2 SNPs in ANKS1B are associated with risk of lung cancer. Here, we showed that ANKS1B is under expressed in ccRCC tumor tissue in comparison to patient-matched normal. Given the role of ANKS1B as an enhancer of apoptosis, down regulation of this gene could be involved in increasing the risk of ccRCC development.

Availability of supporting data
The data supporting the results of this article are available in the Gene Expression Omnibus repository and are accessible through GEO Series accession number GSE46699 [http://www.ncbi.nlm.nih.gov/geo/query/acc.cgi?acc=GSE46699].

Additional file

Additional file 1: Results for stage 1, stage 2 and the combined samples from stage 1 and stage 2. Fold change of expression in smokers relative to non-smokers and p-values are provided. The proband probesets that met our filtering criteria are in bold font; the results for all additional probesets that map to the same gene are provided to demonstrate consistency of results across probesets targeting the same gene.

Competing interests
The authors declare that they have no competing interests.

Authors' contributions

JEP participated in the conception and design, assisted in the statistical analyses and drafted the manuscript. DJS performed the statistical analyses and helped draft the manuscript. BMB participated in the conception and design, performed the statistical analyses and revised the manuscript. RWJ participated in the interpretation and revised the manuscript. JCC reviewed the pathology of all subjects and revised the manuscript. ASP conceived the study, participated in the interpretation, drafting and final approval of the manuscript. All authors read and approved the final manuscript.

Acknowledgements

We thank the Mayo Biospecimen Accessioning and Processing Core and the Mayo Medical Genome Facility Gene Expression Core for sample preparation and microarray services. This work was supported by a Team Science Project grant from the James and Esther King Foundation.

Author details

[1]Division of Biomedical Statistics and Informatics, Mayo Clinic, Rochester, MN, USA. [2]Department of Health Sciences Research, Mayo Clinic, 4500 San Pablo Road, Jacksonville, FL 32224, USA. [3]Statistical Genetics, Sage Bionetworks, Seattle, WA, USA. [4]Department of Hematology and Oncology, Mayo Clinic, Jacksonville, FL, USA. [5]Laboratory Medicine and Pathology, Mayo Clinic, Rochester, MN, USA.

References

1. US Department of Health and Human Services: *The Health Consequences of Smoking: a Report of the Surgeon General.* Atlanta, GA: Department of Health and Human Services, Centers for Disease Control and Prevention, National Center for Chronic Disease Prevention and Health Promotion, Office on Smoking and Health; 2004.
2. Hunt JD, van der Hel O, Mcmillian GP, Boffetta P, Brennan P: **Renal cell carcinoma in relation to cigarette smoking: meta-analysis of 24 studies.** *Int J Cancer* 2005, **114**:101–108.
3. Benichou J: **Population attributable risk of renal cell cancer in Minnesota.** *Am J Epidemiol* 1998, **148**:424–430.
4. McCann J: **Obesity, cancer links prompts new recommendations.** *J Natl Cancer Inst* 2001, **93**:901–902.
5. McGuire BB, Fitzpatrick JM: **BMI and the risk of renal cell carcinoma.** *Curr Opin Urol* 2011, **21**:356–361.
6. Eckel-Passow JC, Serie DJ, Bot BM, Joseph RW, Hart SN, Cheville JC, Parker AS: **Somatic expression of ENRAGE is associated with obesity status among patients with clear cell renal cell carcinoma.** *Carcinogenesis* 2013: DOI:10.1093/carcin/bgt485.
7. McCall MN, Irizarry RA: **Frozen robust multiarray analysis (fRMA).** *Biostatistics* 2010, **11**:242–253.
8. Bot BM, Eckel-Passow JE, LeGrand SN, Hilton T, Cheville JC, Igel T, Parker AS: **Expression of endothelin 2 and localized clear cell renal cell carcinoma.** *Hum Pathol* 2012, **43**:843–849.
9. International Agency for Research on Cancer (IARC): *Monographs on the Evaluation of the Carcinogenic Risk of Chemicals to Humans: Tobacco smoking. Vol. 38.* Lyon: International Agency for Research on Cancer; 1986.
10. Yamasaki E, Ames BN: **Concentration of mutagens from urine by absorption with the nonpolar resin XAD-2: cigarette smokers have mutagenic urine.** *Proc Natl Acad Sci U S A* 1977, **74**:3555–3559.
11. Evan GI, Vousden KH: **Proliferation, cell cycle and apoptosis in cancer.** *Nature* 2001, **411**:342–348.
12. Lin J, Lu C, Stewart DJ, Gu J, Huang M, Chang DW, Lippman SM, Wu X: **Systematic evaluation of apoptotic pathway gene polymorphisms and lung cancer risk.** *Carcinogenesis* 2012, **33**:1699–1706.

2

A comparison of supracostal and infracostal access approaches in treating renal and upper ureteral stones using MPCNL with the aid of a patented system

Difu Fan[1†], Leming Song[1*†], Donghua Xie[1*†], Min Hu[1*†], Zuofeng Peng[1†], Xiaohui Liao[2†], Tairong Liu[1], Chuance Du[1], Lunfeng Zhu[1], Lei Yao[1], Jianrong Huang[1], Zhongsheng Yang[1], Shulin Guo[1], Wen Qin[1], Jiuqing Zhong[1] and Zhangqun Ye[3]

Abstract

Background: There are still disagreements on which is a better approach to choose to establish percutaneous tract for percutaneous nephrolitotomy (PCNL), between supracostal and infracostal approaches. The aim of this study is to investigate the safety, efficacy and practicability of minimally invasive PCNL (MPCNL) with the aid of a patented system either through supracostal or through infracostal access.

Methods: A retrospective study was carried out for 83 patients with renal or upper ureteral stones. Under the guidance of B ultrasound or C-arm, these patients were treated by MPCNL through either 12th rib infracostal (Group 1, 43 cases) or supracostal (Group 2, 40 cases) access approach. These 2 groups were compared for total number of percutaneous tracts, average time in establishing a given percutaneous tract, the number of percutaneous tract used for each case, the average stone clearance time, the clearance rate of all stones by one surgery, and the amount of bleeding using a single percutaneous tract.

Results: There was a significantly smaller total number of percutaneous tracts needed, a smaller number of cases that needed two percutaneous tracts to clear stones completely, a shorter average time in establishing a percutaneous tract, and a smaller average amount of bleeding in infracostal access group. At the same time, there were a significantly larger number of cases in which stones were cleared completely using a single percutaneous tract and a higher renal stone clearance rate by one surgery.

Conclusion: There were several advantages of infracostal access. These included accuracy in establishing a percutaneous tract, safety, quickness, convenience and flexibility in moving the patented sheath, and higher renal and upper ureteral stone clearance rate by one surgery.

Keywords: Patented system, Percutaneous nephrolithotomy, Percutaneous tract access

* Correspondence: xdh888@yahoo.com; xiedh07@gmail.com; gzshm2005@126.com
†Equal contributors
[1]Department of Urology, The Affiliated Ganzhou City People's Hospital of Nanchang University, Ganzhou, Jiangxi 341000, China
Full list of author information is available at the end of the article

Background

Since some scholars [1] first proposed a minimally invasive percutaneous nephrolithotomy (MPCNL) to remove stones, MPCNL has gradually been accepted by many patients and urologists in China, as a significant improvement over standard percutaneous nephrolithotomy (PCNL), and has become one of the most important ways to treat urinary tract stones in China [2–4].

To perform PCNL smoothly and successfully, it is critical to choose a suitable percutaneous tract access approach. A small-sized and highly efficient percutaneous tract is desirable to avoid injury from the puncture and percutaneous tract establishment, and to reduce complications [5]. Currently, most scholars agreed that PCNL through a supracostal access approach can clear stones efficiently with a low rate of complications in treating staghorn renal calculi and upper ureteral stones [6]. From August 2008 to April 2011, 83 patients who met the group inclusion standard underwent the MPCNL with 43 cases of renal stones and 40 cases of ureteral stones either through a 12th rib infracostal access approach (Group 1, 43 cases) or a 10th to 12th rib supracostal access approach (Group 2, 40 cases). All these patients were treated by MPCNL with the aid of a patented stone-breaking and clearance system (patent number ZL200820137434.6). We compared these 2 groups on different markers and reported the results as below.

Patients and Methods

First of all, the study was performed with the approval of ethics committee at the Affiliated Ganzhou City People's Hospital of Nanchang University, China, in compliance with the Helsinki Declaration. Written informed consent was obtained from every patient for publication of this research report and any accompanying images.

Methods

A retrospective study was carried out for the 83 patients with renal or upper ureteral stones. The inclusion standards were as below. Complete or incomplete staghorn renal stones with sizes ≥2.0 cm; renal calyceal stones with co-existing calyceal obstruction and clinical symptoms; ureteral stones above L4 and >1 cm in size, stone has stayed in the ureter for >2 months complicated by ureteral ectasis above the stone, or patients who have previously failed shock wave lithotripsy (SWL) or ureteroscopic lithotripsy. Some of the patients who had anemia which was rectified before inclusion in the study. All patients with hypertension, diabetes, abnormal heart and lung function, or patients who were too obese to tolerate a prone position during surgery were excluded. The stone burden (cm^2) was calculated by multiplying maximal length and maximal width of the stone in plain film of kidney-ureter-bladder (KUB).

Surgery took place under continued epidural anesthesia or general anesthesia. The patient was first placed in a lithotomic position and then a prone position. The abdomen was not boosted, as previously described [7].

Real time ultrasonography or C-arm-guided percutaneous punctures were made with an 18-gauge coaxial needle into the targeted calyx. When using an infracostal access approach the puncture point was located below the 12th rib or at the tip of the 12th rib between the posterior line axillary and linea scapularis. The targeted point was one of the rear group calyces in the lower or middle pole. When using supracostal access approach the puncture point was located between the 11 th rib supracostal and the 12th rib supracostal. The targeted point was one of the rear group calyces in the upper or middle pole. For both access approaches, we always minimized the angle between the long axis of our percutaneous tract and the long axis of the collecting system when we were dealing with renal staghorn stones. The point we preferred to target was the calyx with the stone inside that was closest to our puncturing point. When we were dealing with ureteral stones we always minimized the angle between the long axis of our percutaneous tract and the axis between the proximal to the distal segments of the ureter. The puncture point was in the 11th intercostal space or the 12th subcostal margin, between the posterior axillary line and scapula line. The puncture was judged successful if there was urine overflow or if it touched a stone. Zebra guidewire was inserted and fixed. The puncturing needle was then taken out. After a 0.5–0.7 cm skin incision, the dilatation of the percutaneous tract was performed serially over the guidewire with a fascial dilator to 16 F. A 16 F patented sheath (Fig. 1) was placed at the percutaneous access port and was connected to a vacuum aspiration machine, as previously described [7]. Subsequently, a small diameter nephroscope (12Fr) was inserted through the sheath to explore stones. A holmium laser was used to break the stones and a vacuum suctioning device was used to clear gravel, as previously described [7]. When residual stones found using intraoperative real-time ultrasonography or C-arm needed a second or third percutaneous tract to clear stones, the 2nd and/or 3rd percutaneous tract(s) was/were established using an infracostal approach to target one of the rear group calyces in the lower or middle pole. The amount of intraoperative bleeding was calculated using a hydrogenated high iron hemoglobin method, as previously described [7, 8]. A KUB was taken 3 to 5 days after surgery, and a computerized tomography (CT) was performed for cases with uric acid stones, to check for residual stones. If no residual stones > 4 mm were present, which was defined as stone-free, the nephrostomy tube was removed and no further treatment was pursued. Otherwise, a second-

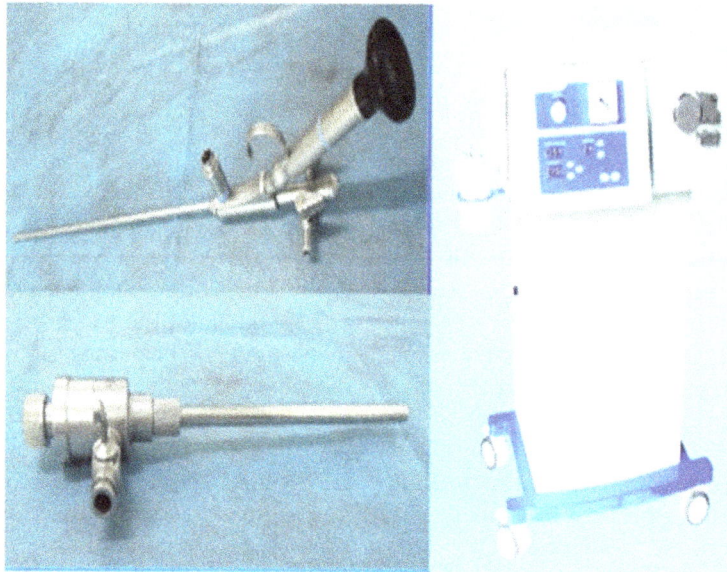

Fig. 1 Lithotripsy and suctioning/clearance system comprised of small diameter percutaneous nephroscope, patented sheath, and irrigation and suctioning system

stage percutaneous nephrolithotomy or SWL treatment was performed, as previously described [7]. Total percutaneous tract number, average time in establishing the percutaneous tract, the number of percutaneous tract used for each case, the average stone clearance time (From the beginning of stone clearance to the end of the nephrostomy tube indwelling), one time stone clearance rate, one stage renal stone clearance rate and bleeding amount using a single percutaneous tract were recorded as data. Complications were evaluated according to the Clavien classification.

Statistics

All data were analyzed using SPSS11.5. A Student's *t*-test was used for quantitative variables and a Chi-square test was used for qualitative variables. $p < 0.05$ was used to indicate statistical significance.

Results

There were 43 cases of renal stones (staghorn stones, stones in a higher positioned kidney, upper renal calyceal stones, complicated middle or lower renal calyceal stones) and 40 cases of ureteral stones above the level of L4. Among these 83 patients, there were 53 males and 30 females. The median age was 43 years old. There were 75 cases with hydronephrosis at varying degrees. There were 13 cases complicated with pyonephrosis. There were 5 cases who had SWL previously. There were no statistical differences in mean stone burden, age, body mass index (BMI), and preoperative hemoglobin level between the 2 groups (see Table 1).

All the patients in these 2 groups were treated successfully. No gastrointestinal damage, pleural or peritoneal effusions, pyemia, or sepsis occurred. There were 2 cases in the supracostal group that were complicated by pleural cavity injury (Clavien Grade 3). However, these 2 cases were cured by conservative therapies including closed drainage of thoracic cavity. Four cases of fever (Clavien Grade 1) were noted in each group (9 % for Group 1 and 10 % for Group 2) without significant difference. No Clavien Grade 2 or 4 complications, and other Grade 1 and 3 complications were noted in either group (see Table 2).

There was a significantly smaller total number of percutaneous tracts needed, a smaller number of cases that

Table 1 General Data Comparison

	Infracostal Access	Supracostal Access	p value
Number of cases number with renal stones	23	20	
Number of cases with ureteral stones	20	20	
Average stone burden (cm²)	7.56 ± 2.35	7.98 ± 2.29	>0.05
Percentage of staghorn stones	11/43(25.6 %)	11/40(27.5 %)	
Mean			
Age (years)	45.3 ± 15.3	42.4 ± 17.5	>0.05
BMI	25.3 ± 0.3	24.4 ± 3.2	>0.05
Mean hemoglobin level (g/dL)	12.2 ± 0.53	13.2 ± 8.2	>0.05

BMI Body mass index

Table 2 Operative Data Comparison

		Infracostal Access	Supracostal Access	p value
Total number of percutaneous tracts (%)		47/43(109.3 %)	53/40(132.5 %)	0.005
Percutaneous tract (%)	Single tract	40/43(93.0 %)	29/40(72.5 %)	0.0165
	Two tracts	2/43(4.7 %)	9/40(22.5 %)	0.0209
	Three tracts	1/43(2.3 %)	2/40(5.0 %)	0.29
Average time needed for establishing a percutaneous tract (min)		(3 ± 1.6)min	(6 ± 3.9)min	0.001
Average time needed for stone clearance (min)	Renal stones	(42 ± 12)min	(61 ± 26)min	0.33
	Ureteral stones	(10 ± 6)min	(11 ± 8)min	0.29
Renal stone clearance rate by one surgery using a single percutaneous tract		18/23(78.26 %)	7/20(35.0 %)	0.002
Stone clearance rate by one surgery	Renal stones	21/23(91.3 %)	18/20(90.0 %)	0.43
	Ureteral stones	100 %	100 %	
Renal stones needing secondary treatment (secondary MPCNL or ESWL) (%)		2/23(8.7 %)	2/20(10.0 %)	0.43
Mean amount of bleeding (ml)		72.8 ± 28.1	86.74 ± 32.6	0.040
Clavien Grade 1 complication		4(9 %)	4(10 %)	0.82
Clavien Grade 2 complication		0(0 %)	0(0 %)	0.001
Clavien Grade 3 complication		0(0 %)	2(5 %)	
Clavien Grade 4 complication		0(0 %)	0(0 %)	

needed two percutaneous tracts to clear stones completely, a shorter average time in establishing a percutaneous tract, and a smaller average amount of bleeding in Group 1 ($p < 0.05$). At the same time, there was a significantly larger number of cases in which stones were cleared completely using a single percutaneous tract, and a higher renal stone clearance rate by one surgery ($p < 0.05$). However, there were no significant differences in the average renal stone clearance time, the average ureteral stone clearance time, ureteral stone clearance rate using a single percutaneous tract by one surgery, renal stone clearance rate by one surgery, and cases in which 3 percutaneous tracts were needed to clear all stones (see Table 2).

Discussion

Currently many scholars believe that a supracostal approach to puncturing renal upper or middle calyces in order to establish the percutaneous tract can maximally break the staghorn renal and upper ureteral stones. This approach makes it easier to find the outlet of the renal pelvis and indwell a double-J pigtail stent. This belief has been based on consideration of the anatomic characteristics of the renal collecting system, because the supracostal approach is on the direction of the long axis of the renal collecting system [6, 9, 10]. In treating renal staghorn calculi using PCNL, we must first consider the safety of the surgery. A secondary consideration is to increase the stone clearance rate by one surgery. The access approach and size of the percutaneous tract, and the efficacy and flexibility of the stone breaking devices are critical factors in determining the safety and efficacy in treating staghorn renal calculi by PCNL [11].

Our patented lithotripsy and suctioning/clearance system is comprised of a patented metal sheath, a small diameter (12 F) nephroscope, and an irrigation and suctioning system (Fig. 1). Previous study indicated that the patented system group had a significantly higher percentage of stone-free outcomes after one surgery and significantly less intraoperative bleeding compared to EMS (Electro Medical System) group [7].

To perform a PCNL, we must first consider how to design the percutaneous tract access approach, in order to achieve the maximal stone clearance rate using a single percutaneous tract and reduce the injury from the establishment of multiple percutaneous tracts [9]. The percutaneous tract must maximally facilitate the movement of the sheath to clear stones and avoid complications, such as bleeding, from the movement of the sheath. Due to the interference of ribs, ultrasound image could be affected when using a supracostal approach. This will affect the accuracy of puncturing. In the meantime, the large number of blood vessels in the upper and middle poles of the kidney will increase the risk of puncturing. In addition, there is potential risk of pleural and lung injury when using a supracostal approach [12, 13]. In our study, we did see this complication in 5 % of our cases in the supracostal group, and none in the infracostal group. Also, by using the supracostal access approach, the narrow intercostal space limited the movement of the sheath. This can affect stone clearance. In our study, we found that there was higher need for multiple percutaneous tracts for stone clearance in the supracostal group.

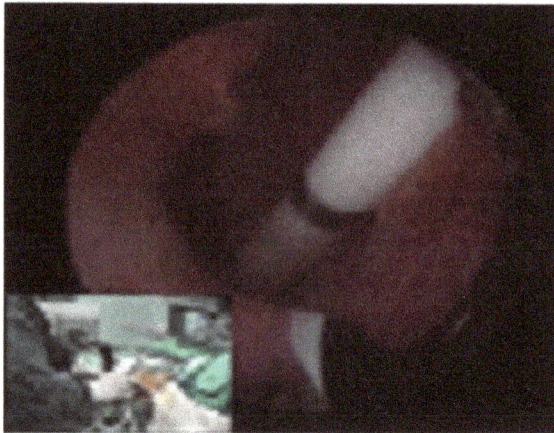

Fig. 2 The outlet of the renal pelvis and upper ureter can be visualized clearly using an infracostal approach

We also found stone clearance to be more efficient when a second or/and third percutaneous tract was/were established using an infracostal approach. In our supracostal group, there were 13 percutaneous tracts established using an infracostal approach. The higher the number of percutaneous tracts needed, the higher the risk of bleeding. Because there are fewer blood vessels in the rear part of the lower renal pole, the risk of serious bleeding from puncturing is lower when using an infracostal approach. The ultrasound images are clearer when using the infracostal approach because there is no interference from the ribs. This makes the puncturing more convenient and more accurate [14]. Our study revealed that there were significant differences in the total number of percutaneous tracts, ratio of cases needing a single percutaneous tract, ratio of cases needing 2 percutaneous tracts, average time in establishing a percutaneous tract, and average amount of bleeding. This indicated the safety and practicability of the infracostal access approach.

Regardless of the approach was used, the principle is to extract stones along the long axis of the kidney. Many urologists have concerns that when using the infracostal access approach it becomes difficult for the scope and sheath to access the outlet of the renal pelvis and the upper segment of the ureter, therefore affecting the indwelling of a double-J pigtail stent or stone clearance of upper ureteral stones. However, the material of our patented sheath is hard, not easily deformed, and small in diameter, maximizing access. For each surgery in the infracostal group, we did not booster the abdomen to immobilize the kidney. The increased ability of the kidney and ureter to move facilitates the hard sheath's access to all target locations. Because the patented sheath is small, and its range of movement is increased, it can easily access most of the renal calyces and the upper ureter in order to explore and remove stones under direct vision, reducing the number of percutaneous tracts required for multiple or staghorn kidney stones, thereby reducing kidney damage. Using the patented system to clear stones in patients with significant hydronephrosis, we can suck away the hydrops and reduce the volume of the kidney easily. Thus the perirenal space is increased, the tension in the renal pelvis is decreased, and the movement of the kidneys and ureter is therefore increased. This will further facilitate access by the sheath to different areas in order to break and remove the

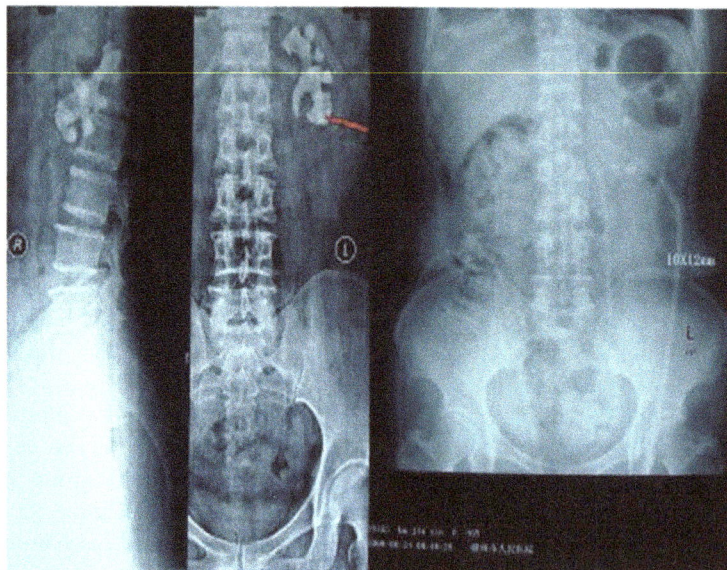

Fig. 3 Comparison of preoperative and postoperative KUBs of a patient with left renal staghorn stone (*Red line* represents the direction of infracostal access approach; *Left*, Preoperative KUB; *Right*, Postoperative KUB)

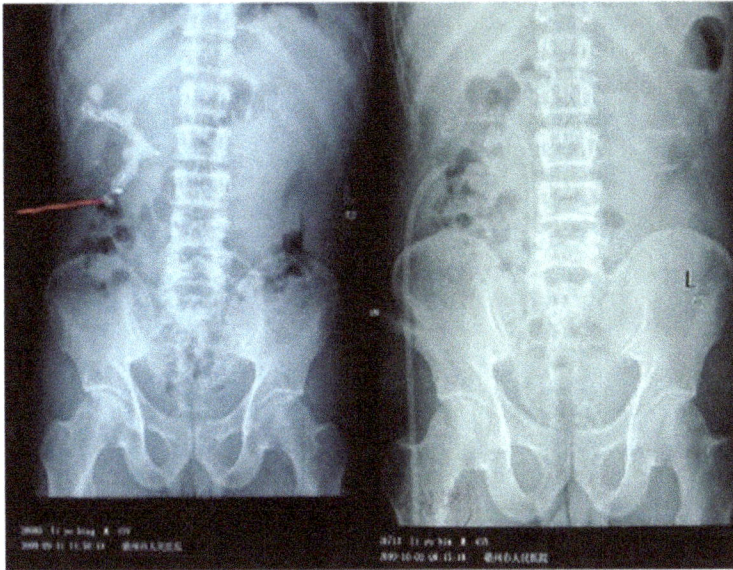

Fig. 4 Comparison of preoperative and postoperative KUBs of a patient with right renal multiple stones (*Red line* represents the direction of infracostal access approach; *Left*, Preoperative KUB; *Right*, Postoperative KUB)

stones. For some staghorn stones with a wide angle, we usually broke the part in the renal pelvis first, in order to create space. Then we moved the stones located in the small calyces using the hard sheath to the renal pelvis under a video monitor to do lithotripsy. For secondary stones impacted inside small calyceal necks, we usually dilated the calyceal neck first, then did lithotripsy inside the calyces or broke and/or sucked stones by putting the sheath immediately outside the calyceal necks. For slush like stone materials, we used the sheath to suck them away quickly. Due the larger movements of the scope, kidney stone clearance rate by one surgery was significantly higher in the infracostal group (Fig. 2, 3, 4, 5).

Conclusions

There were several advantages of infracostal access in treating renal stones and upper ureteral stones. These include accuracy in establishing a percutaneous tract, safety, quickness, convenience and flexibility in moving the patented sheath, and higher renal and upper ureteral

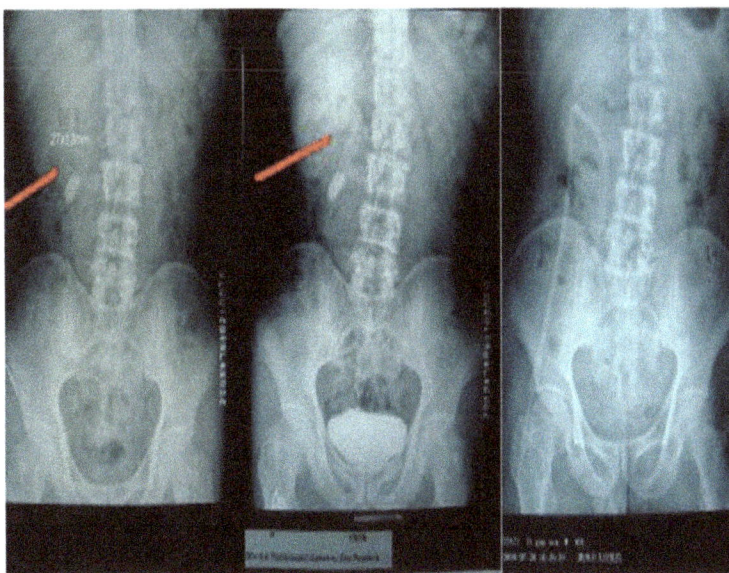

Fig. 5 Comparison of preoperative and postoperative images of a patient with right upper ureteral stone (*Red line* represents the direction of infracostal access approach; *Left*, Preoperative KUB; *Middle*, Preoperative IVU; *Right*, Postoperative KUB)

stone clearance rate by one surgery. However, we do recognize that our sample size was not large. Larger, prospective studies in multiple clinical centers are warranted to further compare the supracostal and infracostal access approaches in treating upper urinary tract stones using MPCNL with the aid of our patented system.

Abbreviations
MPCNL: Minimally invasive percutaneous nephrolithotomy; PCNL: Percutaneous nephrolithotomy; SWL: Shock wave lithotripsy; KUB: Plain film of kidney-ureter-bladder; CT: Computerized tomography; EMS: Electro Medical System.

Competing interests
The authors declare that they have no competing interests.

Authors' contributions
DF, LS, MH, ZP, XL collected the data and participated in drafting the manuscript. DX drafted the manuscript. DX, XL, LS and ZY (Zhangqun Ye) advanced the manuscript by revising it critically. TL, CD, LZ, LY, JH, ZY (Zhongsheng Yang), SG, WQ, and JZ collected the data. All authors read and approved the final manuscript.

Acknowledgements
This work was supported by major scientific and technological project funds of Jiangxi Provincial Health Department, Jiangxi, China (20094015) to L.M.S.

Author details
[1]Department of Urology, The Affiliated Ganzhou City People's Hospital of Nanchang University, Ganzhou, Jiangxi 341000, China. [2]Dermatology Institute of Gan County, Jiangxi 341100, China. [3]Department of Urology, Tongji Hospital, Tongji Medical College, Huazhong University of Science and Technology, Wuhan, Hubei 430030, China.

References
1. Lahme S, Bichler KH, Strohmaier WL, Götz T. Minimally invasive PCNL in patients with renal pelvic and calyceal stones. Eur Urol. 2001;40:619–24.
2. Li X, He ZH, Zeng GH, Chen WZ, Wu KJ, Shan ZC, et al. Treatment methods for upper urinary tract stones in modern era, a report of 5178 cases. J Chinese Clin Urol. 2004;19:325–7.
3. Zeng GH, Zhong W, Li X, Wu K, Chen W, Lei M, et al. Minimally invasive percutaneous nephrolithotomy for staghorn calculi: a novel single session approach via multiple 14-18Fr tracts. Surg Laparosc Endosc Percutan Tech. 2007;17:124–8.
4. Li X, He Z, Wu K, Li SK, Zeng G, Yuan J, et al. Chinese minimally invasive percutaneous nephrolithotomy: the Guangzhou experience. J Endourol. 2009;23:1693–7.
5. Nishizawa K, Yamada H, Miyazaki Y, Kobori G, Higashi Y. Results of treatment of renal calculi with lower-pole fluoroscopically guided percutaneous nephrolithotomy. Int J Urol. 2008;15:399–402.
6. Gupta R, Kumar A, Kapoor R, Srivastava A, Mandhani A. Prospective evaluation of safety and efficacy of the supracostal approach for percutaneous nephrolithotomy. BJU Int. 2002;90:809–13.
7. Song L, Chen Z, Liu T, Zhong J, Qin W, Guo S, et al. The application of a patented system to minimally invasive percutaneous nephrolithotomy. J Endourol. 2011;25:1281–6.
8. Xu GB, Li X, He ZH, He YZ, Lei M. Factors affecting blood loss during minimally invasive percutaneous nephrolithotomy. J Chinese Urol. 2007;28:456–9.
9. Lojanapiwat B, Prasopsuk S. Upper-pole access for percutaneous nephrolithotomy: comparison of supracostal and infracostal approaches. J Endourol. 2006;20:491–4.
10. Kara C, Değirmenci T, Kozacioglu Z, Gunlusoy B, Koras O, Minareci S. Supracostal Approach for PCNL: Is 10th and 11th Intercostal Space Safe According to Clavien Classification System? Int Surg. 2014;99:857-62
11. Honeck P, Nagele U, Michel MS. Technical innovations in endourological stone therapy. Urologe A. 2008;47:587–90.
12. Honey RJ, Wiesenthal JD, Ghiculete D, Pace S, Ray AA, Pace KT. Comparison of supracostal versus infracostal percutaneous nephrolithotomy using the novel prone-flexed patient position. J Endourol. 2011;25:947–54.
13. Mousavi-Bahar SH, Mehrabi S, Moslemi MK. The safety and efficacy of PCNL with supracostal approach in the treatment of renal stones. Int Urol Nephrol. 2011;43:983–7.
14. Osman M, Wendt-Nordahl G, Heger K, Michel MS, Alken P, Knoll T. Percutaneous nephrolithotomy with ultrasonography guided renal access: experience from over 300 cases. BJU Int. 2005;96:875–8.

3

Prospective evaluation of plasma levels of ANGPT2, TuM2PK, and VEGF in patients with renal cell carcinoma

Bishoy A Gayed[1†], Jessica Gillen[2†], Alana Christie[3†], Samuel Peña-Llopis[4], Xian-Jin Xie[3], Jingsheng Yan[3], Jose A Karam[5], Ganesh Raj[1], Arthur I Sagalowsky[1], Yair Lotan[1], Vitaly Margulis[1,6*] and James Brugarolas[2,4]

Abstract

Background: To assess pathological correlations and temporal trends of Angiopoietin-2 (ANGPT2), vascular endothelial growth factor (VEGF) and M2 Pyruvate kinase (TuM2PK), markers of tumor vascular development and metabolism, in patients with renal cell carcinoma (RCC).

Methods: We prospectively collected plasma samples from 89 patients who underwent surgical/ablative therapy for RCC and 38 patients with benign disease (nephrolithiasis, hematuria without apparent neoplastic origin, or renal cysts). In RCC patients, marker levels were compared between at least 1 preoperative and 1 postoperative time point generally 3 weeks after surgery. Marker temporal trends were assessed using the Wilcoxon sign-rank test. Plasma VEGF, ANGPT2, and TuM2PK levels were determined by ELISA and tested for association with pathological variables.

Results: Median age was comparable between groups. 83/89 (93%) of the cohort underwent surgical extirpation. 82% of the tumors were organ confined (T $\leq$2, N0). Only ANGPT2 exhibited significantly elevated preoperative levels in patients with RCC compared to benign disease ($p = 0.046$). Elevated preoperative levels of ANGPT2 and TuM2PK significantly correlated with increased tumor size and advanced grade ($p < 0.05$). Chromophobe RCC exhibited higher levels of ANGPT2 compared to other histologies ($p < 0.05$). A decline in marker level after surgery was not observed, likely due to the timing of the analyses.

Conclusion: Our results suggest that ANGPT2 is a marker of RCC. Additionally, ANGPT2 and TuM2PK significantly correlated with several adverse pathological features. Further studies are needed to determine clinical applicability.

Keywords: Biomarkers, Angiogenesis, Prospective, Renal cell carcinoma, Tumor metabolism

Background

In 2014, 63920 new diagnoses, and 13860 deaths attributed to tumors of the kidney and renal pelvis are expected [1]. 5-year cancer specific survival (CSS) probability rates for patients with localized and locally advanced disease are around 80-90% and 20-50%, respectively [2]. Advances in surgical techniques and the development of targeted therapies have lead to improved oncologic outcomes of patients with RCC, however, survival of patients with advanced disease continues to be deficient [3]. A better understanding of the biology of tumors is required to improve oncological outcomes.

Central to the development of RCC of clear-cell type (ccRCC) is the loss of VHL with activation of a hypoxia-adaptive program that involves metabolic changes and angiogenesis. Our understanding of the nature of ccRCC has led to the development of targeted agents that antagonize VEGF signaling [4]. Currently, therapies target the VEGF ligand or its receptor. Other determinants of angiogenesis are being investigated, including Angiopoietin 2 (ANGPT2) [5,6]. ANGPT2 is found at sites of

---
* Correspondence: Vitaly.Margulis@utsouthwestern.edu
†Equal contributors
[1]Department of Urology, University of Texas Southwestern Medical Center, Dallas, Texas, USA
[6]Department of Urology, UT Southwestern Medical Center at Dallas, 5323 Harry Hines Blvd., Dallas 75390-9110, Texas, USA
Full list of author information is available at the end of the article

vascular remodeling and functions by undermining vascular foundation [7].

Loss of VHL induces profound metabolic changes. For instance, we recently showed that VHL inactivation in the mouse is sufficient to inhibit mitochondrial respiration [8]. Tumor cells often rely on aerobic glycolysis for energy generation, which makes carbon sources available for anabolic processes. One protein that plays a critical role in tumor metabolism is pyruvate kinase. Several isoforms of this enzyme exist, however, the M2 isoform (M2PK) is specifically implicated in oncogenesis, and is overexpressed in tumor cells [9]. Studies have shown that the dimeric form (TuM2PK) may be a marker of malignant renal disease [10]. In addition, TuM2PK may be a useful predictor of recurrence in patients with RCC [11]. However, the current role of TuM2PK continues to be undefined.

Currently, prognostic factors such as stage and grade fail to incorporate the individual biological heterogeneity and clinical behavior of RCC [12]. Thus, there is a strong impetus for detecting and incorporating biomarkers into clinical practice that expose the biological behavior of tumors and aid in risk assessment [13].

In this prospective feasibility study, we analyzed a panel of potential RCC markers (VEGF, TuM2PK, and ANGPT2) in patients with RCC vs. a control group with benign renal disease. We correlated the levels of the marker with pathologic features of the tumor at surgery and evaluated the levels postoperatively.

Methods
Patient selection
Between October 2008 and March 2010, patients presenting to the UT Southwestern Medical Center Urology Clinic with a renal mass suspicious for RCC as well those with presumed benign etiology were enrolled in an UT Southwestern Medical Center IRB approved tissue and blood repository protocol. Patients enrolled in the study signed written consent. Research was carried out in compliance with the Helsinki Declaration. 125 patients were followed from the time of diagnosis to at least 2 preoperative time points and 1 postoperative time point taken more than 24 h after surgery. Of these, 9 presented with metastatic disease and 3 patients developed other malignancies, and were withdrawn, leaving 113 patients (102 underwent surgical nephrectomy and 11 radiofrequency ablation). Benign pathology was reported in 13 surgical patients and 5 additional patients were withdrawn because were not left NED after surgery. 5 patients treated with ablative intervention had either no biopsy, were benign, or insufficient material was available. After applying these criteria, 90 patients qualified for this analysis and 89 underwent ELISA assays. 38 patients qualified as controls with either of

the following benign conditions: nephrolithiasis, hematuria of presumed benign etiology, or simple renal cysts. Computerized tomography (CT) scans were used to evaluate urologic conditions and establish radiologic absence of malignancy. Further, patients with hematuria also underwent complete workup, including cytology, imaging, and cystoscopy to rule out malignancy.

Collection and storage of samples
Peripheral venous blood was collected from patients with RCC at preoperative and postoperative time points. Patients serving as controls had blood drawn at their initial clinic visit. Blood was collected in EDTA tubes, and centrifuged, typically within 15 minutes. Plasma samples were aliquoted and stored at −80°C until analysis.

Elisa assays
Plasma from each pre and postoperative time point was evaluated. Serum samples, collected for other purposes, were not used for this study as platelet degranulation during clotting may lead to falsely elevated levels of the marker [14]. Plasma VEGF and ANGPT2 levels were determined by ELISA according to the manufacturer's instructions (R & D Systems, Minneapolis, MN, USA). Plasma TuM2PK levels were also determined by ELISA according to the manufacturer's instructions (ScheBo, Wettenberg, Germany). Each time point was run in duplicate and all samples for each patient were run on the same plate. Standards and a set of controls were run on each plate. ELISA results for each marker were displayed as heatmaps by normalizing the values of each patient to the number of standard deviations above or below the average.

Statistics
Patient characteristics are displayed using medians, ranges, frequencies, and percentages. Where applicable, marker levels were calculated as the patient's average preoperative draw and the average postoperative draw. To evaluate marker trends over time the Wilcoxon sign-ranks test was used. Wilcoxon rank sum test was used to find if there was a difference between RCC patients and control patients. All statistics were performed using software from GraphPad Prism version 5.03 (GraphPad Software, San Diego, CA, USA) and SAS version 9.3 (SAS Institute Inc., Cary, NC, USA). A p-value < 0.05 was considered significant. False discovery rate control was used for the p-values from the testing between marker levels and pathological variables.

Results
Clinical features
Table 1 outlines the demographic and clinical characteristics of both cohorts. A total of 127 patients were

Table 1 Characteristics of RCC and control patients

Variable	RCC (n = 89)	Controls (n = 38)
Age Median (range)	62 (25-85)	57 (23-89)
Sex - no. (%)		
Male	52 (58.4)	20 (52.6)
Female	37 (41.6)	18 (47.4)
Race - no. (%)		
Caucasian	66 (74.2)	28 (70.0)
African American	9 (10.1)	6 (15.0)
Hispanic	9 (10.1)	6 (15.0)
East Indian	4 (4.5)	0
Asian	1 (1.1)	0
Diagnosis - no. (%)		
RCC	89 (100)	
Stones		27 (71.1)
Hematuria		9 (23.7)
Renal Cyst		2 (5.3)
Approach - no. (%)		
Ablation	6 (6.7)	
Nephrectomy	83 (93.3)	
Open	42 (50.6)	
Laparoscopic	41 (49.4)	
Radical	36 (43.4)	
Partial	47 (56.6)	
AJCC Stage† - no. (%)		
I	60 (73.2)	
II	7 (8.5)	
III	15 (18.3)	
IV	0	
pT Classification† - no. (%)		
T1a	41 (49.4)	
T1b	20 (24.1)	
T2	7 (8.4)	
T3	1 (1.2)	
T3a	5 (6.0)	
T3b	9 (10.8)	
T3c	0	
T4	0	
Pathologic Size† - median (range)	4.1 (1.3-25)	
LN Involvement† - no. (%)		
NX	71 (85.5)	
N0	11 (13.3)	
N1	1 (1.2)	
Histology - no. (%)		
Clear Cell	69 (77.5)	
Papillary	14 (15.7)	

Table 1 Characteristics of RCC and control patients
(Continued)

Chromophobe	5 (5.6)	
Unclassified RCC	1 (1.1)	
Fuhrman Grade† - no. (%)		
1	10 (12.0)	
2	44 (53.01)	
3	26 (31.33)	
4	3 (3.6)	

†Analysis does not include patients treated with RFA.

included in the study, 89 patients underwent treatment of their renal mass and 38 patients presented with benign conditions that served as the control group. The two groups were comparable with respect to age, gender, and race. 83/89 (93%) patients with renal masses underwent extirpative resection, with either partial or radical nephrectomy. 82% of the tumors were organ confined (pT ≤2, N0) and 78% had clear cell histology.

Association of marker levels with malignancy

Median time between the operation and the last postoperative draw was 25 days (interquartile range 18–187 days). ANGPT2 exhibited significantly elevated preoperative levels in patients with RCC ($p = 0.046$) compared to those with benign disease, while preoperative TuM2PK and VEGF levels were comparable between patients with benign and malignant disease (Figure 1).

Temporal changes of markers

Figure 2 is a heatmap representation of the different markers for each patient over time.

Table 2 shows how marker levels are affected over time. We calculated the median difference of 1st postoperative levels vs. the average of all the preoperative levels (which we perceived to be most representative of preoperative levels). Our results showed that ANGPT2 and TuM2PK levels increased significantly. Similar results were observed when all postoperative samples were included in the analysis.

When the first postoperative sample was excluded (despite being ~3 weeks after the surgery), the differences largely disappeared. In keeping with this finding, there was a significant difference in ANGPT2 and TuM2PK levels between the first and remaining postop values. Overall, these data are consistent with the notion that surgery induces plasma ANGPT2 and TuM2PK levels.

Association of pathological features with markers levels

Interestingly, elevated preoperative levels of ANGPT2 and TuM2PK significantly correlated with several adverse pathological features (Figure 3). There was a

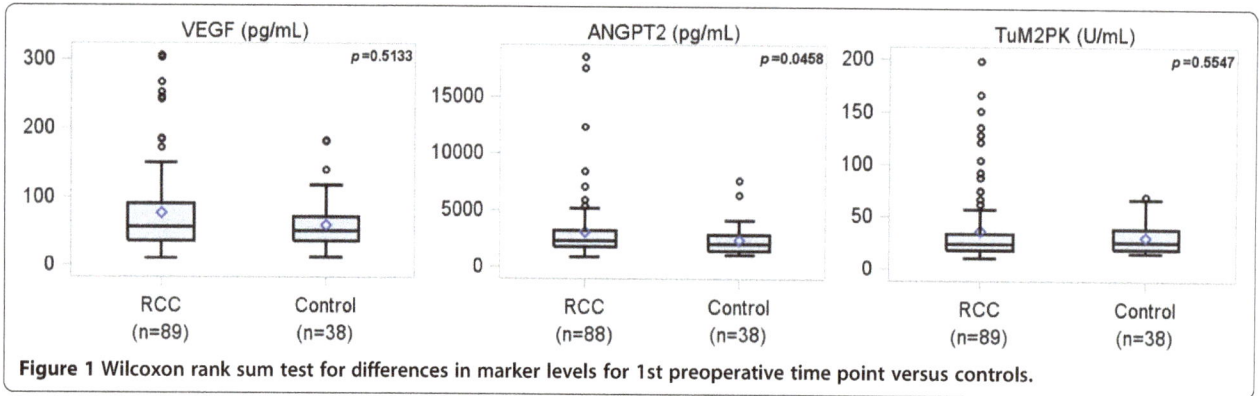

Figure 1 Wilcoxon rank sum test for differences in marker levels for 1st preoperative time point versus controls.

significant correlation between ANGPT2 levels and tumor size ($p = 0.0009$). Similarly, TuM2PK levels were also correlated with tumor size ($p = 0.0009$). In addition, there was a correlation between ANGPT2 and TuM2PK and grade. Higher levels of both ANGPT2 and TuM2PK were observed in grade 4 tumors ($p < 0.05$). In addition, chromophobe RCC exhibited significantly higher levels of ANGPT2 compared to other histologies ($p < 0.05$) (Figure 3). No correlation was seen between VEGF levels and adverse pathological features.

Discussion

Circulating tumor biomarkers may assist with primary diagnosis, determination of recurrence and prognosis. However, no suitable renal cancer biomarkers have been identified and incorporated in clinical practice. In this study, we explored a sensitive paradigm. We evaluated samples from patients with a primary in place and performed comparisons of circulating proteins before and after surgery. Intra-patient comparisons are likely to minimize confounding by other variables. In addition, we compared biomarker levels between renal cancer patients and a group of controls with non-malignant disease. By enrolling surgical candidates, we were able to correlate circulating biomarker levels to the pathological features of the tumor. We focused our studies on VEGF, ANGPT2 and TuM2PK.

One pathway that is being extensively studied is the angiopoietin/Tie-2 pathway. This pathway is comprised not only of angiopoietin 1 (ANGPT1), but also of ANGPT2, and its receptor vascular receptor tyrosine kinase Tie-2. These factors play a significant role in neo-vascularization [15,16]. ANGPT1 has been shown to be involved in vascular development, while ANGPT2 functions to undermine vascular integrity [7,15]. ANGPT2 overexpression has also been shown to augment tumor angiogenesis [17]. Sallinen et al. showed that patients with ovarian carcinoma had significantly higher levels of ANGPT2 than individuals with benign disease. Further,

elevated ANGPT2 levels correlated with advanced stage as well as worse DFS and OS [18]. Others have shown that ANGPT2 to be a biomarker of disease status, adverse pathological features, and worse oncological outcomes [19,20]. While the definitive role of ANGPT2 in RCC remains undefined, studies exist showing that ANGPT2 concentrations appear to be elevated in patients with RCC [21,22]. Efforts are also ongoing to target angiopoietin/Tie-2 system with drugs such as AMG-386 and CVX-060 in patients with RCC [23].

TuM2PK has been implicated as a driver of aerobic glycolysis, and shown to be a marker of malignancy in several neoplasms [9]. Landt et al. revealed that TuM2PK levels can distinguish between malignant and premalignant cervical lesions. Additionally, they showed that increased levels of TuM2PK were associated with node positive as well as metastatic disease [24]. A recent meta-analysis showed that elevated TuM2PK levels correlated with malignancy as well as extent of disease in patients with GI malignancy [25].

Few reports exist regarding the role of TuM2PK in patients with RCC. Nisman et al. showed that elevated levels of TuM2Pk were significantly associated with worse pathological features, including grade and tumor necrosis [11]. Their results also revealed that patients with elevated circulating TuM2PK had worse 5-year RFS than patients with normal marker levels (55% vs. 94% $p < 0.001$). On multivariate analysis, TuM2PK was an independent predictor of disease recurrence ($p = 0.04$) [11]. In an interesting study by Roigas et al. plasma levels of TuM2PK were compared between healthy patients and patients with RCC. Elevated levels of TuM2PK were significantly elevated in patients with RCC than healthy patients [26]. Conversely, Varga et al. concluded that TuM2PK is not an adequate marker for RCC [27].

In our study, we prospectively analyzed the prognostic significance of 3 markers of angiogenesis and metabolism. Most importantly, elevated preoperative levels of ANGTP2 and TuM2PK were significantly associated

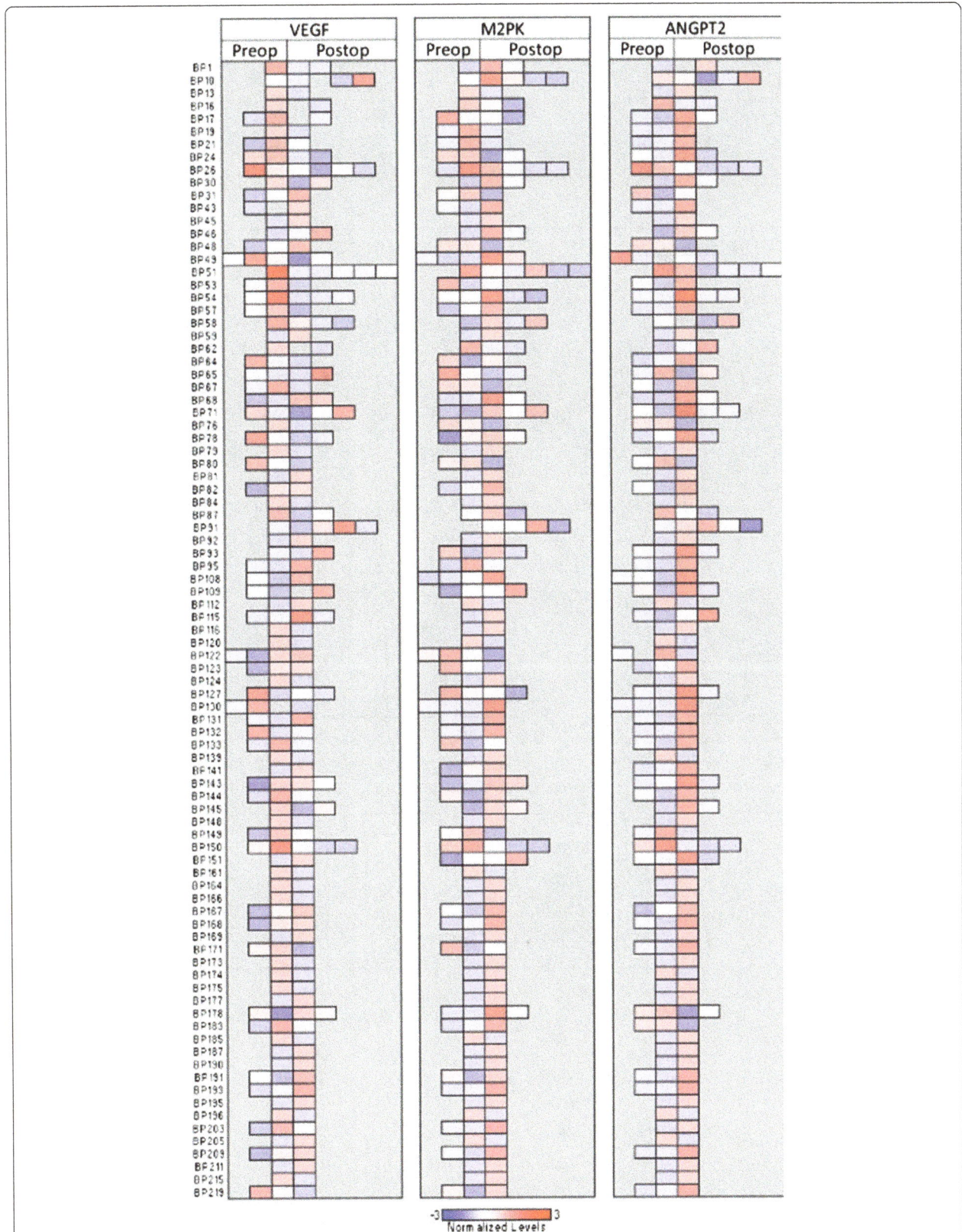

Figure 2 Heatmap representation of VEGF, M2PK, and ANGPT2 plasma levels by patient, over time. For each marker and patient, values were normalized to the number of standard deviations above (red) of below (blue) the average. Samples are arranged in chronological order for each patient. The number of samples available for each patient varies, and isolated gray boxes for a particular patient represent missing values for the particular analysis.

Table 2 Wilcoxon signed rank test for median of difference in marker levels between pairs of time points

	1st post – Avg. Preoperative			Avg. all but 1st post – Avg. preoperative			Avg. all post – Avg. preoperative			Avg. all but 1st Post – 1st postoperative		
	n	Median	p	n	Median	p	n	Median	p	n	Median	p
ANGPT2	88	318.1	0.0004	26	2.4	0.3914	88	253.1	0.0082	26	−300.2	<0.0001
M2PK	89	13.0	<0.0001	27	−2.1	0.2880	89	12.4	<0.0001	27	−8.6	0.0003
VEGF	89	−6.1	0.2021	23	−2.2	0.1973	89	−4.0	0.3581	23	4.0	0.6799

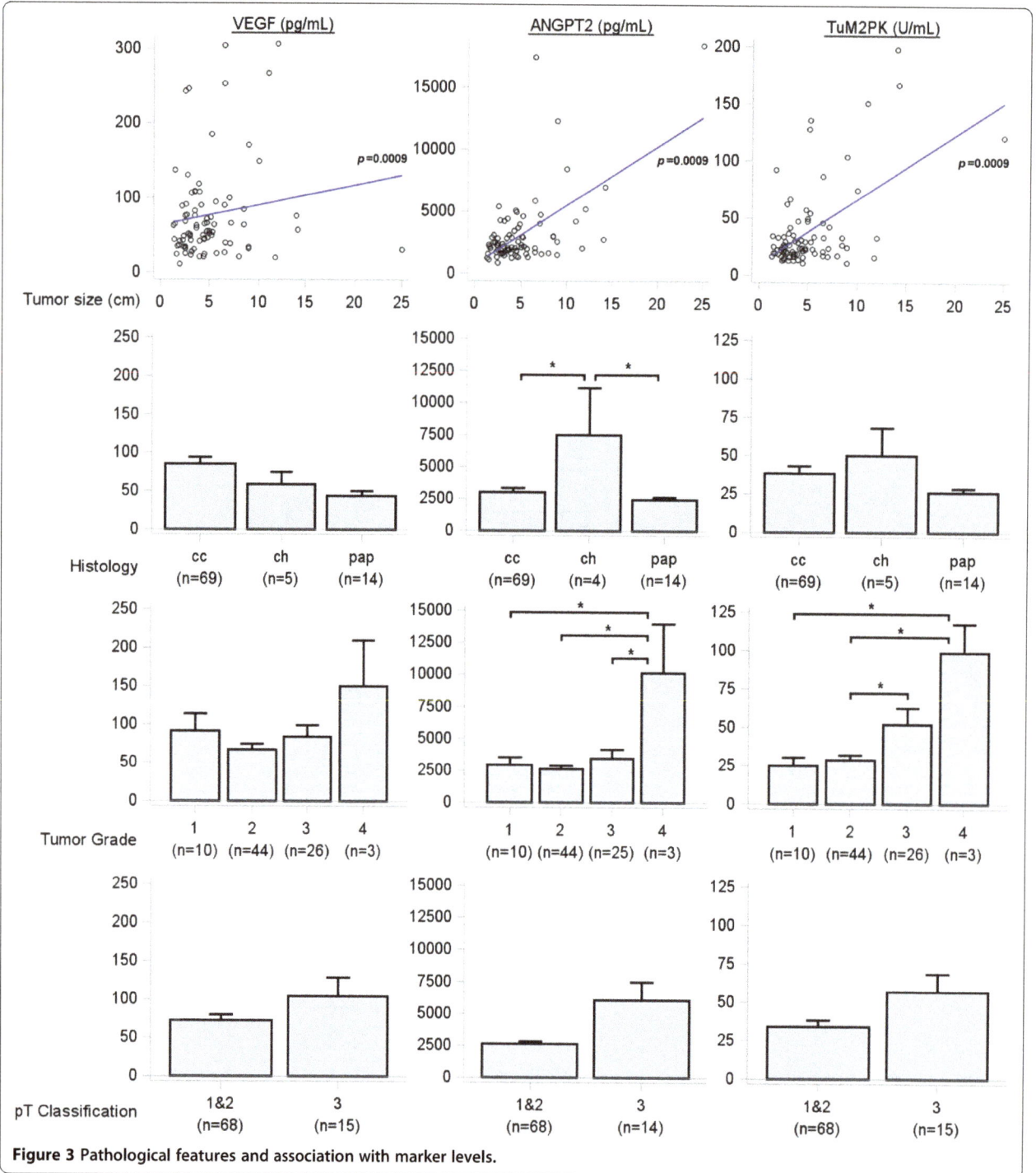

Figure 3 Pathological features and association with marker levels.

with several adverse pathological features, notably size and grade.

While anti-VEGF therapies have become mainstay of treatment for patients with metastatic clear cell RCC, the role and efficacy of targeted therapies in non-clear cell variants remains unclear [28]. Developing therapies based on molecular markers specific for other histologies could improve oncological outcomes. In our study, ANGTP2 levels were significantly higher in patients with chromophobe RCC, than those with either clear cell or papillary RCC, suggesting that ANGPT2/TIE2 system may play a particularly important role in chromophobe tumors and may serve as a target for therapy. However, not all chromophobe samples exhibited the same degree of ANGPT2 elevation.

Disappointingly, temporal trends did not show the predicted decrease in marker levels that we expected. This could be due to several reasons. The short follow-up of the study did not allow for enough time for the marker levels to decrease. Also, the timing of when marker samples were collected could account for the variability in levels. However, currently the timing of when marker samples should be collected remains undefined. Nevertheless, some reports show that it may take 11 weeks for elevated levels of TuM2PK to normalize [10].

The definitive goal of developing novel biomarkers would be incorporation into current prognostic tools. Novel markers, such as ANGPT2 and TuM2PK could improve oncological outcomes in patients with RCC by identifying patients who may benefit from a particular therapy, thus individualizing treatment plans. Biomarker-based scoring algorithms, such as the Bio-Score, which is based on the expression levels of B7-H1, survivin, and Ki67, help to predict the likelihood of RCC specific death [29]. Individuals with high Bio-scores are associated with a higher rate of death from RCC than individuals with low BioScores [29]. Thus, biomarker incorporation into current prognostic models could serve as an excellent risk stratification tool that both individualizes therapy and as well as directs treatment.

Our study has several limitations. The number of patients is modest. While we concluded that elevated marker levels were significantly seen in certain subtypes of RCC, our data is still limited by the number of patients included in the study. As with prospective studies, results are based on availability of samples postoperatively and patient follow up. Despite these challenges, our study does show significant associations between some markers and adverse pathological parameters.

Conclusion

In our preliminary study, plasma levels of ANGPT2 and TuM2PK obtained prior to ablation or surgery for renal masses, were increased compared to controls and were associated with several aggressive pathological features including tumor size and grade. Our findings support further research into the role of circulating proteins as a means to augment current prognostic predictors of outcome in patients with kidney cancer.

Abbreviations

ANGPT2: Angiopoietin-2; VEGF: Vascular endothelial growth factor; TuM2PK: M2 pyruvate kinase; RCC: Renal cell carcinoma; CSS: Cancer specific survival; ccRCC: Clear-cell type.

Competing interests

No authors have any direct or indirect commercial financial incentive associated with publishing the article. The present manuscript or portions thereof are not under consideration by another journal or electronic publication and have not been previously published. All authors declare that they have no competing interests.

Authors' contributions

BG conception/design; analysis/interpretation; writing. JG conception/design; analysis/interpretation; writing. AC analysis/interpretation; writing. SPL - conception/design; analysis/interpretation; writing. XJX - conception/design; analysis/interpretation; writing. JY - conception/design; analysis/interpretation; writing. JK - conception/design; analysis/interpretation; writing. GR - analysis/interpretation; writing. AS - analysis/interpretation; writing. YL - analysis/interpretation; writing. VM - design, analysis/interpretation; writing. JB - conception/design; analysis/interpretation; writing and funding. All authors read and approved the final manuscript.

Acknowledgements

We acknowledge the patients who donated samples. This work was supported by UL1RR024982, titled, North and Central Texas Clinical and Translational Science Initiative from the National Center for Research Resources (NCRR), a component of NIH and NIH Roadmap for Medical Research, and its contents are solely the responsibility of the authors and do not represent official views.

Author details

[1]Department of Urology, University of Texas Southwestern Medical Center, Dallas, Texas, USA. [2]Department Internal Medicine, University of Texas Southwestern Medical Center, Dallas, Texas, USA. [3]Department of Clinical Science, University of Texas Southwestern Medical Center, Dallas, Texas, USA. [4]Department of Developmental Biology, University of Texas Southwestern Medical Center, Dallas, Texas, USA. [5]Department of Urology, MD Anderson Cancer Center, Houston, Texas, USA. [6]Department of Urology, UT Southwestern Medical Center at Dallas, 5323 Harry Hines Blvd., Dallas 75390-9110, Texas, USA.

References

1. Siegel R, Ma J, Zou Z, Jemal A. Cancer statistics, 2014. CA Cancer J Clin. 2014;64(1):9–29.
2. Campbell SC, Lane, BR. Malignant Renal Tumors. In: Campbell-Walsh Urology, 10th Edition. 10th edn. Edited by Kavoussi L, Novick A, Partin A, Peters C; 2012: 1443–1444.
3. Vaishampayan U, Vankayala H, Vigneau FD, Quarshie W, Dickow B, Chalasani S, et al. The Effect of Targeted Therapy on Overall Survival in Advanced Renal Cancer: A Study of the National Surveillance Epidemiology and End Results Registry Database. Clin Genitourin Canc. 2014;12(2):124–9.
4. Haas NB, Uzzo RG. Targeted therapies for kidney cancer in urologic practice. Urol Oncol-Semin Ori. 2007;25(5):420–32.
5. Maisonpierre PC, Suri C, Jones PF, Bartunkova S, Wiegand SJ, Radziejewski C, et al. Angiopoietin-2, a natural antagonist for Tie2 that disrupts in vivo angiogenesis. Science. 1997;277(5322):55–60.
6. Teichert-Kuliszewska K, Maisonpierre PC, Jones N, Campbell AI, Master Z, Bendeck MP, et al. Biological action of angiopoietin-2 in a fibrin matrix

model of angiogenesis is associated with activation of Tie2. Cardiovasc Res. 2001;49(3):659–70.

7. Huang H, Bhat A, Woodnutt G, Lappe R. Targeting the ANGPT-TIE2 pathway in malignancy. Nat Rev Cancer. 2010;10(8):575–85.

8. Kucejova B, Sunny NE, Nguyen AD, Hallac R, Fu X, Pena-Llopis S, et al. Uncoupling hypoxia signaling from oxygen sensing in the liver results in hypoketotic hypoglycemic death. Oncogene. 2011;30(18):2147–60.

9. Christofk HR, Vander Heiden MG, Harris MH, Ramanathan A, Gerszten RE, Wei R, et al. The M2 splice isoform of pyruvate kinase is important for cancer metabolism and tumour growth. Nature. 2008;452(7184):230–3.

10. Wechsel HW, Petri E, Bichler KH, Feil G. Marker for renal cell carcinoma (RCC): the dimeric form of pyruvate kinase type M2 (Tu M2-PK). Anticancer Res. 1999;19(4A):2583–90.

11. Nisman B, Yutkin V, Nechushtan H, Gofrit ON, Peretz T, Gronowitz S, et al. Circulating tumor M2 pyruvate kinase and thymidine kinase 1 are potential predictors for disease recurrence in renal cell carcinoma after nephrectomy. Urology. 2010;76(2):513. e511-516.

12. Shariat SF, Chade DC, Karakiewicz PI, Ashfaq R, Isbarn H, Fradet Y, et al. Combination of multiple molecular markers can improve prognostication in patients with locally advanced and lymph node positive bladder cancer. J Urol. 2010;183(1):68–75.

13. Hernandez-Yanez M, Heymach JV, Zurita AJ. Circulating biomarkers in advanced renal cell carcinoma: clinical applications. Curr Oncol Rep. 2012;14(3):221–9.

14. Banks RE, Forbes MA, Kinsey SE, Stanley A, Ingham E, Walters C, et al. Release of the angiogenic cytokine vascular endothelial growth factor (VEGF) from platelets: significance for VEGF measurements and cancer biology. Br J Cancer. 1998;77(6):956–64.

15. Mita AC, Takimoto CH, Mita M, Tolcher A, Sankhala K, Sarantopoulos J, et al. Phase 1 study of AMG 386, a selective angiopoietin 1/2-neutralizing peptibody, in combination with chemotherapy in adults with advanced solid tumors. Clin Cancer Res. 2010;16(11):3044–56.

16. Augustin HG, Koh GY, Thurston G, Alitalo K. Control of vascular morphogenesis and homeostasis through the angiopoietin-Tie system. Nat Rev Mol Cell Biol. 2009;10(3):165–77.

17. Ahmad SA, Liu W, Jung YD, Fan F, Wilson M, Reinmuth N, et al. The effects of angiopoietin-1 and –2 on tumor growth and angiogenesis in human colon cancer. Cancer Res. 2001;61(4):1255–9.

18. Sallinen H, Heikura T, Laidinen S, Kosma VM, Heinonen S, Yla-Herttuala S, et al. Preoperative angiopoietin-2 serum levels: a marker of malignant potential in ovarian neoplasms and poor prognosis in epithelial ovarian cancer. Int J Gynecol Cancer. 2010;20(9):1498–505.

19. Bhaskar A, Gupta R, Vishnubhatla S, Kumar L, Sharma A, Sharma MC, et al. Angiopoietins as biomarker of disease activity and response to therapy in multiple myeloma. Luek Lymphoma. 2013;54(7):1473–8.

20. Srirajaskanthan R, Dancey G, Hackshaw A, Luong T, Caplin ME, Meyer T. Circulating angiopoietin-2 is elevated in patients with neuroendocrine tumours and correlates with disease burden and prognosis. Endocr Relat Cancer. 2009;16(3):967–76.

21. Currie MJ, Gunningham SP, Turner K, Han C, Scott PA, Robinson BA, et al. Expression of the angiopoietins and their receptor Tie2 in human renal clear cell carcinomas; regulation by the von Hippel-Lindau gene and hypoxia. J Pathol. 2002;198(4):502–10.

22. Bullock AJ, Zhang L, O'Neill AM, Percy A, Sukhatme V, Mier JW, et al. Plasma angiopoietin-2 (ANG2) as an angiogenic biomarker in renal cell carcinoma (RCC). [Abstract] J Clin Oncol. 2010;28:15s. suppl; abstr 4630.

23. Pal SK, Williams S, Josephson DY, Carmichael C, Vogelzang NJ, Quinn DI. Novel therapies for metastatic renal cell carcinoma: efforts to expand beyond the VEGF/mTOR signaling paradigm. Mol Cancer Ther. 2012;11(3):526–37.

24. Landt S, Jeschke S, Koeninger A, Thomas A, Heusner T, Korlach S, et al. Tumor-specific correlation of tumor M2 pyruvate kinase in pre-invasive, invasive and recurrent cervical cancer. Anticancer Res. 2010;30(2):375–81.

25. Hathurusinghe HR, Goonetilleke KS, Siriwardena AK. Current status of tumor M2 pyruvate kinase (tumor M2-PK) as a biomarker of gastrointestinal malignancy. Ann Surg Oncol. 2007;14(10):2714–20.

26. Roigas J, Schulze G, Raytarowski S, Jung K, Schnorr D, Loening SA. Tumor M2 pyruvate kinase in plasma of patients with urological tumors. Tumour Biol. 2001;22(5):282–5.

27. Varga Z, Hegele A, Stief T, Heidenreich A, Hofmann R. Determination of pyruvate kinase type tumor M2 in human renal cell carcinoma: a suitable tumor marker? Urol Res. 2002;30(2):122–5.

28. Singer EA, Gupta GN, Marchalik D, Srinivasan R. Evolving therapeutic targets in renal cell carcinoma. Curr Opin Oncol. 2013;25(3):273–80.

29. Parker AS, Leibovich BC, Lohse CM, Sheinin Y, Kuntz SM, Eckel-Passow JE, et al. Development and evaluation of BioScore: a biomarker panel to enhance prognostic algorithms for clear cell renal cell carcinoma. Cancer. 2009;115(10):2092–103.

4

Ureteroscopic management of asymptomatic and symptomatic simple parapelvic renal cysts

XiaWa Mao, Gang Xu, HuiFeng Wu and JiaQuan Xiao[*]

Abstract

Background: To investigate feasibility and safety of treating simple parapelvic renal cysts using flexible ureteroscopy with the Holmium laser.

Methods: Between February 2010 and July 2013, a total of 21 patients, aging from 29 to 71 (49.00 ± 13.23), were diagnosed with parapelvic renal cysts by ultrasonography in combination with contrast-enhanced computer tomography (CT) and intravenous urography (IVU) in the Department of Urology Surgery, People's Hospital of the Zhejiang province. Fifteen patients were asymptomatic and 6 patients were symptomatic with flank pain. All patients underwent drainage of the cysts using flexible ureteroscopy with Holmium laser. Patients were followed up 1, 3 and 12 months after the operation.

Results: The intervention was successful in 20 patients and failed in 1 patient who, subsequently successfully underwent a laparoscopic cyst removal. There were no intra-operative and post-operative complications reported. The mean operation time was 27 min (range: 15 to 45 min). The mean hospital stay was 2.6 days (range: 1 to 5 days). Twenty patients were followed up until 15 months after surgery. After such ureteroscopic management, there were no renal cysts detected in 7 patients (35 %) and a reduction in size of the renal cysts was found in 13 patients (65 %). Flank pain subsided in all 6 (100 %) previously symptomatic patients.

Conclusions: Flexible ureteroscopy with the Holmium laser may be a feasible and effective treatment option in selected patients with simple parapelvic renal cysts. Further prospective randomized studies that compare the procedure to laparoscopic treatments are needed.

Keywords: Parapelvic renal cyst, Flexible ureterscopy, Holmium laser

Background

At least 20 % of adults will have formed simple renal cysts by the age of 40 and up to 33 % will have developed renal cysts at the age of 60 [1]. Most parapelvic renal cysts are found by chance and are generally symptomless but as they are closely associated with the hilar vessels and the collecting system they can produce symptoms of renal obstruction. If symptomatic, the most commonly reported symptoms are lumbar discomfort (followed by urinary tract infection (9.5 %) and hematuria (4.8 %) [2]. Other possible consequences of parapelvic cysts include stone formation, vascular compression, renin-mediated hypertension and spontaneous hemorrhage. A successful diagnosis can be achieved by ultrasonography and contrast-enhanced computer tomography examinations [3].

The management of parapelvic renal cysts has evolved over the past decades from open exploration for marsupilation or nephrectomy to laparoscopic renal-sparing cyst excision, unroofing, decortication and ablation [4, 5]. Percutaneous aspiration and sclerotherapy are contraindicated for parapelvic cysts since potentially serious complications such as extravasation of sclerosing agents from the renal cyst into the retroperitoneum may lead to local inflammation and consequent ureteropelvic junction obstruction, fever, pain and high possibility of cyst recurrence [6, 7]. Successful endoscopic management of renal cysts by antegrade percutaneous nephroscopic

* Correspondence: Jiaquanxiao@hotmail.com
Department of Urology, The Second Affiliated Hospital of Zhejiang University School of Medicine, Hangzhou, P.R. China

ablation and retrograde flexible ureteroscopy have recently been reported [8–10]. The retrograde approach is effective and has a low complication rate. Other benefits include its minimally invasive nature and a short hospital stay after surgery. Basiri et al. reported the successful ureteroscopic treatment of parapelvic renal cysts in 2 cases, while they could not report the long-term follow-up details [9]. In a recent study by Luo et al., treatment of renal parapelvic cysts with a flexible ureteroscope could make 10 of 15 patients cyst free after 6 or 12 months [11]. Despite these promising results, there have only been very few reports describing the management of renal cysts with retrograde flexible ureteroscopy. Furthermore, little information can be found regarding the long-term results of this treatment. The objective of our study was to report the long-term results of management of renal cysts with retrograde flexible ureteroscopy using holmium laser.

Methods

Between February 2010 and July 2013, 21 patients from the Department of Urology of People's Hospital of Zhejiang Province participated in this investigation. Patients included in this study met the following criteria: presence of a simple renal parapelvic cyst greater than 3 cm in size; no history of ureteral stricture; and presence of a parapelvic cyst wall close to the pelvic wall. Those whose cysts were suspected for malignant in imaging and those who were less than 18 years old or more than 80 years old were excluded from the study. A total of 15 patients were asymptomatic and the cysts were incidental findings during routine medical examination. Six patients were symptomatic with flank pain. Patients were informed in detail about the ureteroscopic operation and possible complications and all patients provided written informed consent before enrollment in the study. Urine analysis, urine culture, serum electrolytes, ultrasonography, intravenous urography (IVU) and contrast-enhanced computed tomography (CT) were performed in all patients prior to the operation. We defined simple parapelvic renal cysts as

circular renal cysts, filled with clear fluid and without any connection to the pyelocaliceal system. Ureteral stenting was performed 2 weeks before the operation in each patient to facilitate ureteroscopic access. All data was collected in a prospectively maintained database. Patients were invited for follow-up examinations at 1, 3 and 12 months postoperation. The Ethics Committee of People's Hospital of Zhejiang Province had agreed to the study.

The procedure was performed while the patient was under general anesthesia in lithotomy position. All patients were given a prophylactic dose of cefatriaxone (1.0 g) 30 min before the operation. Initially, a rigid diagnostic ureteroscopy with an 8.5 F instrument was performed to dilate and explore the ureter in order to confirm a normal ureter (Fig. 1a). Then, a 12 F ureteral access sheath was introduced over a guidewire. Afterwards, the flexible ureteroscope was advanced into the renal pelvis to identify the location of peripelvic cyst (Fig. 1b). Incision and drainage of the renal cyst wall were performed using a holmium laser with a 200 um fiber (Fig. 1c). If stones were present, lithotripsy was performed during the same session. A window in the cyst as large as possible was opened with a holmium laser (Lumenis, VersaPulse®, PowerSuite™, 60 W, two wavelength for adequate drainage. The laser setting were 0.8 J and a frequency of 25 Hz, a combination which is less likely to injure adjacent tissue we find more accurate. Finally, a 6double J stent was placed in the ureter with upper end inside the cyst... The stent was removed one month after the operation.

Patients' demographic characteristics,, the operative time, surgical time and length of hospital stay were recorded. The cyst size was measured before the operation, and during the follow-up period in an outpatient clinic at 1, 3 and 12 months after the surgery. The follow-up examination included a CT scan and ultrasound. Lack of detection of the cyst or a decrease in size to less than 50 % of the original mass was considered evidence of a successful operation [12].

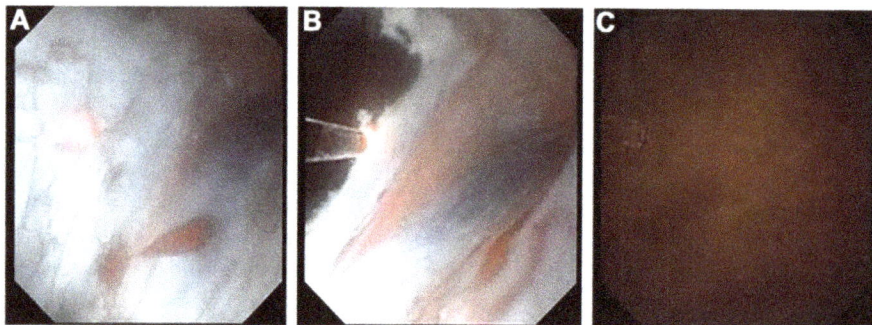

Fig. 1 Video screenshots flexible ureteroscopic surgery with Holmium laser for a simple parapelvic renal cysts. **a** A rigid diagnostic ureteroscopy with an 8.5 F instrument is used to dilate and visualize the ureter. **b** A flexible ureteroscope is advanced into the renal pelvis to identify the location of peripelvic cyst. **c** A holmium laser with a 200 um fiber is used to incise and drain the renal cyst wall

Results

Patients' basic characteristics are detailed in Table 1. A total of 21 patients underwent flexible ureteroscopic drainage of simple renal parapelvic cysts using a holmium laser. The patient population included 12 males and 9 females and the mean age was 49 years (range from 29 to 71 years). Additional patient details are presented in Table 1. The mean cyst size was 4.5 cm (range from 3 to 7 cm) and stones were found inside the renal cysts (mean size 0.8 cm) of 3 patients.

The ureteroscopic procedure was successful in 20 patients with no major complications and no trauma to adjacent organs and great vessels; no pneumothorax or hemothorax were detected. The mean operation time was 27 min (range: 15-45 min) and the mean hospital stay was 2.6 days (range: 1-5 days). One operation failed as the renal cyst wall could not be found endoscopically. The procedure was converted to laparoscopy which made renal cyst unroofing possible.

Postoperativ fever was noted in one female patient 2 h after the operation (38.5 °C temperature, with a low blood pressure 85/65 mmHg). The patient's parapelvic renal cyst contained tens of small stones with sizes ranging from 2 to 4 mm and the pre-operative urine culture had demonstrated the presence of Escherichia coli. After antibiotic treatment, the urosepsis settled in 3 days.

Patients underwent follow-up examinations at 1, 3 and 12 months post operation. One month after the operation, there was no evidence of renal cysts in 7 (35 %) patients and 13 (65 %) patients experienced a mean reduction in cyst size of 49.2 ± 12.6 mm to 20.0 ± 7.1 mm. The mean size of the renal cysts of the 13 patients further decreased to 16.5 ± 5.5 mm 3 months after the operation. The renal cysts of 5 patients were no longer detected 12 months after the operation, indicating no detection in 12 patients in total; and the mean size of the renal cysts in the remaining 8 patients further decreased to 11.9 ± 5.3 mm 12 months after the operation. Patients' outcomes are detailed in Table 1. Complete resolution of flank pain occurred in all 6 (100 %) previously symptomatic patients. A typical CT scan of a non detectable renal cyst 1 month after the operation (Fig. 2).

Discussion

The terms parapelvic and peripelvic cysts generally describe cysts around the renal pelvis or renal sinus [13].

Table 1 Patients' characteristics

Patient number	Gender	Age	Preoperative cyst size (cm)	Surgical time (min)	Hospital stay (day)	Cyst size at 1 month after the surgery (cm)	Cyst size at 3 months after the surgery (cm)	Cyst size at 1 year after the surgery (cm)
1	Male	35	4	24	2	1	0.5	0.5
2	Male	41	5	30	2	2	2	1
3	Male	29	4	33	1	2	1	1
4	Male	59	6	15	3	3	2	1
5	Male	68	4	30	4	2	2	2
6	Male	26	5	18	2	2	2	2
7	Male	43	4.5	22	2	0	0	0
8	Male	47	4	22	4	0	0	0
9	Male	29	3	25	2	0	0	0
10	Male	70	4	45	5	2	2	1
11	Male	38	3	24	1	1	1	1
12	Male	54	5	23	4	2	2	0
13	Female	62	3	20	2	0	0	0
14	Female	71	4	37	2	0	0	0
15	Female	33	4	29	3	1	1	0
16	Female	41	4	27	4	0	0	0
17	Female	45	6	35	2	3	2	0
18	Female	56	7	30	2	2	2	0
19	Female	60	3	34	3	0	0	0
20	Female	50	7	17	2	3	2	0
21	Female (switch to laparoscopic surgery)	72	5	59	3	0		

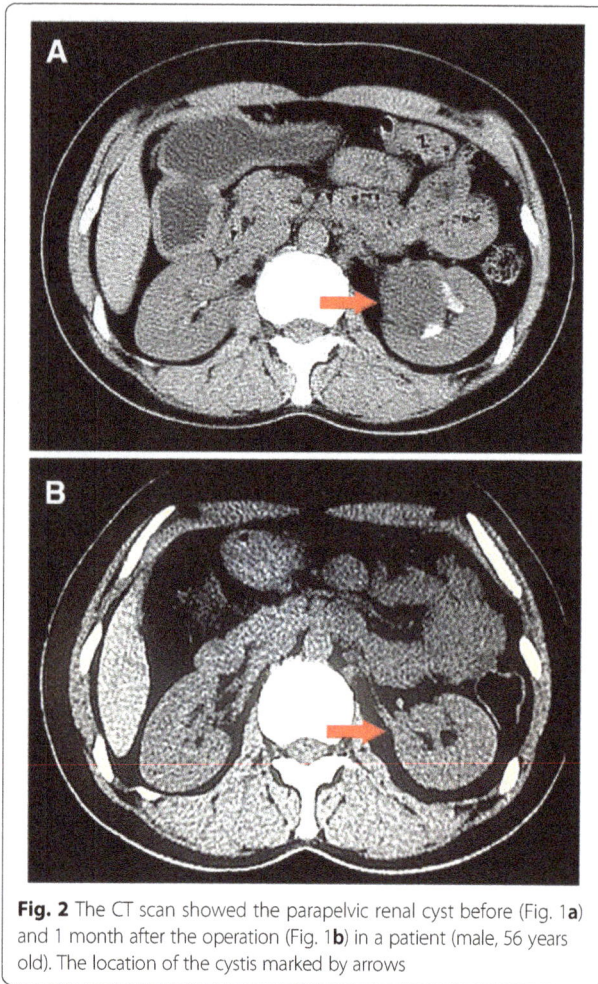

Fig. 2 The CT scan showed the parapelvic renal cyst before (Fig. 1**a**) and 1 month after the operation (Fig. 1**b**) in a patient (male, 56 years old). The location of the cystis marked by arrows

renal vessels. Sclerotherapy is considered to be contraindicated in the treatment of parapelvic renal cyst because it can provoke perirenal inflammation and subsequently, ureteropelvic junction obstruction. Laparoscopic unroofing requires advanced surgical skills, is considerable invasive and unavoidably leads to comparatively more blood loss. However, it is a common treatment for cysts which are not parapelvic or those who are not suitable for ureteroscopy for example because of ureteral stenosis. Percutaneous ablation has results similar to laparoscopic treatment and has better results than aspiration with or without using sclerosing agents. This from of treatmen however, is invasive and requires the help of radiologist in the operating room.

Liaconis and Basiri first reported ureteroscopic treatment of parapelvic renal cyst with flexible and semirigid ureteroscopy [9, 10]. Both were preliminary studies with only one or two patients and a short follow-up period (3 and 6 months). Luo et al. reported disappearance of parapelvic renal cyst in 10 of 15 patients at 6 or 12 months after flexible ureterescopy [11]. To our knowledge, the current study evaluating the efficacy of ureteroscopic treatment of parapelvic renal cyst included the largest number of patients with a relative long follow-up. Compared with other methods, management of parapelvic renal cysts by flexible ureteroscopic with a holmium laser is characterized by its minimally invasive nature and a low complication rate. A major disadvantage of the treatment is that it cannot provide a pathological specimen. This suggests that a laparoscopic operation should be considered in patients with complicated parapelvic renal cysts that may be malignant in order to achieve an accurate pathological diagnosis.

The key point of this operation is to identify the renal cyst wall in order not to injure the renal parenchyma or renal vessels. The typical renal cyst looks transparent and is black and blue in some areas injecting methylene blue into the cyst can help the surgeon to identify the cyst wall more accurately. We encountered a low complication rate. In our study urosepsis was found in one patient with a parapelvic cyst containing stones. This finding implies that special attention must be paid to such patients. In addition, it should be noted that one operation failed in our study due to the difficulty in identifying the wall of the renal cyst. In the study by Luo et al., the mean total operation time, and mean duration of hospitalization were 31 ± 8 min and 3 days, respectively [11]. In the present study iopertive time was 27 min (range: 15 to 45 min) and hospital stay was2.6 days (range: 1 to 5 days), respectively.

Apart form a short operative time and a short hospital stary, retrograde intrarenal surgery may have further advantages compared with laparoscopic unrrofing: A possible serious complication of laparoscopy is formation of

They do not communicate with the collecting system and are believed to be lymphatic in origin secondary to obstruction. Generally, most of renal cysts are symptomless, but they can occasionally cause lumbar discomfort, haematuria, hypertension and hydronephrosis. On IVU, parapelvic renal cysts can show stretching and compression of calyces, similar to the appearance of renal sinus lipomatosis which involves proliferation of sinus fat leading to a mass effect on the intrarenal collecting system [14]. CT scan does not show enhancement following the administration of intravenous contrast dye and there is usually no hydroureter. On ultrasounds those renal cysts are generally centrally-placed and may be mistaken for hydronephrosis. Therefore, imaging with contrast dye in form of an IVU or a CT urogram should be performed for differential diagnosis.

Until now, various treatments of simple renal cyst have been proposed with varying outcomes, including sclerotherapy, laparoscopic unroofing and percutaneous ablation [8, 15, 16]. Compared with the treatment of simple renal cyst, the treatment of parapelvic renal cysts can be more difficult because of the location near the renal hilum and a urinary fistula due to inability to differentiate a parapelvic renal cyst and the renal collecting system. Moreover, laparoscopy has shown to have a greater significant estimated blood loss, increased operative time, and increased length of hospitalizationas opposed to the truly mini-invasive retrograde intrarenal surgery. Limitations of our study were that we had no comparison group and that a longer follow-up would be beneficial.

Conclusion

Flexible ureteroscopic treatment of parapelvic renal cyst is a feasible and effective treatment for parapelvic renal cysts. Compared to previous similar studies, this report represents the largest number of patients with the longest follow up period. A large prospective randomized study comparing this procedure to laparoscopic operation is warranted to confirm these results.

Abbreviations
CT: Computed tomography; IVU: Intravenous urography.

Competing interests
The authors declare that they have no competing interest.

Authors' contributions
XWM designed the study. GX recorded patients' information. HFW analysed the data. JQX contributed to the writing of the manuscript. All authors read and approved the final manuscript.

Acknowledgements
No funding assisted with the study.

References
1. Laucks Jr SP, McLachlan MS. Aging and simple cysts of the kidney. Br J Radiol. 1981;54:12–4.
2. Camargo AH, Cooperberg MR, Ershoff BD, Rubenstein JN, Meng MV, Stoller ML. Laparoscopic management of peripelvic renal cysts: University of California, San Francisco, experience and review of literature. Urology. 2005;65:882–7.
3. Tarzamni MK, Sobhani N, Nezami N, Ghiasi F. Bilateral parapelvic cysts that mimic hydronephrosis in two imaging modalities: a case report. Cases J. 2008;1:161.
4. Yoder BM, Wolf Jr JS. Long-term outcome of laparoscopic decortication of peripheral and peripelvic renal and adrenal cysts. J Urol. 2004;171:583–7.
5. Amar AD, Das S. Surgical management of benign renal cysts causing obstruction of renal pelvis. Urology. 1984;24:429–33.
6. Lang EK. Renal cyst puncture and aspiration: a survey of complications. Am J Roentgenol. 1977;128:723–7.
7. Camacho MF, Bondhus MJ, Carrion HM, Lockhart JL, Politano VA. Ureteropelvic junction obstruction resulting from percutaneous cyst puncture and intracystic isophendylate injection: an unusual complications. J Urol. 1980;124:713–4.
8. Korets R, Mues AC, Gupta M. Minimally invasive percutaneous ablation of parapelvic renal cysts and caliceal diverticula using bipolar energy. J Endourol Endourol Soc. 2011;25:769–73.
9. Basiri A, Hosseini SR, Tousi VN, Sichani MM. Ureteroscopic management of symptomatic, simple parapelvic renal cyst. J Endourol. 2010;24:537–40.
10. Liaconis H, Pautler SE, Razvi HA. Ureteroscopic decompression of an unusual uroepithelial cyst using the holmium:YAG laser. J Endourol. 2001;15:295–7.
11. Luo Q, Zhang X, Chen H, Liu Z, Chen X, Dai Y, et al. Treatment of renal parapelvic cysts with a flexible ureteroscope. Int Urol Nephrol. 2014;46:1903–8.
12. Glassberg K. Renal dysplasis and cystic disease of the kidney. Campbell's Urol. 2002;8:1443–95.
13. Wilson SR, Withers C, Wilson S, Charboneau W. The Urinary Tract. Diagnostic Ultrasound. 2005;1:373.
14. Rha SE, Byun JY, Jung SE, Oh SN, Choi YJ, Lee A, et al. The renal sinus: pathologic spectrum and multimodality imaging approach. Radiographics. 2004;24 Suppl 1:S117–131.
15. Kabala J, Roobottom C. The kidneys and ureters. London: Textbook of Radiology and Imaging Churchill Livingstone; 2003. p. 953.
16. Bean WJ. Renal cysts: treatment with alcohol. Radiology. 1981;138:329–31.

5

Xp11.2 translocation renal cell carcinomas in young adults

Linfeng Xu[†], Rong Yang[†], Weidong Gan[*], Xiancheng Chen, Xuefeng Qiu, Kai Fu, Jin Huang, Guancheng Zhu and Hongqian Guo[*]

Abstract

Background: Little is known about the biological behavior of Xp11.2 translocation renal cell carcinomas (RCCs) as few clinical studies have been performed using a large sample size.

Methods: This study included 103 consecutive young adult patients (age ≤ 45 years) with RCC who underwent partial or radical nephrectomy at our institution from 2008 to 2013. Five patients without complete clinical data were excluded. Of the 98 remaining patients, 16 and 82 patients were included in the Xp11.2 translocation and non-Xp11.2 translocation groups, respectively. Clinicopathologic data were collected, including age, gender, tumor size, laterality, symptoms at diagnosis, surgical procedure, pathologic stage, tumor grade, time of recurrence and death.

Results: Xp11.2 translocation RCCs were associated with higher tumor grade and pathologic stage ($P < 0.05$, Fisher's exact test). During the median follow-up of 36 months (range: 3–71 months), the number of cancer-related deaths was 4 (4.9 %) and 3 (18.7 %) in the non-Xp11.2 translocation and Xp11.2 translocation groups, respectively. The Kaplan-Meier cancer specific survival curves revealed a significant difference between non-Xp11.2 translocation RCCs and Xp11.2 translocation RCCs in young adults ($P = 0.042$).

Conclusions: Compared with non-Xp11.2 translocation RCCs, the Xp11.2 translocation RCCs seemingly showed a higher tumor grade and pathologic stage and have similar recurrence-free survival rates but poorer cancer-specific survival rates in young adults.

Keywords: Xp11.2 translocation, Renal cell carcinomas, TFE3, FISH

Background

Renal cell carcinoma (RCC) is the most common type of kidney cancer in adults and accounts for approximately 3 % of adult malignancies and 90–95 % of neoplasms arising from the kidney [1]. The morbidity and mortality of RCC is still growing. RCC can be histologically classified into several subtypes, among which clear cell RCC is the most prevalent and represents 70–80 % of kidney cancers [2].

Xp11.2 translocation RCC was first listed as a specific disease entity in the World Health Organization Classification of Tumors in 2004 [3]. This RCC subtype is defined by different translocations involving chromosome Xp11.2, all of which result in transcription factor E3 (TFE3) gene fusions. Several fusions of the TFE3 gene with different genes have been identified to date, including ASPL(17q25), PRCC(1q21), PSF(1q34), NonO(Xq12) and CLTC(17q23) [4]. Another subset of RCC is associated with transcription factor EB (TFEB) resulting from t(6;11)(p21;q12). PRCC-TFE3 RCCs [5] and ASPL-TFE3 RCCs [6] are the most frequent kinds of Xp11.2 translocation RCCs.

Recent reports have shown that the incidence of Xp11.2 translocation RCC is low. Approximately one-third of pediatric RCCs are estimated to be Xp11.2 translocation RCCs associated with TFE3 gene fusion [7]. Several studies have recently evaluated its incidence as 0.9 % (6/632) in adult RCCs [8], 15 % (4/26) in young adult RCCs [9], and 54 % (7/13) in child RCCs [10].

A meta-analysis by Rao et al. [11] demonstrated that TFE3 + pediatric RCCs were associated with a poorer outcome and higher stage (III/IV) than TFE3-RCCs.

* Correspondence: gwd@nju.edu.cn; doctorghq@gmail.com
[†]Equal contributors
Department of Urology, The Affiliated Drum Tower Hospital of Medical College of Nanjing University, Zhongshan Road 321, Nanjing, Jiangsu Province 210008, China

Komai et al. [12] reported that young patients (≤45 years) with RCC had similar recurrence-free survival rates but better cause-specific survival rates compared with older patients. In that study, Xp11.2 translocation RCCs accounted for at least one half of the young patients with RCC who had developed recurrence.

Until now, few clinical studies have examined the biological behavior of Xp11.2 translocation RCCs in young adults (≤45 years). In this study, we aimed to better define the biological behavior of Xp11.2 translocation RCCs and to determine whether its clinical outcomes differ from those of non-Xp11.2 translocation RCCs in young adults.

We hypothesized that Xp11.2 translocation RCCs have poorer prognosis than non-Xp11.2 translocation RCCs in young adults. The objectives of this study were as follows: (1) to compare the clinicopathologic data of Xp11.2 translocation RCCs with that of non-Xp11.2 translocation RCCs and obtain the clinicopathologic features that correlated with Xp11.2 translocation RCCs, and (2) confirm if cancer-specific survival (CSS) and recurrence-specific survival (RFS) of Xp11.2 translocation RCCs were significantly different from those of non-Xp11.2 translocation RCCs.

Methods

Study population

Of the 879 consecutive adult RCCs in our institution from 2008 to 2013, 103 patients were in the age range of 18–45 years. Five cases without complete clinical data were excluded. Of the remaining 98 patients, there were 16 with Xp11.2 translocation RCCs, 61 with clear cell RCCs, 10 with papillary RCCs, 9 with chromophobe RCCs and 2 with unclassified RCCs. In this study, we defined young age as ≤ 45 years according to definitions used in previous studies [9, 12]. We diagnosed Xp11.2 translocation RCCs with positive fluorescence in situ hybridization (FISH) after initial screening according to medical history, age, pathologic morphology and subsequent TFE3 immunostaining. The study was approved by the Committee on Medical Ethics of Nanjing Drum Tower Hospital, Jiangsu, China. All patients provided written informed consent.

Immunostaining

To investigate the incidence of Xp11.2 translocation RCC, TFE3 immunostaining was performed on paraffin-embedded tissue with the primary antibody TFE3 (Millipore, Billerica MA, US) using the manual overnight incubation methodology (using heat-induced epitope retrieval and the Dako Envision detection system).

FISH

A dual-color break-apart FISH assay for TFE3 gene rearrangement at the Xp11.2 region was performed on the TFE3 positively stained tissue using a self-designed polyclonal break-apart probe. In brief, FISH of interphase nuclei was performed on 4-μm-thick paraffin-embedded sections. The telomere sides of TFE3 gene cloning fragments (CTD-2516D6, CTD-2522 M13, and RP11-416B14) were labeled with fluorescein-12-dUTP and the centromeric sides of TFE3 gene cloning fragments (CTD-2312C1, CTD-2248C21, and RP11-959H17) were labeled with tetramethylrhodamine-5-dUTP. After sample preparation, hybridization with labeled DNA was performed overnight. Slides were counterstained with 4, 6-diamidino-2-phenylindole (DAPI, Vysis, Abbott Park, IL, USA) and analyzed using an Olympus BX-51 fluorescence microscope (Center Valley, PA, USA). Co-localization of red and green signals in tumor nuclei was considered negative, and a split signal in more than 10 % tumor nuclei was regarded positive for TFE3 rearrangement.

Assessment

The collected clinicopathologic data were as follows: age, gender, tumor size, laterality, symptoms at diagnosis, surgical procedure, pathologic stage, and tumor grade. All patients presented with tumor-free status after nephrectomy because no surgery was conservative or cytoreductive.

All patients had undergone a thorough medical history interview, physical examination, radiographic staging according to the computed tomography and/or magnetic resonance imaging of the abdomen as well as chest radiography. If warranted by the patient symptoms or physical examination findings, bone scans and brain imaging were performed.

The characteristics of the 98 patients are summarized in Table 1. The patients were followed up every 3–12 months with imaging studies. At each consultation, the patient's status (alive or dead) and the degree of tumor progression were determined. In the present study, the endpoints of follow-up were CSS and RFS.

Statistical analysis

The intergroup differences in the categorical and continuous variables were analyzed using Fisher's exact test and Student's t test, respectively. The CSS and RFS curves were obtained for Xp11.2 translocation and non-Xp11.2 translocation groups using the Kaplan-Meier method and compared using a log-rank test. All statistical analyses were performed using SPSS, version 17. In all analyses, calculated P values of < 0.05 were considered to indicate significance.

Results

Patients' outcome and pathologic results are shown in Table 1. The Xp11.2 translocation RCCs were significantly associated with higher tumor grade and pathologic stage

Table 1 Patient and tumor characteristics

Variable	non-Xp11.2 translocation group ($n = 82$)	Xp11.2 translocation group ($n = 16$)	P value
Age(y)			0.296
Media(Range)	40 (18–45)	27 (21–40)	
Gender(n)			0.086
Male	56 (68.3 %)	7 (43.8 %)	
Female	25 (31.7 %)	9 (56.3 %)	
Size(cm)			0.588
Media(Range)	4.6 (1.8–17.0)	4.5 (3.0–11.5)	
Laterality(n)			1.000
Left	39 (47.6 %)	7 (43.8 %)	
Right	43 (52.4 %)	9 (56.3 %)	
Symptoms(n)			
Asymptomatic	57 (69.5 %)	11 (68.8 %)	
Symptomatic	25 (30.5 %)	5 (31.3 %)	1.000
Nephrectomy (n)			0.156
Radical	49 (59.8 %)	13 (81.3 %)	
Partial	33 (40.2 %)	3 (18.8 %)	
Overall stage(n)			0.026
I	57 (69.5 %)	10 (62.5 %)	
II	22 (26.8 %)	2 (12.5 %)	
III	2 (2.4 %)	3 (18.8 %)	
IV	1 (1.2 %)	1 (6.3 %)	
TNM(2010AJCC)			
T(n)			0.026
T1	57 (69.5 %)	10 (62.5 %)	
T2	22 (26.8 %)	2 (12.5 %)	
T3	2 (2.4 %)	3 (18.8 %)	
T4	1 (1.2 %)	1 (6.3 %)	
N(n)			0.013
N_0	81 (98.8 %)	13 (81.3 %)	
N_1	1 (1.2 %)	3 (18.8 %)	
M(n)			
M_0	82 (100 %)	16 (100 %)	
M_1	0 (0)	0 (0)	
Tumor grade (n)			0.011
Low	25 (30.5 %)	0 (0 %)	
Medium	38 (46.3 %)	9 (56.3 %)	
High	19 (23.2 %)	7 (43.8 %)	
Follow-up (mo)			0.464
Media(Range)	33.5 (7–71)	29 (3–70)	

($P < 0.05$, Fisher's exact test). No statistically significant difference was observed in age, gender, tumor size, laterality, symptoms at diagnosis, or surgical procedure.

The number of cancer-related deaths was 4 (4.9 %) and 3 (18.7 %) in the non-Xp11.2 translocation and Xp11.2 translocation groups, respectively. Analyses of CSS curves indicated that Xp11.2 translocation RCCs were significantly more frequently associated with a poorer outcome than non-Xp11.2 translocation RCCs ($P = 0.042$, Fig. 1a).

A total of 12 (14.6 %) and 3 patients (18.7 %) in non-Xp11.2 translocation and Xp11.2 translocation groups developed recurrence, respectively. The Kaplan-Meier RFS curves revealed no difference between these two groups ($P = 0.505$, Fig. 1b).

Discussion

Xp11.2 translocation RCC has been recognized as a distinct entity in the World Health Organization renal tumor classification scheme for 11 years. Its diagnosis is usually based on microscopic appearance and TFE3 immunostaining. Further diagnostic testing is difficult because fresh tissue collection for cytogenetics and molecular analysis is not routinely performed in adult RCCs. Polymerase chain reaction can also be used to confirm a specific gene translocation on formalin-fixed, paraffin-embedded tissue, but it is infrequently used as a clinical diagnostic tool and is more often used in the research setting. At present, the TFE3 break-apart FISH assay has been used to further confirm diagnosis of Xp11.2 translocation RCC [13–16].

The incidence of Xp11.2 translocation RCC is low. Previous studies have revealed an incidence of 0.9 (6/632) [8] to 5 %(6/121) [17] in all adult RCCs and 15 % (4/26) in young adult RCCs [9]. According to age at the time of surgery, the incidence values of TFE3 positivity in the age ranges of 0–10, 11–20, 21–30, and 31–40 years were 67 (2/3), 75 (3/4), 29 (2/7), and 14 % (6/44), respectively ($P < 0.001$) [18]. Because RCC is more commonly encountered in the adult population, the amount of Xp11.2 translocation RCCs in adults may exceed that in the pediatric group. Our study revealed an incidence of 1.8 % (16/879) in all adult RCCs and 15.5 % (16/103) in young adult RCCs, which was consistent with previous reports.

Currently little is known concerning the biological behavior of Xp11.2 translocation RCCs because few clinical studies have been performed with a large sample size.

Based on the available data, the pediatric Xp11.2 translocation RCC is relatively inert, and its prognosis is better than that of adult Xp11.2 translocation RCC [19, 20]. Song et al. [21] reported that pediatric Xp11.2 translocation RCC easily invaded regional lymph nodes and was highly malignant. However, patients with N + M0 maintained a favorable prognosis following surgery alone.

Xp11.2 translocation RCCs that occur in adults may be more aggressive than those in children. Argani et al. [22] investigated 28 adult patients with Xp11 translocation

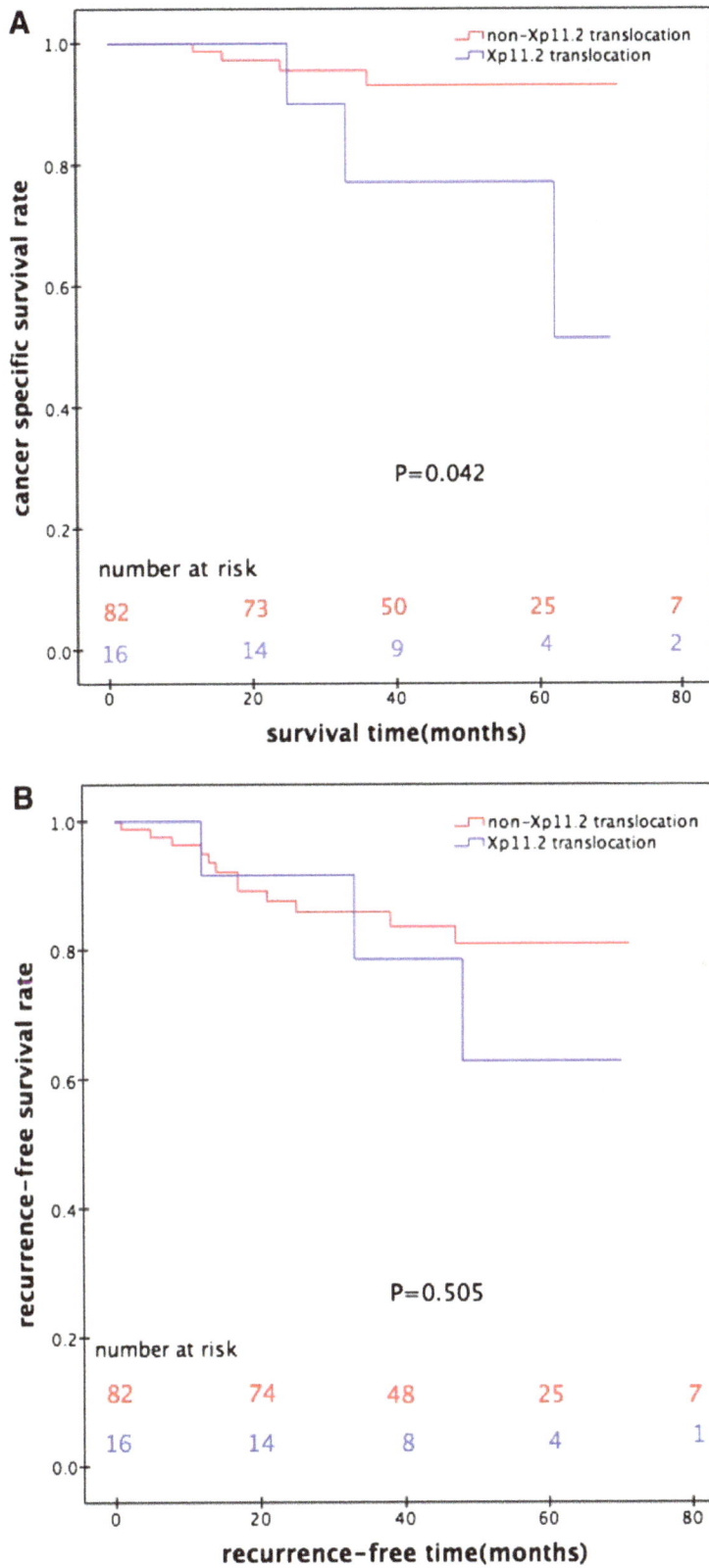

Fig. 1 Cancer-specific survival (**a**) and recurrence-specific survival (**b**) analyses were computed comparing non-Xp11.2 translocation renal cell carcinomas (RCCs) with Xp11.2 translocation RCCs in young adults. Red line: non-Xp11.2 translocation RCC; blue line: Xp11.2 translocation RCC

RCC, including 16 patients with stage III–IV cancers. Lymph node metastasis occurred in 11 of 13 patients who could be evaluated. Meyer [23] examined 5 adult patients with Xp11.2 translocation RCC, all of whom were in the late stage of their disease with distant metastasis, rapid disease course, and poor outcomes with an average survival of 18 months. Of the 7 adult patients with Xp11.2 translocation RCC that Komai et al. [9] investigated, 5 were classified as stages III–IV and 2 died within 1 year. In a study by Zou et al. [24], the authors reported that 5 out of 9 Xp11.2 RCC patients presented with TNM stages 3–4, and 6 died 10 months to 7 years after their operation. According to the review by Armah and Parwani [20], clinical and pathological heterogeneity may exist between pediatric Xp11.2 translocation RCC and adult Xp11.2 translocation RCC. Xp11.2 translocation RCCs had a high degree of invasiveness, rapid disease course, and poor prognosis in adolescents and adults over the age of 16 years, compared to that in children.

Xp11.2 translocation RCCs were extremely uncommon after 45 years of age, but this is likely an underestimation. Four patients reported by Arnoux [25] were older than 45 years, including three women (53, 71, and 75 years old) and one man (86 years old). One patient was metastatic at diagnosis. Radical nephrectomy was first performed in all cases. TNM staging was T3aN2R0, T3bN0R0, T2N2R0, and T3aN2R2, with a Furhman grade of 4. Two patients progressed with metastasis 5 and 7 months after surgery, and two with lymphatic invasion 2 and 9 months after nephrectomy. One patient died during follow-up. Ellis et al. [26] confirmed that older age or advanced stage at presentation predicted death through multivariate analysis.

In this study, among 16 young adults with Xp11.2 translocation RCCs, 4 (25 %) were classified stage III–IV and 7 (43.8 %) were Furman's grade 3–4. The Kaplan-Meier CSS curve revealed a significant difference between non-Xp11.2 translocation and Xp11.2 translocation groups. The results of the present study indicated that Xp11.2 translocation RCCs are associated with higher tumor grade and pathologic stage and poorer CCS in young adults.

Based on morphological appearance, RCC is subdivided into clear cell (70–80 %), papillary (10–15 %), chromophobe (3–5 %), collecting duct (1 %), and unclassified (1 %) subtypes [27]. Several studies have shown age to influence the distribution of histological subtypes [12, 28]. A more consistent finding across several studies is that the proportion of tumors with chromophobe histology decreases with increasing age [12, 29, 30]. The clinical behavior of chromophobe RCCs is less aggressive than that of clear cell RCCs, independent of Fuhrman grade or tumor size [31]. The change of histological subtypes may be associated with better prognosis of non-Xp11.2 translocation RCCs.

Similar to conventional RCCs, radical nephrectomy is recommended for Xp11.2 translocation RCCs. Nephron-sparing surgery is an alternative with favorable outcomes in symptomless small RCCs [32]. For the treatment of adult metastatic Xp11.2 translocation RCCs, VEGF-targeted agents appear to demonstrate some efficacy [33].

Our study had several limitations. The sample size was small due to low incidence of this rare disease and the follow-up time was relatively short. The calculation was weak to answer the hypothesis. Thus, we should interpret the CSS curve with some caution before further follow-up is performed.

Conclusions

Our study showed that Xp11.2 translocation RCCs were seemingly associated with higher tumor grade and pathologic stage in young adults. Moreover, it seemed that Xp11.2 translocation RCCs had similar RFS rates but poorer CSS rates than non-Xp11.2 translocation RCCs in young adults. Our findings suggest that Xp11.2 translocation RCCs should be treated more actively and monitored by follow up.

Abbreviations
RCC: Renal cell carcinoma; TFE3: Transcription factor E3; TFEB: Transcription factor EB; FISH: Fluorescence in situ hybridization; CSS: Cancer specific survival; RFS: Recurrence-free survival.

Competing interests
The authors declare that they have no competing interests.

Authors' contributions
LX and RY participated in the sequence alignment and drafted the manuscript. XC carried out the immunoassays. KF and GZ participated in the sequence alignment. XQ and JH participated in the design of the study and performed the statistical analysis. WG and HG conceived the study, participated in its design and coordination, and helped draft the manuscript. All authors read and approved the final manuscript.

Acknowledgements
We received financial support from National Natural Science Foundation of China (ID: 21377052), Natural Science Foundation of Jiangsu Province (ID: BK20131281), "Summit of the Six Top Talents" Program of Jiangsu Province (ID:WSN-005) and Nanjing health distinguished youth fund (ID:JQX12004).

References
1. Siegel R, Naishadham D, Jemal A. Cancer statistics, 2013. CA Cancer J Clin. 2013;63(1):11–30. doi:10.3322/caac.21166.
2. Rini BI, Campbell SC, Escudier B. Renal cell carcinoma. Lancet. 2009;373(9669):1119–32. doi:10.1016/S0140-6736(09)60229-4.
3. Argani P, Ladanyi M. Renal carcinomas associated with Xp11.2 translocations / TFE3 gene fusions. In: Eble JNSG, Epstein JI, Sesterhenn IA, editors. Pathology and genetics of tumors of the urinary system and male genital organs. Lyon: IARC Press; 2004. p. 37.
4. Kuroda N, Mikami S, Pan CC, Cohen RJ, Hes O, Michal M, et al. Review of renal carcinoma associated with Xp11.2 translocations/TFE3 gene fusions with focus on pathobiological aspect. Histol Histopathol. 2012;27(2):133–40.
5. Argani P, Antonescu CR, Couturier J, Fournet JC, Sciot R, Debiec-Rychter M, et al. PRCC-TFE3 renal carcinomas: morphologic, immunohistochemical, ultrastructural, and molecular analysis of an entity associated with the t(X;1)(p11.2;q21). Am J Surg Pathol. 2002;26(12):1553–66.

6. Argani P, Antonescu CR, Illei PB, Lui MY, Timmons CF, Newbury R, et al. Primary renal neoplasms with the ASPL-TFE3 gene fusion of alveolar soft part sarcoma: a distinctive tumor entity previously included among renal cell carcinomas of children and adolescents. Am J Pathol. 2001;159(1):179–92. doi:10.1016/S0002-9440(10)61684-7.

7. Argani P, Ladanyi M. Translocation carcinomas of the kidney. Clin Lab Med. 2005;25(2):363–78. doi:10.1016/j.cll.2005.01.008.

8. Sukov WR, Hodge JC, Lohse CM, Leibovich BC, Thompson RH, Pearce KE, et al. TFE3 rearrangements in adult renal cell carcinoma: clinical and pathologic features with outcome in a large series of consecutively treated patients. Am J Surg Pathol. 2012;36(5):663–70. doi:10.1097/PAS.0b013e31824dd972.

9. Komai Y, Fujiwara M, Fujii Y, Mukai H, Yonese J, Kawakami S, et al. Adult Xp11 translocation renal cell carcinoma diagnosed by cytogenetics and immunohistochemistry. Clin Cancer Res. 2009;15(4):1170–6. doi:10.1158/1078-0432.CCR-08-1183.

10. Ramphal R, Pappo A, Zielenska M, Grant R, Ngan BY. Pediatric renal carcinoma: clinical, pathologic, and molecular abnormalities associated with the members of the mit transcription factor family. Am J Clin Pathol. 2006;126(3):349–64. doi:10.1309/98YE9E442AR7LX2X.

11. Qiu R, Bing G, Zhou XJ. Xp11.2 Translocation renal cell carcinomas have a poorer prognosis than non-Xp11.2 translocation carcinomas in children and young adults: a meta-analysis. Int J Surg Pathol. 2010;18(6):458–64. doi:10.1177/1066896910375565.

12. Komai Y, Fujii Y, Iimura Y, Tatokoro M, Saito K, Otsuka Y, et al. Young age as favorable prognostic factor for cancer-specific survival in localized renal cell carcinoma. Urology. 2011;77(4):842–7. doi:10.1016/j.urology.2010.09.062.

13. Kim SH, Choi Y, Jeong HY, Lee K, Chae JY, Moon KC. Usefulness of a break-apart FISH assay in the diagnosis of Xp11.2 translocation renal cell carcinoma. Virchows Archiv. 2011;459(3):299–306. doi:10.1007/s00428-011-1127-5.

14. Mosquera JM, Dal Cin P, Mertz KD, Perner S, Davis IJ, Fisher DE, et al. Validation of a TFE3 break-apart FISH assay for Xp11.2 translocation renal cell carcinomas. Diagn Mol Pathol. 2011;20(3):129–37. doi:10.1097/PDM.0b013e31820e9c67.

15. Rao Q, Williamson SR, Zhang S, Eble JN, Grignon DJ, Wang M, et al. TFE3 break-apart FISH has a higher sensitivity for Xp11.2 translocation-associated renal cell carcinoma compared with TFE3 or cathepsin K immunohistochemical staining alone: expanding the morphologic spectrum. Am J Surg Pathol. 2013;37(6):804–15. doi:10.1097/PAS.0b013e31827e17cb.

16. Green WM, Yonescu R, Morsberger L, Morris K, Netto GJ, Epstein JI, et al. Utilization of a TFE3 break-apart FISH assay in a renal tumor consultation service. Am J Surg Pathol. 2013;37(8):1150–63. doi:10.1097/PAS.0b013e31828a69ae.

17. Zhong M, De Angelo P, Osborne L, Paniz-Mondolfi AE, Geller M, Yang Y, et al. Translocation renal cell carcinomas in adults: a single-institution experience. Am J Surg Pathol. 2012;36(5):654–62. doi:10.1097/PAS.0b013e31824f24a6.

18. Klatte T, Streubel B, Wrba F, Remzi M, Krammer B, de Martino M, et al. Renal cell carcinoma associated with transcription factor E3 expression and Xp11.2 translocation: incidence, characteristics, and prognosis. Am J Clin Pathol. 2012;137(5):761–8. doi:10.1309/AJCPQ6LLFMC4OXGC.

19. Geller JI, Argani P, Adeniran A, Hampton E, De Marzo A, Hicks J, et al. Translocation renal cell carcinoma: lack of negative impact due to lymph node spread. Cancer. 2008;112(7):1607–16. doi:10.1002/cncr.23331.

20. Armah HB, Parwani AV. Xp11.2 translocation renal cell carcinoma. Arch Pathol Lab Med. 2010;134(1):124–9.

21. Song HC, Sun N, Zhang WP, He L, Fu L, Huang C. Biological characteristics of pediatric renal cell carcinoma associated with Xp11.2 translocations/TFE3 gene fusions. J Pediatr Surg. 2014;49(4):539–42. doi:10.1016/j.jpedsurg.2013.10.005.

22. Argani P, Olgac S, Tickoo S, Goldfischer M, Moch H, Chan DY, et al. Adult Xp11 translocation renal cell carcinoma (RCC): Expanded clinical, pathologic, and genetic spectrum. Lab Invest. 2007;87:135a–a.

23. Meyer PN, Clark JI, Flanigan RC, Picken MM. Xp11.2 translocation renal cell carcinoma with very aggressive course in five adults. Am J Clin Pathol. 2007;128(1):70–9. doi:10.1309/Lr5g1vmxpy3g0cuk.

24. Zou H, Kang X, Pang LJ, Hu W, Zhao J, Qi Y, et al. Xp11 translocation renal cell carcinoma in adults: a clinicopathological and comparative genomic hybridization study. Int J Clin Exp Pathol. 2014;7(1):236–45.

25. Arnoux V, Long JA, Fiard G, Pasquier D, Bensaadi L, Terrier N, et al. Xp11.2 translocation renal carcinoma in adults over 50 years of age: about four cases. Prog Urol. 2012;22(15):932–7. doi:10.1016/j.purol.2012.06.009.

26. Ellis CL, Eble JN, Subhawong AP, Martignoni G, Zhong M, Ladanyi M, et al. Clinical heterogeneity of Xp11 translocation renal cell carcinoma: impact of fusion subtype, age, and stage. Mod Pathol. 2014;27(6):875–86. doi:10.1038/modpathol.2013.208.

27. Störkel S, Eble JN, Adlakha K, Amin M, Blute ML, Bostwick DG, et al. Classification of renal cell carcinoma: Workgroup No. 1. Union Internationale Contre le Cancer (UICC) and the American Joint Committee on Cancer (AJCC). Cancer. 1997;80(5):987–9.

28. Verhoest G, Veillard D, Guille F, De La Taille A, Salomon L, Abbou CC, et al. Relationship between age at diagnosis and clinicopathologic features of renal cell carcinoma. Eur Urol. 2007;51(5):1298–304. doi:10.1016/j.eururo.2006.11.056. discussion 304–5.

29. Jeong IG, Yoo CH, Song K, Park J, Cho YM, Song C, et al. Age at diagnosis is an independent predictor of small renal cell carcinoma recurrence-free survival. J Urol. 2009;182(2):445–50. doi:10.1016/j.juro.2009.04.013.

30. Suh JH, Oak T, Ro JY, Truong LD, Ayala AG, Shen SS. Clinicopathologic features of renal cell carcinoma in young adults: a comparison study with renal cell carcinoma in older patients. Int J Clin Exp Pathol. 2009;2(5):489–93.

31. Steffens S, Roos FC, Janssen M, Becker F, Steinestel J, Abbas M, et al. Clinical behavior of chromophobe renal cell carcinoma is less aggressive than that of clear cell renal cell carcinoma, independent of Fuhrman grade or tumor size. Virchows Arch. 2014;465(4):439–44. doi:10.1007/s00428-014-1648-9.

32. Xu L, Yang R, Wang W, Zhang Y, Gan W. Laparoscopic radiofrequency ablation-assisted enucleation of Xp11.2 translocation renal cell carcinoma: A case report. Oncol Letters. 2014;8(3):1237–9. doi:10.3892/ol.2014.2267.

33. Choueiri TK, Lim ZD, Hirsch MS, Tamboli P, Jonasch E, McDermott DF, et al. Vascular endothelial growth factor-targeted therapy for the treatment of adult metastatic Xp11.2 translocation renal cell carcinoma. Cancer. 2010;116(22):5219–25. doi:10.1002/cncr.25512.

6

Panobinostat synergizes with bortezomib to induce endoplasmic reticulum stress and ubiquitinated protein accumulation in renal cancer cells

Akinori Sato[*], Takako Asano, Makoto Isono, Keiichi Ito and Tomohiko Asano

Abstract

Background: Inducing endoplasmic reticulum (ER) stress is a novel strategy used to treat malignancies. Inhibition of histone deacetylase (HDAC) 6 by the HDAC inhibitor panobinostat hinders the refolding of unfolded proteins by increasing the acetylation of heat shock protein 90. We investigated whether combining panobinostat with the proteasome inhibitor bortezomib would kill cancer cells effectively by inhibiting the degradation of these unfolded proteins, thereby causing ubiquitinated proteins to accumulate and induce ER stress.

Methods: Caki-1, ACHN, and 769-P cells were treated with panobinostat and/or bortezomib. Cell viability, clonogenicity, and induction of apoptosis were evaluated. The in vivo efficacy of the combination was evaluated using a murine subcutaneous xenograft model. The combination-induced ER stress and ubiquitinated protein accumulation were assessed.

Results: The combination of panobinostat and bortezomib induced apoptosis and inhibited renal cancer growth synergistically (combination indexes <1). It also suppressed colony formation significantly (p <0.05). In a murine subcutaneous tumor model, a 10-day treatment was well tolerated and inhibited tumor growth significantly (p <0.05). Enhanced acetylation of the HDAC6 substrate alpha-tubulin was consistent with the suppression of HDAC6 activity by panobinostat, and the combination was shown to induce ER stress and ubiquitinated protein accumulation synergistically.

Conclusions: Panobinostat inhibits renal cancer growth by synergizing with bortezomib to induce ER stress and ubiquitinated protein accumulation. The current study provides a basis for testing the combination in patients with advanced renal cancer.

Keywords: Panobinostat, Bortezomib, Endoplasmic reticulum stress, Ubiquitinated protein, Histone acetylation, Renal cancer, Combination therapy

Background

A new therapeutic approach to advanced renal cancer is urgently needed because there is presently no curative treatment, and one innovative treatment strategy used against cancer is to induce endoplasmic reticulum (ER) stress and ubiquitinated protein accumulation [1]. Protein unfolding rates that exceed the capacity of protein chaper-ones cause ER stress, and chronic or unresolved ER stress can lead to apoptosis [2]. On the other hand, unfolded proteins that fail to be repaired by chaperones are then ubiquitinated and the accumulation of these ubiquitinated proteins is also cytotoxic [3].

Histone deacetylase (HDAC) 6 inhibition acetylates heat shock protein (HSP) 90 and suppresses its function as a molecular chaperon, increasing the amount of un-folded proteins in the cell [4]. Because these unfolded proteins are then ubiquitinated and degraded by the pro-teasome [5], HDAC6 inhibition alone is thought to cause no or only slight ER stress and ubiquitinated protein

* Correspondence: zenpaku@ndmc.ac.jp
Department of Urology, National Defense Medical College, 3-2 Namiki, Tokorozawa, Saitama 359-8513, Japan

accumulation if the proteasome function is normal. We thought that combining an HDAC inhibitor with the proteasome inhibitor bortezomib would cause ER stress and ubiquitinated protein accumulation synergistically because the increased ubiquitinated proteins would not be degraded by the inhibited proteasome.

Panobinostat is a novel HDAC inhibitor that has been clinically tested not only in patients with hematological malignancies [6,7] but also patients with solid tumors, including renal cell carcinoma [8,9]. Bortezomib has been approved by the FDA and widely used for the treatment of multiple myeloma [10].

In the present study using renal cancer cells, we investigated whether the combination of panobinostat and bortezomib induces ER stress and ubiquitinated protein accumulation, and kills cancer cells effectively in vitro and in vivo.

Methods
Cell lines
Renal cancer cell lines (Caki-1, ACHN, and 769-P) were purchased from the American Type Culture Collection (Rockville, MD). Caki-1 cells were maintained in MEM, ACHN cells in DMEM, and 769-P cells in RPMI medium, all supplemented with 10% fetal bovine serum and 0.3% penicillin-streptomycin (Invitrogen, Carlsbad, CA).

Reagents
Panobinostat and bortezomib were obtained from Cayman Chemical (Ann Arbor, MI) and LC Laboratories (Woburn, MA), respectively, dissolved in dimethyl sulfoxide (DMSO), and stored at $-20°C$ until use.

Evaluating effect of the combination of panobinostat and bortezomib on cell viability and colony formation
For cell viability assay, 5×10^3 cells were plated in a 96-well culture plate one day before treatment and treated with panobinostat (25–50 nM) and/or bortezomib (5–15 nM) for 48 hours. Cell viability was evaluated by MTS assay (Promega, Madison, WI) according to the manufacturer's protocol. For colony formation assay, 1×10^2 cells were plated in 6-well plates one day before treatment and cultured for 48 hours in media containing 50 nM panobinostat and/or 10 nM bortezomib. They were then given fresh media and allowed to grow for 1–2 weeks, depending on the cell line. The number of colonies was then counted after fixing the cells with 100% methanol and staining them with Giemsa's solution.

Evaluating effect of the combination of panobinostat and bortezomib on induction of apoptosis
1.5×10^5 cells were plated in a 6-well culture plate one day before being cultured for 48 hours in medium containing 50 nM panobinostat and/or 10 nM bortezomib.

Induction of apoptosis was evaluated, using flow cytometry, by annexin-V assay and cell cycle analysis. For annexin-V assay the harvested cells were stained with annexin V according to the manufacturer's protocol (Beckman Coulter, Marseille, France). For cell cycle analysis the harvested cells were resuspended in citrate buffer and stained with propidium iodide. They were then analyzed by flow cytometry using CellQuest Pro Software (BD Biosciences, San Jose, CA).

Murine xenograft model
The animal protocol for this experiment has been approved by the institutional Animal Care and Use Committee of National Defense Medical College. 5-week-old male nude mice (strain BALB/c Slc-nu/nu) were purchased from CLEA (Tokyo, Japan). The animals were housed under pathogen-free conditions and had access to standard food and water ad libitum. 1×10^7 Caki-1 cells were subcutaneously injected into the flank and treatments were initiated 4 days after the injection (day 1), when the tumors became palpable. The mice were divided into 4 groups of 5, the control group receiving intraperitoneal injections of DMSO and the other groups receiving either panobinostat (2 mg/kg) or bortezomib (60 μg/kg) or both. Injections were given once a day, 5 days a week, for 2 weeks. Tumor volume was estimated as one half of the product of the length and the square of the width (i.e., volume = $0.5 \times$ length $\times$ width^2).

Western blotting
Cells were treated under the indicated conditions for 48 hours and whole-cell lysates were obtained using RIPA buffer. Equal amounts of protein were subjected to SDS-PAGE and transferred onto nitrocellulose membranes that were then probed with antibodies specific for glucose-regulated protein (GRP) 78, ubiquitin (Santa Cruz Biotechnology, Santa Cruz, CA), actin (Millipore, Billerica, MA), HSP70, endoplasmic reticulum resident protein (ERp) 44, endoplasmic oxidoreductin-1-like protein (Ero1-L)α, cleaved poly(ADP-ribose) polymerase (PARP) (Cell Signaling Technology, Danvers, MA), acetylated α-tubulin (Enzo Life Sciences, Farmingdale, NY), and acetylated histone (Abcam, Cambridge, UK). This probing was followed by treatment with horseradish-peroxidase-tagged secondary antibodies (Bio-Rad, Hercules, CA) and visualization by chemiluminescence (ECL, Amersham, Piscataway, NJ).

Statistical analyses
The combination indexes were calculated using the Chou-Talalay method and CalcuSyn software (Biosoft, Cambridge, UK). The statistical significance of observed differences between samples was determined using the Mann-Whitney U test (StatView software, SAS Institute,

Cary, NC). Differences were considered significant at p <0.05.

Results

Combination of panobinostat and bortezomib inhibited renal cancer growth synergistically

We first investigated the combined effect of panobinostat and bortezomib on renal cancer cell viability by MTS assay. Panobinostat and bortezomib each inhibited the growth of renal cancer cells in a dose-dependent fashion, and the combination did so more effectively than either did by itself (Figure 1A). Analysis using the Chou-Talalay method indicated that the effect of the combination was synergistic (combination index <1) in many of the treatment conditions (Table 1). We then investigated whether the combination affects the clonogenic survival of renal cancer cells. Colony formation

assay revealed that the combination suppressed colony formation significantly and did so significantly more than did either panobinostat or bortezomib alone (Figure 1B).

We also used a subcutaneous xenograft mouse model to test the efficacy of the combination therapy in vivo. A 10-day treatment with panobinostat and bortezomib was well tolerated and suppressed tumor growth significantly (Figure 2). The p values at day 12 were 0.0283 for the control group and combination group, 0.0283 for the bortezomib group and combination group, and 0.0472 for the panobinostat group and combination group. The average tumor size at day 15 was 520 ± 175 mm^3 (mean $\pm$ SE) in the vehicle-treated mice and was 266 ± 39 mm^3 in the combination-treated mice. Thus the combination of panobinostat and bortezomib was shown to be effective for suppressing renal cancer growth both in vitro and in vivo.

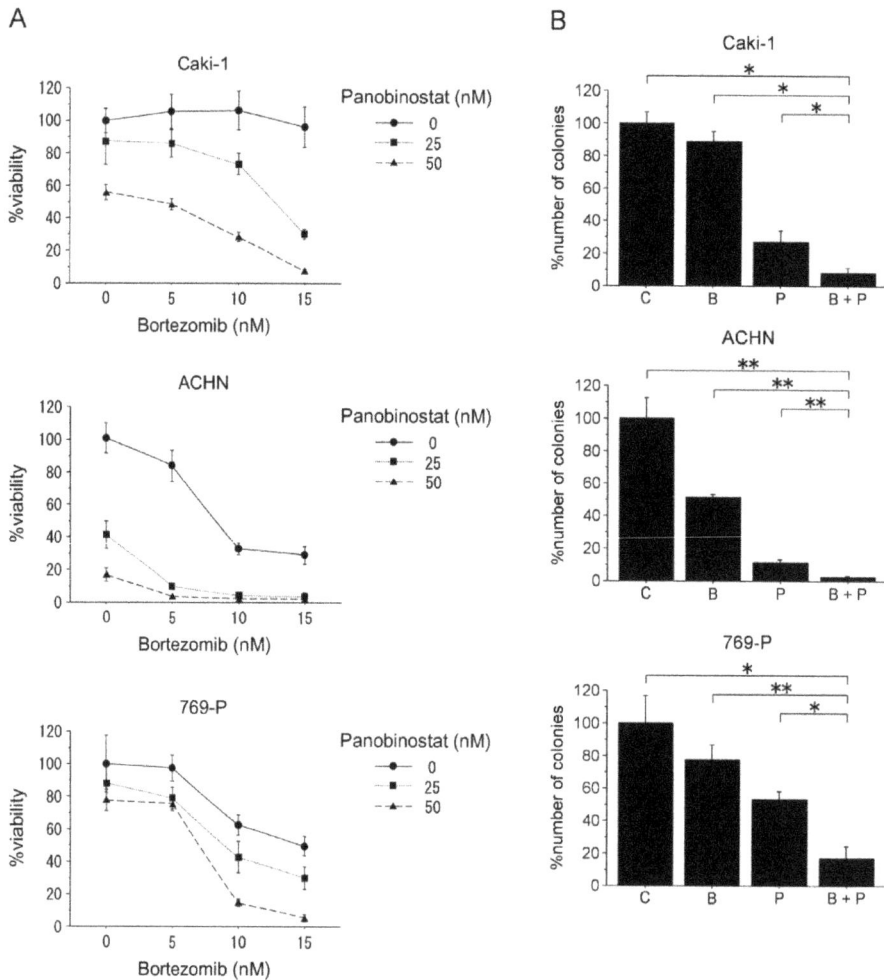

Figure 1 The combination of panobinostat and bortezomib inhibited renal cancer growth effectively. A, MTS assay results (mean ± SD, n = 6) after cells were treated for 48 hours either with bortezomib or panobinostat alone or with bortezomib and panobinostat together. **B**, Colony formation assay results (mean ± SD, n = 3) after 1–2 week incubation in control media (C) or media containing 50 nM panobinostat (P) and/or 10 nM bortezomib (B). *p = 0.0495; **p = 0.0463.

Table 1 Combination indexes for the combination of panobinostat and bortezomib in renal cancer cells

Panobinostat (nM)	Bortezomib (nM)		
	5	10	15
Caki-1			
25	0.927	0.581	0.791
50	1.186	0.737	0.808
ACHN			
25	0.557	0.458	0.553
50	0.463	0.394	0.544
769-P			
25	1.074	0.803	0.946
50	1.41	0.512	0.519

Combination of panobinostat and bortezomib induced apoptosis

The combination increased the annexin-V fluorescence intensity (up to 19.4-fold compared with control vehicle) (Figure 3A) and also increased the number of the cells in the sub-G1 fraction (up to 70.5%) (Figure 3B). Thus the combination of panobinostat and bortezomib was demonstrated to induce apoptosis in renal cancer cells.

Combination of panobinostat and bortezomib induced ER stress and ubiquitinated protein accumulation synergistically

The combination induced ER stress synergistically as indicated by the increased expression of ER stress markers such as GRP78, HSP70, ERp44, and (except in 769-P cells) Ero1-Lα (Figure 4A). As expected, the

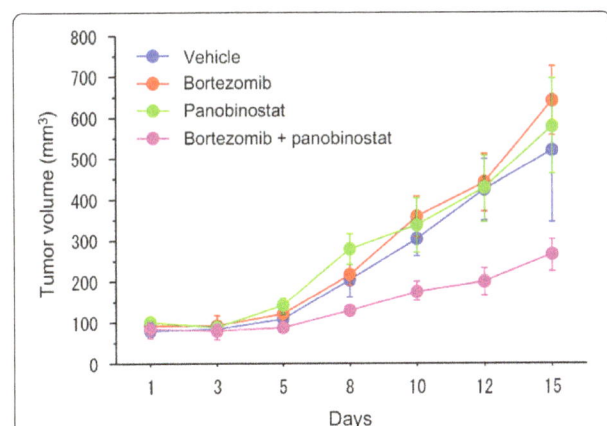

Figure 2 The combination of panobinostat and bortezomib suppressed tumor growth in vivo. A murine subcutaneous tumor model was made using Caki-1 cells, and the control group received intraperitoneal injections of DMSO, while other groups received either panobinostat (2 mg/kg) or bortezomib (60 μg/kg) or both. Injections were given once a day, 5 days a week, for 2 weeks. The 10-day treatment was well tolerated and suppressed tumor growth significantly (mean ± SE; p = 0.0283 at day 12).

combination induced ubiquitinated protein accumulation synergistically (Figure 4B): in Caki-1 and 769-P cells, 10 nM bortezomib alone did not cause ubiquitinated proteins to accumulate but in combination with 50 nM panobinostat increased the accumulation of ubiquitinated proteins markedly. In ACHN cells, 10 nM bortezomib caused ubiquitinated protein accumulation and the accumulation was synergistically enhanced by 50 nM panobinostat. Acetylation of α-tubulin by panobinostat is consistent with HDAC6 inhibition because α-tubulin is one of the important substrates of HDAC6. Interestingly, the combination also enhanced the acetylation of histone and α-tubulin synergistically in Caki-1 and ACHN cells. In 769-P cells, the combination enhanced the acetylation of α-tubulin but not that of histone.

Histone acetylation was a consequence of ubiquitinated protein accumulation

We then investigated the relationship between histone acetylation and ubiquitinated protein accumulation. Panobinostat caused histone acetylation in a dose-dependent fashion in all the cell lines but did not induce ubiquitinated protein accumulation (Figure 5A). Bortezomib, on the other hand, caused both ubiquitinated protein accumulation and histone acetylation in a dose-dependent fashion in Caki-1 and ACHN cells but did not cause histone acetylation in 769-P cells (Figure 5B). This is in accordance with the result that the combination did not enhance histone acetylation in 769-P cells despite inducing ubiquitinated protein accumulation in them (Figure 4B). We inferred from these results that the histone acetylation the combination caused in Caki-1 and ACHN cells was a consequence of ubiquitinated protein accumulation.

Discussion

Inducing ER stress and ubiquitinated protein accumulation is a novel approach to cancer therapy. The combination of an HDAC inhibitor and bortezomib is one of the combinations that might be expected to do it. The combination of panobinostat and bortezomib has recently been investigated mainly in hematological malignancies [11,12]. It has been reported that the combination of bortezomib and the HDAC inhibitor suberoylanilide hydroxamic acid inhibits renal cancer growth by causing accumulation of ubiquitinated proteins and histone acetylation [13], but that study did not show the relationship between ubiquitinated protein accumulation and histone acetylation. In the present study, using panobinostat, a more potent HDAC inhibitor (acting at nanomolar concentrations, whereas suberoylanilide hydroxamic acid acts at micromolar concentrations), we investigated the effect of the bortezomib-panobinostat combination on renal cancer growth as well as further mechanisms of the combination of bortezomib and an HDAC inhibitor.

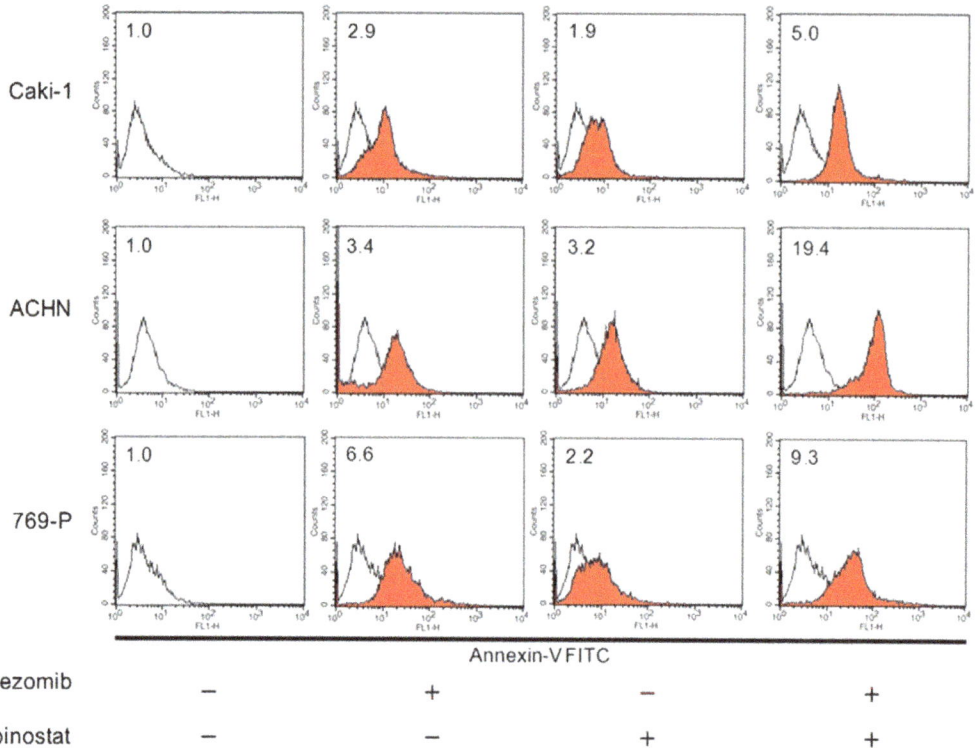

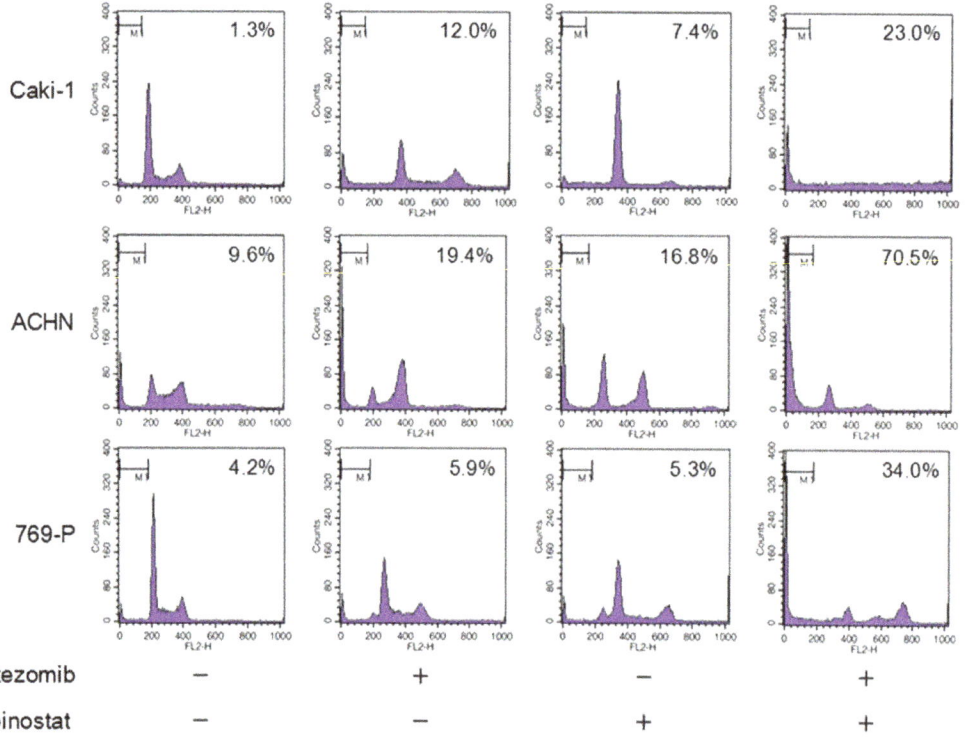

Figure 3 (See legend on next page.)

Inhibition of HDAC6 acetylates HSP90, abrogating its function and increasing the amount of unfolded proteins [4]. We think that bortezomib inhibits degradation of unfolded proteins increased by panobinostat, which induces ER stress and ubiquitinated protein accumulation. Accumulation of unfolded proteins, or ER stress, activates a signaling pathway known as the unfolded protein response (UPR), which leads to increased transcription of ER folding and quality-control factors [14]. In the present study we showed the induction of ER stress by detecting the increased expression of UPR-related proteins: GRP78, HSP70, Ero1-Lα, and ERp44. GRP78 is a master regulator for ER stress because of its role as a major ER chaperone as well as its ability to control the activation of UPR signaling [15]. HSP70 is a molecular chaperone localized in the cytoplasm but associated with

the regulation of the UPR by forming a stable protein complex with the cytosolic domain of inositol-requiring enzyme 1α [16]. Ero1-Lα regulates oxidative protein folding by selectively oxidizing protein disulfide isomerase [17], one of the key players in the control of disulfide bond formation [18]. ERp44 forms mixed disulfides with Ero1-Lα and may be involved in the control of oxidative protein folding [19]. The increased expression of these ER stress-related proteins thus confirmed that ER stress was induced by the combination of panobinostat and bortezomib.

Acetylation of α-tubulin, one of the important substrates of HDAC6 [20], is consistent with the inhibition of HDAC6 by panobinostat. Interestingly, panobinostat itself did not cause marked ER stress even though it inhibited HDAC6 function. This may be because the

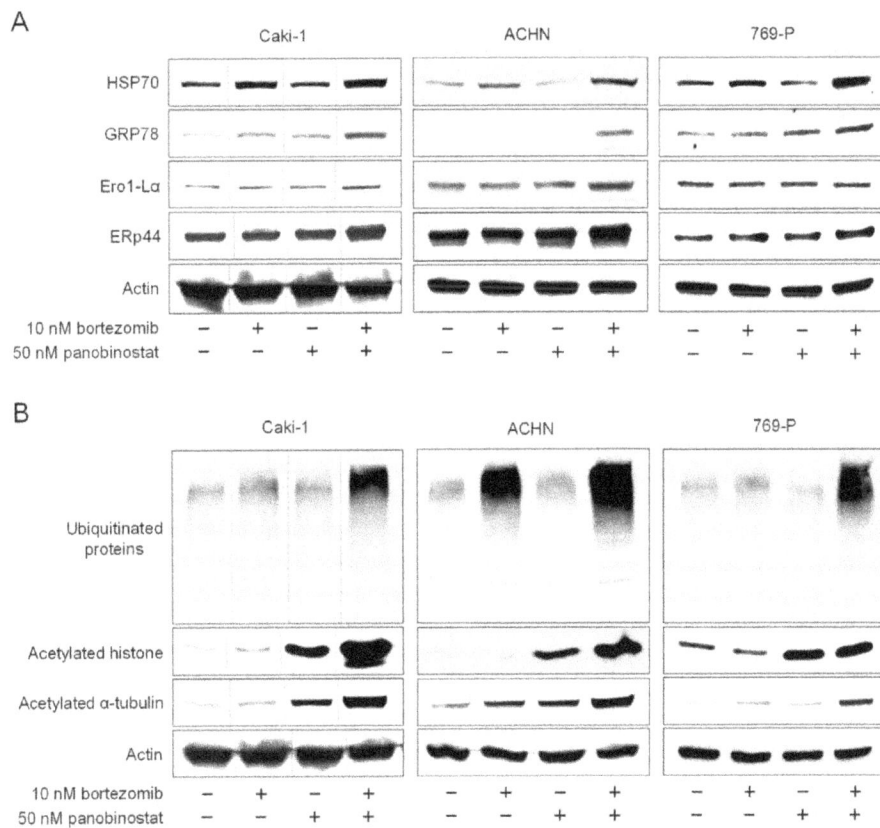

Figure 4 The combination therapy induced ER stress and histone acetylation in renal cancer cells. The 48-hour treatment with the combination of panobinostat and bortezomib induced ER stress synergistically as indicated by the increased expression of GRP78, HSP70, ERp44, and Ero1-Lα **(A)**. It also caused ubiquitinated protein accumulation in all the cell lines synergistically and enhanced histone and also α-tubulin acetylation in Caki-1 and ACHN cells. In 769-P cells, the combination enhanced the acetylation of α-tubulin but not that of histone **(B)**. The dashed lines in the Caki-1 results in parts A and B indicate that the order of the bands has been rearranged from the original gel.

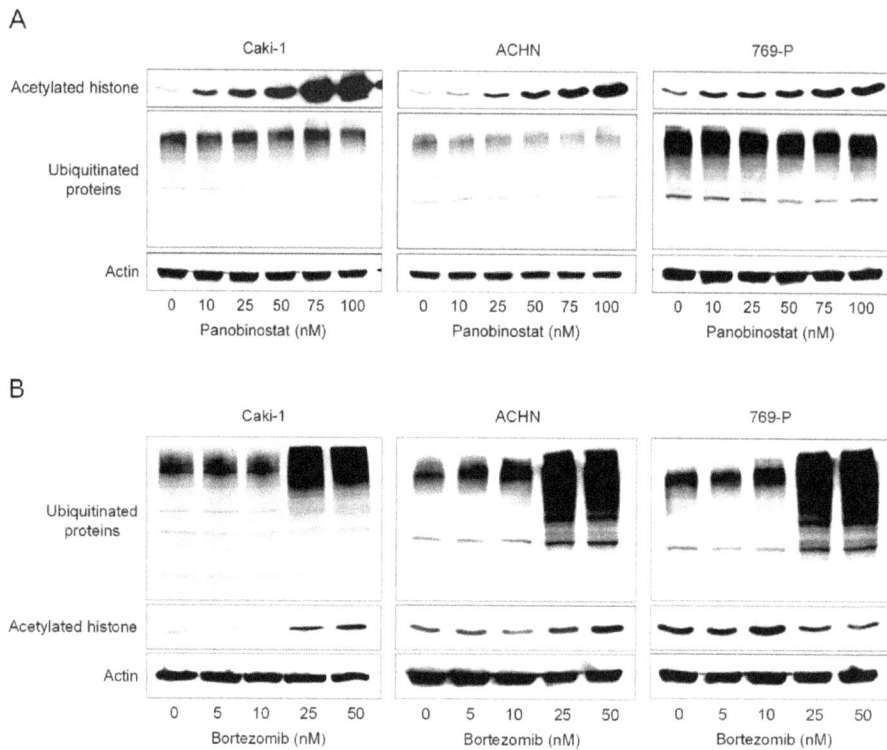

Figure 5 **Histone acetylation was a consequence of ubiquitinated protein accumulation. A**, 48-hour treatment with panobinostat caused dose-dependent histone acetylation in all the cell lines but did not cause ubiquitinated protein accumulation. **B**, 48-hour treatment with bortezomib, on the other hand, caused both histone acetylation and ubiquitinated protein accumulation in Caki-1 and ACHN cells and caused only ubiquitinated protein accumulation in 769-P cells.

unfolded proteins increased by panobinostat can be degraded immediately by the proteasome if its function is not suppressed. This explanation is consistent with the result that panobinostat induced marked ER stress only when combined with bortezomib.

The combination induced ubiquitinated protein accumulation synergistically. This is because panobinostat increased unfolded proteins, which were then ubiquitinated, and bortezomib inhibited their degradation. The ubiquitinated protein accumulation is also in accordance with the above-discussed enhanced ER stress induced by the combination because ER stress is induced by the accumulation of unfolded proteins in the cell, and many of these unfolded proteins are ubiquitinated. Not only are ubiquitinated proteins themselves toxic to tumor cells [3], some of them may be important molecules for cancer cell survival (such as transcription factors and signal transduction molecules) that have lost their function because of unfolding and ubiquitination, presumably leading to the inhibition of multiple signal transduction pathways. Furthermore, the inhibition of NF-kB is thought to play an important role in the combination therapy with panobinostat and bortezomib because of the accumulation of undegraded IkB, a suppressor of NF-kB [21]. Jiang XJ et al. reported that the combination of panobinostat and

bortezomib activated caspases and down-regulated antiapoptotic proteins such as XIAP and Bcl-2 through inhibition of the AKT and NF-kB pathways [11]. The combination is thus thought to inhibit cancer growth by diverse mechanisms other than the induction of ER stress and ubiquitinated protein accumulation.

In Caki-1 and ACHN cells the combination of panobinostat and bortezomib not only caused ubiquitinated protein accumulation but also enhanced histone acetylation. In these cell lines, panobinostat alone caused histone acetylation but not ubiquitinated protein accumulation, whereas bortezomib alone induced both ubiquitinated protein accumulation and histone acetylation. We therefore think the histone acetylation in these cell lines is a consequence of ubiquitinated protein accumulation, which is consistent with the results of a previous study using prostate cancer cells [22]. In 769-P cells, on the other hand, the combination enhanced ubiquitinated protein accumulation but not histone acetylation. This is, however, also in accordance with the result that bortezomib alone did not cause histone acetylation in 769-P cells. In Caki-1 and ACHN cells, HDAC function decreased by ubiquitination may be one explanation. In 769-P cells, bortezomib alone seems to even decrease histone acetylation. Ubiquitination may result in the HDAC activity in 769-P cells being higher than the histone acetyl-transferase activity there. However, further study will be needed to clarify the exact mechanism of this decreased histone acetylation.

The combination of panobinostat and bortezomib has also been tested clinically, mainly in patients with hematological malignancies. In the most recent phase-II study enrolling 55 patients with relapsed and bortezomib-refractory myeloma [23], the patients were treated with eight 3-week cycles of 20 mg panobinostat three times a week and 1.3 mg/m^2 bortezomib twice a week with 20 mg of dexamethasone four times a week on weeks 1 and 2. If the patients showed clinical benefit, then they were treated with 6-week cycles of panobinostat three times a week and bortezomib once a week on weeks 1, 2, and 4 with dexamethasone on the days of and after bortezomib. In that study the overall response rate was 34.5%, the clinical benefit rate was 52.7%, and grade 3 or 4 adverse events were thrombocytopenia (63.6%), fatigue (20.0%), and diarrhea (20.0%). Two limitations of our in-vivo study are that it could not provide information about whether the doses we used in mice were equivalent to those used in humans and that it lacked a proper assessment of side effects. This study is, however, the first to show the beneficial combined effect of panobinostat and bortezomib in renal cancer cells, and it provides a basis for testing the combination in clinical settings.

Conclusions

Panobinostat inhibits renal cancer growth by synergizing with bortezomib to induce ER stress and ubiquitinated protein accumulation. Histone acetylation may be another important mechanism of action. This is the first study to demonstrate the combination's effect on renal cancer cells both in vitro and in vivo, and it provides a basis for testing the combination in patients with advanced renal cancer.

Competing interests
The authors declare that they have no competing interests.

Authors' contributions
AS contributed to design and interpretation of all experiments, drafting of the manuscript and execution of western blotting, colony formation assay and animal experiments. TA collected and assembled data and performed MTS assay, cell cycle analysis, annexin-V assay and animal experiments. MI participated in the study design, performed statistical analysis and helped to draft the manuscript. KI contributed to design and interpretation of all experiments and drafting of the manuscript. TA participated in the study design and coordination and helped to draft the manuscript. All authors read and approved the final manuscript.

References

1. Liu Y, Ye Y: Proteostasis regulation at the endoplasmic reticulum: a new perturbation site for targeted cancer therapy. *Cell Res* 2011, **21**:867–883.
2. Tabas I, Ron D: Integrating the mechanisms of apoptosis induced by endoplasmic reticulum stress. *Nat Cell Biol* 2011, **13**:184–190.
3. Mimnaugh EG, Xu W, Vos M, Yuan X, Isaacs JS, Bisht KS, Gius D, Neckers L: Simultaneous inhibition of hsp 90 and the proteasome promotes protein ubiquitination, causes endoplasmic reticulum-derived cytosolic vacuolization, and enhances antitumor activity. *Mol Cancer Ther* 2004, **3**:551–566.
4. Bali P, Pranpat M, Bradner J, Balasis M, Fiskus W, Guo F, Rocha K, Kumaraswamy S, Boyapalle S, Atadja P, Seto E, Bhalla K: Inhibition of histone deacetylase 6 acetylates and disrupts the chaperone function of heat shock protein 90: a novel basis for antileukemia activity of histone deacetylase inhibitors. *J Biol Chem* 2005, **280**:26729–26734.
5. Glickman MH, Ciechanover A: The ubiquitin-proteasome proteolytic pathway: destruction for the sake of construction. *Physiol Rev* 2002, **82**:373–428.
6. Duvic M, Dummer R, Becker JC, Poulalhon N, Ortiz Romero P, Grazia Bernengo M, Lebbé C, Assaf C, Squier M, Williams D, Marshood M, Tai F, Prince HM: Panobinostat activity in both bexarotene-exposed and -naïve patients with refractory cutaneous T-cell lymphoma: results of a phase II trial. *Eur J Cancer* 2013, **49**:386–394.
7. Wolf JL, Siegel D, Goldschmidt H, Hazell K, Bourquelot PM, Bengoudifa BR, Matous J, Vij R, de Magalhaes-Silverman M, Abonour R, Anderson KC, Lonial S: Phase II trial of the pan-deacetylase inhibitor panobinostat as a single agent in advanced relapsed/refractory multiple myeloma. *Leuk Lymphoma* 2012, **53**:1820–1823.
8. Morita S, Oizumi S, Minami H, Kitagawa K, Komatsu Y, Fujiwara Y, Inada M, Yuki S, Kiyota N, Mitsuma A, Sawaki M, Tanii H, Kimura J, Ando Y: Phase I dose-escalating study of panobinostat (LBH589) administered intravenously to Japanese patients with advanced solid tumors. *Invest New Drugs* 2012, **30**:1950–1957.
9. Hainsworth JD, Infante JR, Spigel DR, Arrowsmith ER, Boccia RV, Burris HA: A phase II trial of panobinostat, a histone deacetylase inhibitor, in the treatment of patients with refractory metastatic renal cell carcinoma. *Cancer Invest* 2011, **29**:451–455.
10. Kane RC, Farrell AT, Sridhara R, Pazdur R: United States Food and Drug Administration approval summary: bortezomib for the treatment of progressive multiple myeloma after one prior therapy. *Clin Cancer Res* 2006, **12**:2955–2960.
11. Jiang XJ, Huang KK, Yang M, Qiao L, Wang Q, Ye JY, Zhou HS, Yi ZS, Wu FQ, Wang ZX, Zhao QX, Meng FY: Synergistic effect of panobinostat and bortezomib on chemoresistant acute myelogenous leukemia cells via AKT and NF-κB pathways. *Cancer Lett* 2012, **326**:135–142.
12. Rao R, Nalluri S, Fiskus W, Savoie A, Buckley KM, Ha K, Balusu R, Joshi A, Coothankandaswamy V, Tao J, Sotomayor E, Atadja P, Bhalla KN: Role of CAAT/enhancer binding protein homologous protein in panobinostat-mediated potentiation of bortezomib-induced lethal endoplasmic reticulum stress in mantle cell lymphoma cells. *Clin Cancer Res* 2010, **16**:4742–4754.
13. Sato A, Asano T, Ito K, Sumitomo M, Asano T: Suberoylanilide hydroxamic acid (SAHA) combined with bortezomib inhibits renal cancer growth by enhancing histone acetylation and protein ubiquitination synergistically. *BJU Int* 2012, **109**:1258–1268.
14. Mori K: Tripartite management of unfolded proteins in the endoplasmic reticulum. *Cell* 2000, **101**:451–454.
15. Lee AS: The ER chaperone and signaling regulator GRP78/BiP as a monitor of endoplasmic reticulum stress. *Methods* 2005, **35**:373–381.
16. Gupta S, Deepti A, Deegan S, Lisbona F, Hetz C, Samali A: HSP72 protects cells from ER stress-induced apoptosis via enhancement of IRE1alpha-XBP1 signaling through a physical interaction. *PLoS Biol* 2010, **8**:e1000410.
17. Mezghrani A, Fassio A, Benham A, Simmen T, Braakman I, Sitia R: Manipulation of oxidative protein folding and PDI redox state in mammalian cells. *EMBO J* 2001, **20**:6288–6296.
18. Bulleid NJ, Freedman RB: Defective co-translational formation of disulphide bonds in protein disulphide-isomerase-deficient microsomes. *Nature* 1988, **335**:649–651.
19. Anelli T, Alessio M, Mezghrani A, Simmen T, Talamo F, Bachi A, Sitia R: ERp44, a novel endoplasmic reticulum folding assistant of the thioredoxin family. *EMBO J* 2002, **21**:835–844.
20. Hubbert C, Guardiola A, Shao R, Kawaguchi Y, Ito A, Nixon A, Yoshida M, Wang XF, Yao TP: HDAC6 is a microtubule-associated deacetylase. *Nature* 2002, **417**:455–458.
21. Mitsiades N, Mitsiades CS, Poulaki V, Chauhan D, Fanourakis G, Gu X, Bailey C, Joseph M, Libermann TA, Treon SP, Munshi NC, Richardson PG, Hideshima T, Anderson KC: Molecular sequelae of proteasome inhibition

in human multiple myeloma cells. *Proc Natl Acad Sci U S A* 2002, **99:**14374–14379.

22. Sato A, Asano T, Ito K, Asano T: Vorinostat and bortezomib synergistically cause ubiquitinated protein accumulation in prostate cancer cells. *J Urol* 2012, **188:**2410–2418.

23. Richardson PG, Schlossman RL, Alsina M, Weber DM, Coutre SE, Gasparetto C, Mukhopadhyay S, Ondovik MS, Khan M, Paley CS, Lonial S: PANORAMA 2: panobinostat in combination with bortezomib and dexamethasone in patients with relapsed and bortezomib-refractory myeloma. *Blood* 2013, **122:**2331–2337.

7

Renal vein thrombosis mimicking urinary calculus: a dilemma of diagnosis

Yimin Wang[1], Shanwen Chen[1*], Wei Wang[1], Jianyong Liu[2] and Baiye Jin[1]

Abstract

Background: Renal vein thrombosis (RVT) with flank pain, and hematuria, is often mistaken with renal colic originating from ureteric or renal calculus. Especially in young and otherwise healthy patients, clinicians are easily misled by clinical presentation and calcified RVT.

Case presentation: A 38-year-old woman presented with flank pain and hematuria suggestive of renal calculus on ultrasound. She underwent extracorporeal shock wave lithotripsy that failed, leading to the recommendation that percutaneous lithotomy was necessary to remove the renal calculus. In preoperative view of the unusual shape of the calculus without hydronephrosis, noncontrast computed tomography was taken and demonstrated left ureteric calculus. However computed tomography angiography revealed, to our surprise, a calcified RVT that was initially thought to be a urinary calculus.

Conclusion: This case shows that a calcified RVT might mimic a urinary calculus on conventional ultrasonography and ureteric calculus on noncontrast computed tomography. Subsequent computed tomography angiography disclosed that a calcified RVT caused the imaging findings, thus creating a potentially dangerous clinical pitfall. Hence, it is suggested that the possibility of a RVT needs to be considered in the differential diagnosis whenever one detects an uncommon shape for a urinary calculus.

Keywords: Renal calculus, Diagnosis, Renal vein thrombosis, Computed tomography

Background

The clinical manifestations of renal vein thrombosis (RVT) in adult patients vary, along with the rapidity and degree of venous occlusion. Symptoms of RVT can include acute flank pain, hematuria, and deterioration of renal function, although RVT is usually asymptomatic. RVT with flank pain and hematuria is often misdiagnosed as renal colic originating from a ureteric or renal calculus, especially in young and otherwise healthy patients. This report describes an unusual patient with RVT, who presented with flank pain and calcified RVT mimicking a urinary calculus.

Case presentation

A 38-year-old woman presented to the emergency room in a regional hospital with nausea and left flank pain that had suddenly started 12 h earlier. She had a history of left flank trauma, having fallen from 2-meter- height 5 years earlier. Physical examination revealed no tenderness over the abdomen or flank and normal chest auscultation. Blood analysis was within normal limits, except for leukocytosis (12.7×10^9/L). Routine urine analysis showed microscopic hematuria without white blood cells or proteins. Abdominal ultrasonography showed an enlarged kidney and a 16-mm hyperechoic focus in the left renal pelvis, suggesting a diagnosis of renal calculus. The patient was therefore administered extracorporeal shock wave lithotripsy at the regional hospital. A follow-up ultrasound examination 2 weeks later showed that the shape and size of the hyperechoic focus had not changed.

Due to left lower back pain and the persistent left hyperechoic focus in the renal area, the patient was referred to our hospital for further evaluation and treatment. Urine analysis and ultrasound examination showed the same results as in the regional hospital (Fig. 1a). An abdominal plain film showed a left-sided renal calcification (Fig. 2a), but there was no evidence of a palpable tender mass or an audible abdominal bruit. Laboratory data, except for

* Correspondence: chensw123@126.com
[1]Department of Urology, the First Affiliated Hospital of Medical College, Zhejiang University, No. 79 Qing Chun Road, 310003 Hangzhou, China
Full list of author information is available at the end of the article

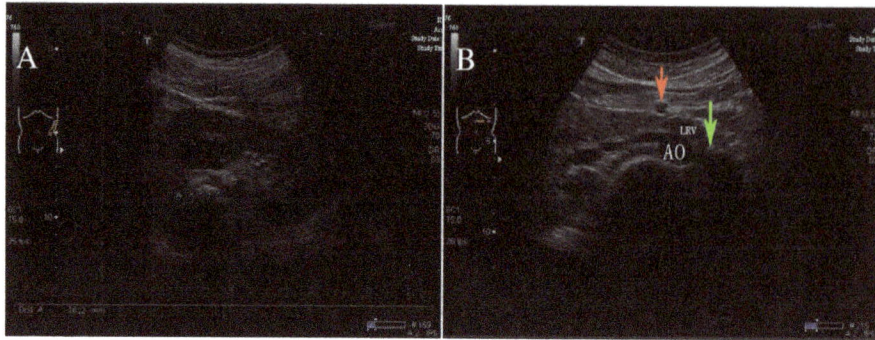

Fig.1 The images from the ultrasonography. **a** An abdominal ultrasonography demonstrated 16-mm hyperechoic, echogenic focus in the left renal pelvis. **b** A color Doppler ultrasonography indicated the hyperechoic focus (*green arrow*) in the left renal vein (LRV). Aorta (AO); left renal vein (LRV); superior mesenteric artery (*red arrow*)

urinalysis results, were within normal limits. Because of the failure of extracorporeal shock wave lithotripsy, percutaneous lithotomy was recommended.

Because the shape of the calculus was unusual and there was no evidence of hydronephrosis, the diagnosis of calculus was questioned. Further evaluation to determine the true nature of the hyperechoic lesion included computed tomography (CT) without contrast, which showed the calculus in the left ureter (Fig. 3a). In addition, intravenous pyelography showed that the pelvic areas around both kidneys were normal, although a patchy shadow was observed above the left renal pelvis (Fig. 2b). Color Doppler ultrasonography showed the hyperechoic focus in the left renal vein (Fig. 1b). CT angiography indicated a hyperdense mass in the left renal vein, suggesting a calcified thrombus, as well as occlusion of the left renal vein, varicosity in the left ovarian vein, and peripheral veins around the left renal hilum (Fig. 3b–d).

The patient was actively monitored. Three months later, there was satisfactory regression of microscopic hematuria and left lower back pain. After 15 months, the patient remained asymptomatic. Routine urine analysis, serum creatinine and glomerular filtration rate were normal. Periodic ultrasound examination also revealed no morphologic changes in the affected kidney, with RVT remaining in situ.

Discussion

RVT is defined as thrombus formation in the main and/or branch renal veins. This may result in full or partial blockage of renal veins and, subsequently, to a series of pathological changes and clinical manifestations [1–3]. RVT is the most frequent vascular abnormality in newborns. In most infants, RVT is bilateral and is accompanied by dehydration after diarrhea or vomiting [4]. RVT is rarely observed in healthy adults; in most affected adults, it is unilateral and may be accompanied in 15–20 % of patients by nephrotic syndrome. RVT is associated with abdominal surgery, including laparoscopic cholecystectomy, trauma, tumor invasion of the renal vein or invasion by primary retroperitoneal diseases.

The pathophysiology of venous thrombosis has been reported to involve a combination of three interrelated factors: endothelial damage, stasis, and hypercoagulability. Although a single abnormality may precipitate thrombosis,

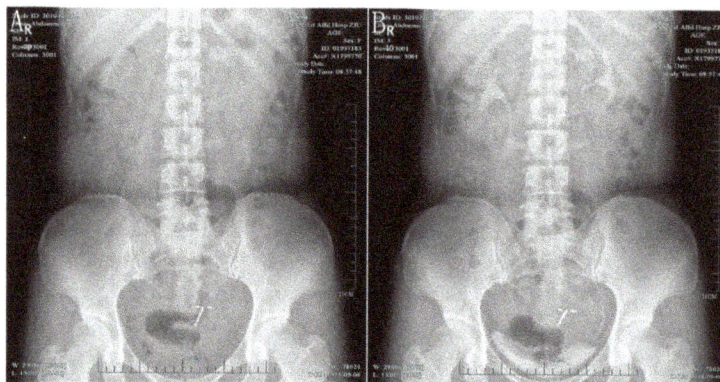

Fig. 2 The images from the abdominal plain film and intravenous pyelography. **a** An abdominal plain film showed a left-sided renal calcification. **b** After injecting contrast medium, intravenous pyelography showed normal renal pelvis and a patchy shadow within the left kidney contour

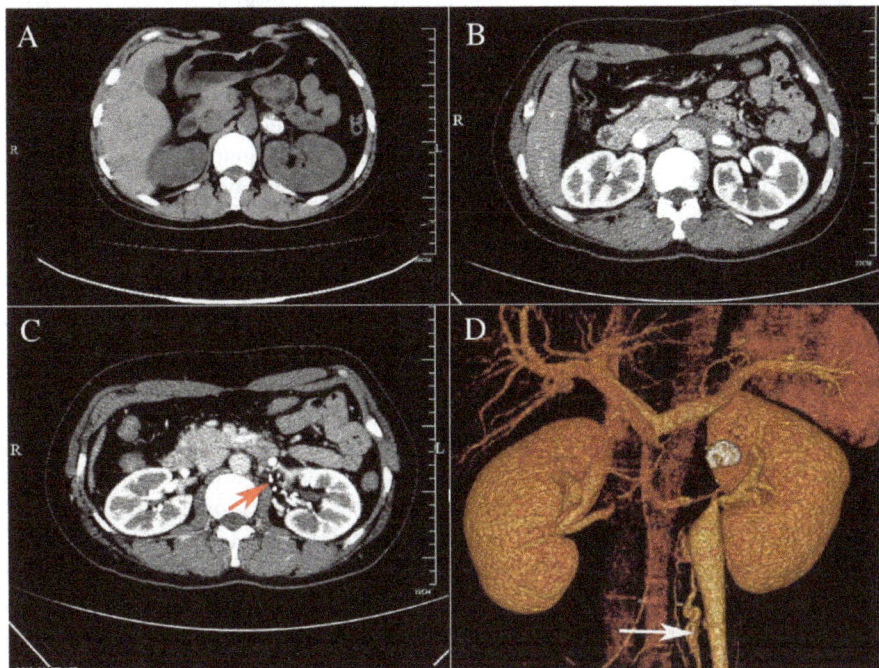

Fig. 3 The images from the computed tomography (CT). **a** The noncontrast CT demonstrated left ureter calculus. **b** The contrast enhanced CT indicated a hyperdense mass in the left renal vein. **c** The contrast enhanced CT indicated peripheral veins (*red arrow*) around the left renal hilum. **d** Three-dimensional CT clearly displayed the calcified RVT with varicose ovary vein (*white arrow*)

most venous thromboses are triggered by at least two of these factors. The causes and mechanisms of RVT are no different from venous thromboses elsewhere in the body (Table 1).

RVT often commences in small intrarenal veins and subsequently extends via larger interlobar veins to the main renal veins and even to the inferior vena cava, where it may cause pulmonary embolism [5]. The clinical presentation of RVT in adults depends on the rate, extent, and completeness of thrombus formation. Patients may be asymptomatic, have minor nonspecific symptoms such as nausea and weakness, or have more major nonspecific symptoms such as upper abdominal pain, flank pain, and hematuria [6]. RVT is likely underreported, as some

Table 1 Causes of renal vein thrombosis

Endothelial damage [18, 19]	Stasis [18, 20]	Hypercoagulability [18, 21]
Blunt trauma	Severe volume losses e.g., GI fluid loss, haemorrhage, dehydration	Nephrotic Syndrome: Membranous glomerulonephritis, Membranoproliferative glomerulonephritis, Focal segmental glomerulosclerosis, Minimal change disease
Trauma during venography	Post transplant distortion/kink of renal vein	Sepsis: Generalized/Localized (in and around kidney)
Renal transplant	Primary retroperitoneal processes with renal vein compression	Puerperium
Infiltration by tumour	Severe volume losses e.g., GI fluid loss, haemorrhage, dehydration	Disseminated malignancy
Acute rejection		Oral contraceptives
Vasculitis		Puerperium
Spontaneous micro-trauma to the endothelium e.g., in homocystinuria		Intrinsic Hypercoagulability: Factor V Leiden (Resistance to activated protein C), Prothrombin gene mutation (G20210A), Deficiency of Protein S, Deficiency of Protein C, Deficiency of anti-thrombin, Unknown/Poorly Understood causes, Anti-phospholipid Syndrome, Primary & Secondary e.g., SLE, Behcet's disease, AIDS-associated nephropathy

patients may go undiagnosed due to a lack of clinical manifestations. Establishing the diagnosis is essential because of the possible sequelae, including pulmonary embolism and progressive renal impairment related to vascular compromise, and the risks of potentially harmful treatment (anticoagulation or thrombolysis). In young patients, flank pain and hematuria are usually regarded as symptoms of renal and ureteric calculi; and similar clinical presentation due to other causes is often overlooked in the emergency room. Pulmonary thrombosis may occur in as many as 50 % of patients with RVT, and RVT complicated by pulmonary embolism can have similar symptoms, suggesting a high index of differential diagnosis not to miss the diagnosis of RVT [7].

In the absence of specific diagnostic laboratory tests and the paucity of clinical manifestations, imaging remains the cornerstone of diagnosing RVT. The gold standard method for diagnosing RVT is selective renal venography, but this is not often performed because of the invasiveness of this procedure, including exposure to high levels of radiation, injection of iodinated contrast, and the potential risk of venous injury causing de novo RVT [8].

In diagnosing RVT, ultrasound imaging and Doppler ultrasonography are not recommended because their results are inconsistent and operator-dependent. Ultrasound scans may show an enlarged kidney, and a hyperechogenic kidney is observed in approximately 90 % of patients during the early phase of acute RVT [9]. Color Doppler ultrasound is ineffective in detecting segmental venous thrombosis, but is superior to conventional ultrasound and abdominal plain film in detecting flow in the renal artery and vein. Although color Doppler ultrasound is highly sensitive when performed by an experienced operator, but remains highly operator-dependent [8]. Rarely, the calcified vessel walls of the renal venous branches coursing through the sinus may be mistaken for a renal calculus on ultrasonography. In the patient described here, there was no evidence of turbulent flow within the calcified RVT. Thus, RVT was not considered in the initial evaluation, although subsequent color Doppler yielded results suggestive of RVT.

CT is currently the imaging method of choice for diagnosing RVT, as it is non-invasive, is somewhat less expensive than other methods, can be performed quickly, and has a high diagnostic accuracy. CT scans have shown high sensitivity (92 %) and specificity (100 %) in diagnosing these lesions and is therefore recommended as an initial diagnostic tool [3]. Our findings showed that a renal calcified RVT may mimic a ureter calculus on noncontrast CT scans, with subsequent CT angiography used in the definitive diagnosis of a calcified RVT. CT angiography has shown nearly 100 % sensitivity in diagnosing RVT [2]. The diagnostic accuracy of CT angiography is similar to that of renal venography, with CT angiography having additional benefits, being a rapid, cost-effective, non-invasive method for evaluating the renal vasculature and for detecting renal tumors and other renal pathologies simultaneously. The disadvantages of CT include exposure to radiation and use of nephrotoxic iodinated contrast media, a potential risk factor in patients with impaired renal function [10].

The treatment modalities for patients with RVT have changed over the past decades, from surgical to predominantly medical management, consisting of initial intravenous and subsequent oral anticoagulation [11]. Asymptomatic patients with unilateral RVT may not require any specific treatment [12]. Rather, active surveillance, along with supportive measures including salt and protein restriction, may partially reverse the hypercoagulability, as in this patient. However, if a patient's condition deteriorates due to either the progression of thrombosis or embolism, active intervention should be considered.

RVT may be diagnosed incorrectly as renal colic or renal cell carcinoma on abdominal ultrasonography [12–14]. Results in our patients showed that a calcified RVT may mimic a urinary calculus on conventional ultrasonography, abdominal plain film and noncontrast CT. Renal stones may also resemble paragonimus calcified ova [15], renal artery aneurysms [16] and acute renal infarctions [17]. Thus, awareness of the conditions that could mimic those observed during the generation of a urinary calculus is important, particularly if a percutaneous procedure is considered. Ultrasonography alone is not sufficient to rule out RVT in these patients, suggesting the need for CT angiography in evaluating our patients.

Conclusions

Results in this patient showed that a calcified RVT might mimic a urinary calculus on conventional ultrasonography, abdominal plain film and noncontrast CT. Subsequent CT angiography revealed a calcified RVT, changing the course of diagnosis, treatment and follow-up. Examination of an unusual or uncommon shape for a calcified mass suggests the need to include a calcified RVT in the differential diagnosis.

Consent

Written informed consent was obtained from the patient for publication of this manuscript and accompanying images. A copy of the written consent is available for review by the Editor-in-Chief of this journal.

Abbreviations
RVT: Renal vein thrombosis; CT: Computed tomography.

Competing interests
The authors declare that they have no competing interests.

Authors' contributions

YW cared for the patients and drafted the report. WW, JL and BJ cared for the patient. SC revised and approved the final version of the manuscript. All authors reviewed the report and approved the final version of the manuscript.

Acknowledgements

Language editor Keer Chen edited our manuscript.

Author details

[1]Department of Urology, the First Affiliated Hospital of Medical College, Zhejiang University, No. 79 Qing Chun Road, 310003 Hangzhou, China. [2]Sidney kimmel Comprehensive Cancer Center, Johns Hopkins University School of Medicine, 21128 Baltimore, USA.

References

1. Li SJ, Guo JZ, Zuo K, et al. Thromboembolic complications in membranous nephropathy patients with nephrotic syndrome-a prospective study. Thromb Res. 2012;130(3):501–5.

2. Asghar M, Ahmed K, Shah SS, Siddique MK, Dasgupta P, Khan MS. Renal vein thrombosis. Eur J Vasc Endovasc Surg. 2007;34(2):217–23.

3. Singhal R, Brimble KS. Thromboembolic complications in the nephrotic syndrome: pathophysiology and clinical management. Thromb Res. 2006;118(3):397–407.

4. Andersen G, Fisker RV, Lauridsen KN. Renal vein thrombosis in the neonatal period. Ugeskr Laeger. 1993;155(41):3301–2. PubMed Nyrevenetrombose i neonatalperioden.

5. Ito T, Takabatake T. Renal vein thrombosis: Pathogenesis, pathophysiology, and therapy. Nihon Rinsho. 2006;64 Suppl 2:477–80.

6. Witz M, Kantarovsky A, Morag B, Shifrin EG. Renal vein occlusion: a review. J Urol. 1996;155(4):1173–9.

7. Mzayen K, Al-Said J, Nayak-Rao S, Catacutan MT, Kamel O. Unusual presentation of renal vein thrombosis with pulmonary artery embolism. Saudi J Kidney Dis Transpl. 2013;24(3):566–70.

8. Kanagasundaram NS, Bandyopadhyay D, Brownjohn AM, Meaney JF. The diagnosis of renal vein thrombosis by magnetic resonance angiography. Nephrol Dial Transplant. 1998;13(1):200–2.

9. Ricci MA, Lloyd DA. Renal venous thrombosis in infants and children. Arch Surg. 1990;125(9):1195–9.

10. Alvarez-Castells A, Sebastia Cerqueda C, Quiroga Gomez S. Computerized tomography angiography of the renal vessels. Arc Esp Urol. 2001;54(6):603–15.

11. Suto M, Aviles DH. Treatment of inferior vena cava and renal vein thrombosis with low-molecular-weight heparin in a child with idiopathic membranous nephropathy. Clin Pediatr. 2004;43(9):851–3.

12. Hidas G, Chervinsky L, Rozenman Y, Zelichtnko G, Shental Y. Renal vein thrombosis–renal colic with unusual course. Harefuah. 2006;145(8):597–600. 29. PubMed.

13. Takayama H, Kinouchi T, Meguro N, et al. Renal vein thrombosis misdiagnosed as a renal cell carcinoma with a tumor thrombus in the inferior vena cava. Int J Urol. 1998;5(1):94–5.

14. Decoster T, Schwagten V, Hendriks J, Beaucourt L. Renal colic as the first symptom of acute renal vein thrombosis, resulting in the diagnosis of nephrotic syndrome. Eur J Emerg Med. 2009;16(4):170–1.

15. Lin CM, Chen SK. Paragonimus calcified ova mimicking left renal staghorn stone. J Urol. 1993;149(4):819–20.

16. Chen S, Meng H, Cao M, Shen B. Renal artery aneurysm mimicking renal calculus with hydronephrosis. Am J Kidney Dis. 2013;61(6):1036–40.

17. Salih SB, Al Durihim H, Al Jizeeri A, Al Maziad G. Acute renal infarction secondary to atrial fibrillation - mimicking renal stone picture. Saudi J Kidney Dis Transpl. 2006;17(2):208–12.

18. Kau E, Patel R, Fiske J, Shah O. Isolated renal vein thrombosis after blunt trauma. Urology. 2004;64(4):807–8.

19. Busi N, Capocasale E, Mazzoni MP, et al. Spontaneous renal allograft rupture without acute rejection. Acta Biomed. 2004;75(2):131–3.

20. Verhaeghe R, Vermylen J, Verstraete M. Thrombosis in particular organ veins. Herz. 1989;14(5):298–307.

21. Laville M, Aguilera D, Maillet PJ, Labeeuw M, Madonna O, Zech P. The prognosis of renal vein thrombosis: a re-evaluation of 27 cases. Nephrol Dial Transplant. 1988;3(3):247–56.

8

Treatment of renal angiomyolipoma: pooled analysis of individual patient data

Teele Kuusk[1], Fausto Biancari[1], Brian Lane[2], Conrad Tobert[2], Steven Campbell[3], Uri Rimon[4], Vito D'Andrea[1], Aare Mehik[1] and Markku H. Vaarala[1*]

Abstract

Background: This study was performed to evaluate the impact of baseline characteristics and treatment methods on the outcome of sporadic renal angiomyolipoma (AML).

Methods: This was a pooled analysis of individual data of 441 patients with AML retrieved from 58 studies and 3 institutional series.

Results: Ninety-three patients underwent nephrectomy, 163 partial nephrectomy/enucleation, 128 embolisation, 19 cryoablation, 6 radiofrequency ablation, and 32 conservative treatment. Their mean follow-up period was 44.5 months. Patients who experienced major bleeding at presentation had significantly larger tumours than did those without bleeding (mean diameter, 10.1 vs. 5.9 cm, respectively; $p < 0.0001$). A total of 9.4 % and 26.4 % of bleeding tumours had a diameter of <4 and <6 cm, respectively. A tumour diameter of ≥8.0 cm (hazard ratio, 2.07; 95 % confidence interval, 1.20–4.77) and the treatment method ($p = 0.001$) were independent predictors of re-intervention. The risk of re-intervention was significantly higher after embolisation, particularly for large tumours (5-year rate of freedom from re-intervention: diameter of ≥8.0 cm, 49.2 %; diameter of <8.0 cm, 74.8 %; $p = 0.018$). Conservatively treated AMLs had a mean baseline diameter of 3.2 ± 2.7 cm; after 41 months, their mean diameter was 3.7 ± 3.1 cm ($p = 0.109$).

Conclusions: The prevalence of major bleeding is high in sporadic AMLs with a diameter of >6 cm. These results suggest that conservative treatment can be considered in AMLs of <6 cm in diameter. Among current treatment methods, embolisation was associated with a significantly higher risk of re-intervention. Further studies are needed to define risk factors for bleeding and assess the relative benefits of different treatment modalities.

Keywords: Angiomyolipoma, Bleeding, Radiofrequency ablation, Surgery, Embolisation, Re-intervention

Background

Renal angiomyolipomas (AMLs) are frequent benign renal tumours composed of fat cells, smooth muscle cells, and blood vessels [1–3]. These tumours belong to a family of perivascular epithelioid cell tumours [4]. AMLs occur sporadically in 80 % of cases, whilst the remaining cases are associated with various genetic disorders [2]. The incidence of AMLs in the general population is 0.4 % [5], but this tumour has been reported in 5.7 % to 6.9 % of partially resected, preoperatively presumed cases of renal carcinoma [6, 7]. The most severe complication related to renal AML is retroperitoneal bleeding, which has been reported in 15 % of patients [2] and may lead to shock in 20 % to 30 % of these patients [8, 9].

According to the current guidelines of the European Association of Urology [10], the primary indications for treatment of renal AML are the presence of symptoms or suspected malignancy. Biopsy may guide the treatment decisions for lesions with unusual growth and imaging characteristics [3]. The Level C recommendations for prophylactic intervention include large AMLs, women of childbearing age, and patients for whom follow-up or access to emergency care may be inadequate [10]. The treatment threshold for AML tumours with a diameter of ≥4 cm has recently been disputed.

---
* Correspondence: markku.vaarala@oulu.fi
[1]Department of Surgery and Medical Research Center Oulu, Oulu University Hospital and University of Oulu, PO Box 21, 90029 OYS Oulu, Finland
Full list of author information is available at the end of the article

Indeed, a recent study showed that treating all AMLs of >4 cm may lead to an over-treatment rate of 65 % [11]. Additionally, the optimal treatment method for bleeding tumours has not yet been defined [2, 11–14]. The aim of this study was to evaluate the impact of baseline characteristics, particularly tumour diameter, and treatment methods on the outcome of sporadic renal AML.

Methods

A literature search of PubMed and Scopus was performed in March 2014 using the key words 'renal' and 'angiomyolipoma'. The Preferred Reporting Items for Systematic Reviews and Meta-Analyses (PRISMA) criteria were followed [15, 16]. Adult patients who received any conservative or invasive treatment for renal AML were included in the analysis. Articles reporting on patients with tuberous sclerosis complex or epithelioid AML were excluded. Only articles written in the English language were included in this analysis. Two of the authors individually reviewed the abstracts of the retrieved citations to select relevant series. Data from each series were independently extracted by the two authors and subsequently cross-checked. This literature search identified a number of small studies with heterogeneous treatment strategies and a lack of treatment-specific data on survival and freedom from re-intervention, which prevented the performance of an aggregate survival meta-analysis. Because of these limitations, a pooled analysis of individual patient data was performed. Retrieved articles were reviewed for any data at the individual level that provided information regarding sex, symptoms, indications for invasive or conservative treatment, type of treatment, freedom from re-intervention, and survival. The definition criterion for major bleeding was any sign of retroperitoneal bleeding on imaging examination.

Authors of case series were asked to provide these data in a dedicated Excel spreadsheet. After permission was granted by the Oulu University Hospital's medical director, data on patients treated at the Oulu University Hospital were retrieved from the electronic records and included in the present analysis. The study was conducted according to the principles of the Helsinki Declaration. For this retrospective chart review, no written informed consent for participation in the study was obtained from participants.

Statistical analysis

Data were analysed at the individual patient level using SPSS statistical software, version 22.0 (IBM Corp., Armonk, NY, USA). Nominal variables are summarised as counts and percentages, whereas continuous variables are reported as means and standard deviations. Univariate analysis was performed using the Kruskal–Wallis, Mann–Whitney, Wilcoxon, and Fisher exact tests, as appropriate. Freedom from re-intervention and survival were estimated using the Kaplan–Meier method. The impact of different baseline characteristics and operative variables on late outcomes was evaluated using the log-rank test and the Cox proportional hazards method. Tumour size was first included in the multivariate analysis as a continuous variable and then dichotomised according to incremental threshold values from 4.0 to 10.0 cm, respectively. A p-value of <0.05 was considered statistically significant.

Results

Fifty-eight studies met the inclusion criteria and were suitable for inclusion in the present analysis (Fig. 1). Individual patient data were obtained from the authors of two studies [17, 18] and from the Oulu University Hospital (7 patients). In overall, this dataset included 441 patients with sporadic renal AML who were the subjects of this analysis. Patient characteristics and their outcomes are summarised in Table 1. Ninety-three patients underwent nephrectomy, 163 partial nephrectomy or enucleation, 128 embolisation, 19 cryoablation, 6 radiofrequency ablation, and 32 conservative treatment (Table 1). Their mean follow-up period was 44.5 ± 35.8 months.

Patients presenting with major retroperitoneal bleeding (54 of 441 patients) had significantly larger tumours than did patients without bleeding (mean maximal tumour diameter, 10.1 ± 5.9 vs. 5.9 ± 4.7 cm, respectively; $p < 0.0001$) (Fig. 2). Among the bleeding tumours, 5 of 54 (9.4 %) and 14 of 54 (26.4 %) had maximal diameters of <4 and <6 cm, respectively.

A Cox proportional hazards model including sex ($p = 0.29$), age ($p = 0.38$), tumour size ($p = 0.24$), presence of major bleeding ($p = 0.86$), and treatment modality ($p = 0.003$) showed that the treatment method was the only independent predictor of re-intervention. When the baseline tumour diameter was dichotomised with an 8.0-cm cutoff, the regression analysis showed that the treatment modality ($p = 0.001$) (Fig. 3) and a baseline tumour diameter of ≥8.0 cm ($p = 0.013$; hazard ratio [HR], 2.07; 95 % confidence interval [95 % CI], 1.20–4.77) were independent predictors of re-intervention. The risk of re-intervention was particularly evident in patients who had undergone embolisation (Fig. 3). Because of this, further analyses were performed only in the subset of patients who underwent embolisation treatment.

Among 128 patients who underwent embolisation, a Cox proportional hazards model including age, sex, baseline tumour diameter, major bleeding, and tumour diameter showed that only a tumour diameter of ≥8.0 cm was an independent predictor of re-intervention ($p = 0.017$; HR, 2.36; 95 % CI, 1.17–4.79). The 5-year actuarial estimate of freedom from re-intervention after embolisation

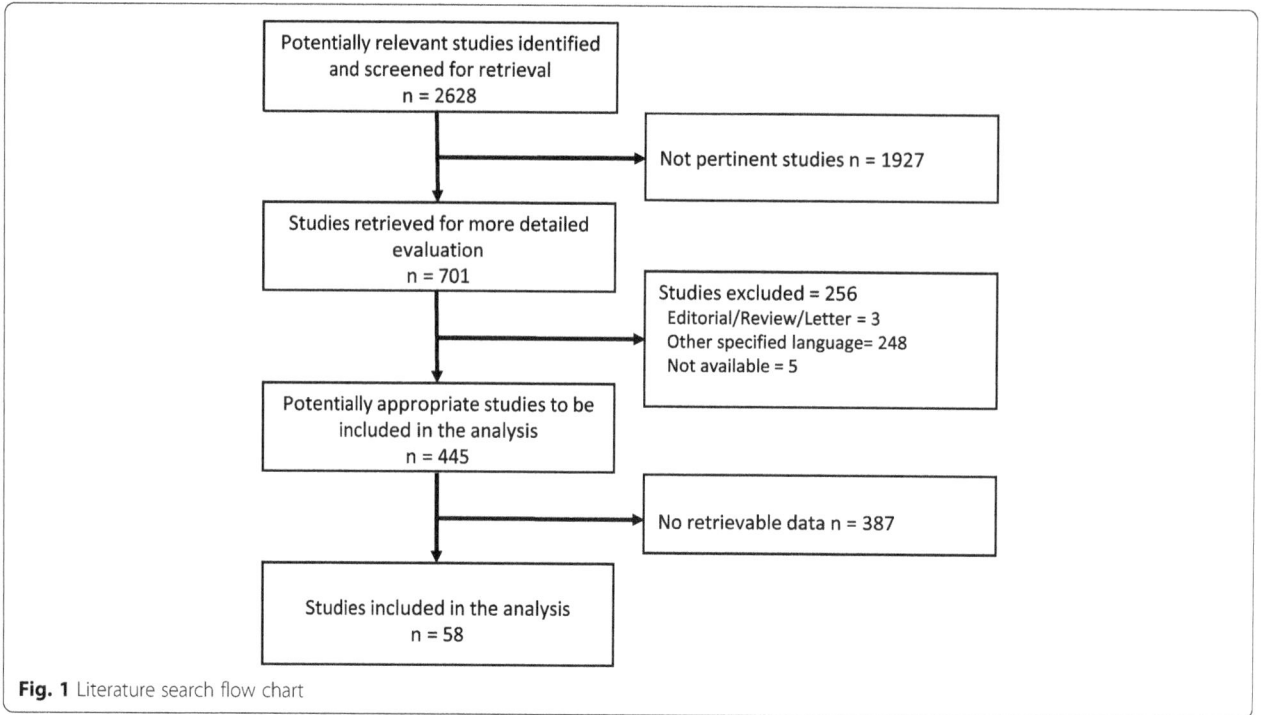

Fig. 1 Literature search flow chart

in patients with a tumour diameter of ≥8.0 cm was 49.2 %, whereas it was 74.8 % for patients with smaller tumours (log-rank test, $p = 0.013$).

Among the 32 patients who were treated conservatively, the mean initial diameter was 3.2 ± 2.7 cm (range, 1.5–14.0 cm), whereas it was 3.7 ± 3.1 cm (range, 1.5–14.0 cm) at the end of the mean follow-up period (41 ± 38 months) (Wilcoxon test, $p = 0.109$). Only 3 of these patients presenting with tumour diameters of 2.5, 4.0, and 7.0 cm demonstrated tumour growth to 6.5, 7.8, and 9.0 cm, respectively. The latter tumours were still treated conservatively at the last follow-up.

Table 1 Baseline characteristics and outcomes of patients with renal angiomyolipomas

Variables	Overall	Conservative treatment	Cryoablation	Embolisation	Radiofrequency ablation	Partial nephrectomy/ enucleation	Nephrectomy	P-value
No. of patients	441	32	19	128	6	163	93	
Age (years)	51.5 ± 14.5	53.2 ± 15.0	53.6 ± 14.8	47.9 ± 14.7	60.4 ± 6.9	52.9 ± 13.7	52.4 ± 14.9	0.020
Females	353 (80.4)	24 (75.0)	18 (94.7)	103 (80.5)	5 (80)	129 (79.6)	74 (79.6)	0.494
Imaging method								<0.0001
US	9 (9.4)	3 (9.4)	0	2 (1.6)	0	2 (1.2)	2 (2.2)	
CT	411 (93.6)	26 (81.3)	8 (42.1)	125 (97.7)	6 (100)	160 (98.2)	86 (94.5)	
MRI	8 (1.8)	3 (9.4)	0	1 (0.8)	0	1 (0.6)	3 (3.3)	
CT/MRI	11 (2.5)	0	11 (57.9)	0	0	0	0	
Tumour diameter (cm)	6.5 ± 5.0	4.4 ± 5.1	2.6 ± 1.6	9.1 ± 4.8	3.9 ± 2.5	4.7 ± 4.1	7.6 ± 6.0	<0.0001
Bleeding	54 (12.2)	4 (12.5)	0	32 (25.0)	0	7 (4.3)	10 (10.8)	<0.0001
3-year survival	97.9 %	100 %	94.7 %	100 %	100 %	95.6 %	98.4 %	0.037
Reintervention	41 (9.4)	1 (3.1)	0	38 (29.7)	0	2 (1.2)	0	<0.0001
Surgery	18 (4.1)	0	0	17 (13.3)	0	0	0	<0.0001
3-year freedom from reintervention	87.8 %	96.9 %	100 %	63.5 %	100 %	98.2 %	100 %	<0.0001

Data were obtained from the overall series, based on treatment strategy. Nominal variables are reported as counts and proportions; continuous variable are reported as mean and standard deviation

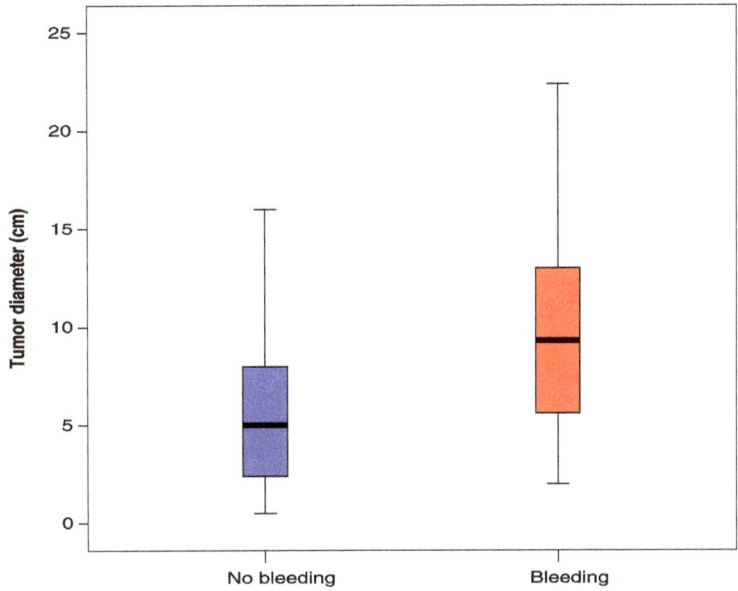

Fig. 2 Box plot showing impact of baseline tumour size on severe bleeding. Fifty-four of 441 patients had severe bleeding at presentation ($p < 0.0001$)

Discussion

The treatment strategy for renal AMLs is based mainly on evidence acquired during the 1980s [8]. Because major bleeding is the most severe complication of AML, prophylactic treatment may be indicated to avoid this haemorrhagic event. For many years, the threshold diameter for prophylactic treatment has been 4 cm [8]; however, this threshold has recently been disputed [11, 19]. Indeed, the diagnostic methods for AMLs have improved significantly during recent years, and the indication and efficacy of invasive treatment strategies for AML should be re-evaluated in light of

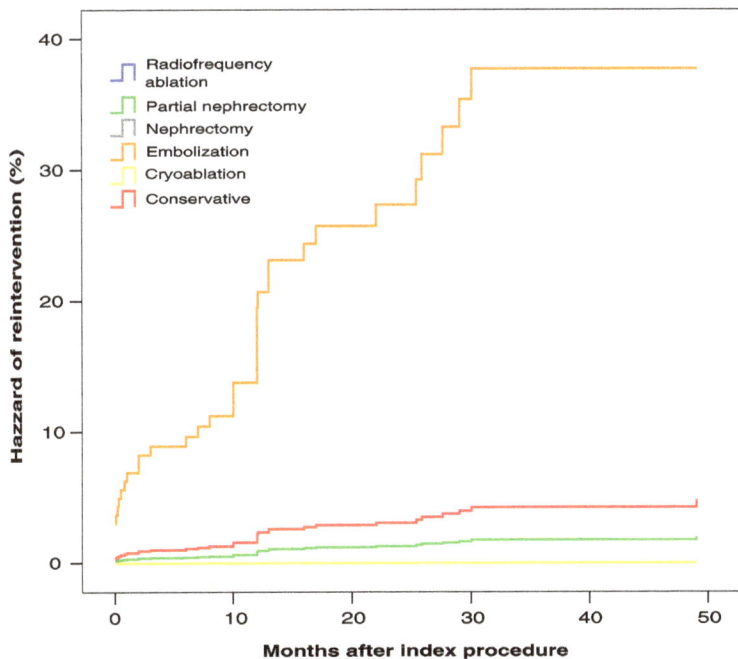

Fig. 3 Cox proportional hazards model for repeat intervention. The model was created according to different treatment strategies and adjusted for tumour diameter, presence of bleeding, age, and sex. The freedom from re-intervention curves after radiofrequency ablation and nephrectomy are behind the cryoablation curve in the figure

recent studies. We performed a literature review covering the era of modern diagnostic modalities to obtain detailed patient data on the efficacy of the current treatment strategies. Most of the published data were heterogeneous and presented significant biases. Therefore, we proceeded with a pooled analysis of all individual patient data available in the literature and included data from two patient series [17, 18] along with patient data from the Oulu University Hospital, Finland.

The present analysis showed that the risk of bleeding is associated with a large tumour diameter. Although even small AMLs are known to bleed, only 10 % of bleeding tumours in our analysis were below the traditional prophylactic treatment threshold of 4 cm. In fact, among bleeding tumours, 5 of 54 (9.4 %) and 14 of 54 (26.4 %) were <4 and <6 cm in diameter, respectively. This suggests that a diameter cutoff for treatment could be appropriately set at >6 cm. Indeed, a recent study suggested that only 34 % of patients with tumours of ≥4 cm required intervention [11]. Moreover, 67 % of symptomatic patients were managed with active surveillance and without late intervention [11]. Minimal or no growth of sporadic AMLs was similarly observed in earlier studies [8, 19, 20].

The prediction of severe bleeding events associated with AML is an important clinical issue and may dictate the prophylactic treatment strategy. A number of studies have suggested that the risk of bleeding is related to the vascularity and size of the tumour [21–23]. Rimon et al. [21] concluded that large (>4 cm) AMLs with minimal vascularity are less likely to bleed and that a grading system, based on tumour vascularity determined using digital subtraction angiography, may help to select patients needing embolisation. AMLs with a dominant large feeding vessel may be optimal for embolisation.

Although several studies [12, 24–26] have shown excellent outcomes with different treatment modalities, the present results suggest suboptimal outcomes after AML embolisation. In the past, embolisation was the treatment of choice for AMLs [19] probably because analyses of different treatment modalities have shown that embolisation is effective for bleeding tumours [19]. Preservation of the renal parenchyma [27, 28], effective occlusion of bleeding vessels [26], and surgery prevention [2] are considered the main benefits of embolisation. However, in our study, the 3-year rate of freedom from re-intervention after embolisation was 63.5 %, whereas it approached 100 % for all other treatment modalities. Embolisation was performed in 128 tumours, 30.5 % of which were asymptomatic and 25.0 % of which were bleeding. Tumours treated by embolisation also had the largest mean diameter (9.1 ± 4.8 cm). Remarkably, only the treatment modality was associated with a risk of re-intervention, consistent with the results of

other series [12, 19, 24–26, 28]. We observed that the risk of re-intervention was lower if embolisation was performed for bleeding tumours with a diameter of <8 cm. Embolisation is less effective than partial nephrectomy for tumours of >8 cm likely because of their high vascularity, making embolisation of these large tumours more complex and less efficacious.

Although the number of patients who underwent invasive methods in our included studies was rather small, no re-interventions after either cryoablation or radiofrequency ablation were reported (Table 1). Castle et al. [29] reported no recurrence after radiofrequency ablation of AMLs with a mean diameter of 2.6 cm. It has been suggested that radiofrequency ablation may also be a valid treatment option for larger tumours [30]. However, post-treatment retroperitoneal bleeding due to fracture of the tumour mass during the procedure may be a significant concern if larger AMLs are treated with cryoablation [31, 32].

The data presented herein support the current strategy for surveillance in asymptomatic patients. Based on our results and those presented earlier [11], aggressive use of prophylactic treatment should be avoided to prevent over-treatment. Based on the present data and a prior study [33], surgery provides good results for larger bleeding AMLs. A 3.4 % recurrence rate among surgically treated patients was observed during a median follow-up of 8 years [33]. However, the risk of major postsurgical complications (range, 7 % to 12 %) [33, 34] is far higher than that of severe adverse events after embolisation [12]. Elective surgical treatment after emergency embolisation performed to stop bleeding may be the treatment of choice for patients not at high risk for major surgery. Additional data are needed to assess the efficacy and durability of radiofrequency ablation and cryoablation in this setting. Prospective studies are warranted to better evaluate the natural course of renal AML, assess the risk factors for bleeding, and compare the different treatment modalities. AMLs that tend to bleed, even small AMLs, may have different radiological and vasculature characteristics [35]. Prospective patient series are needed to reliably evaluate these aspects.

The results of this study may be affected by a number of limitations that should be acknowledged. All studies included in this study were of a retrospective nature with limited follow-up. Data on major bleeding were from non-consecutive, non-longitudinal studies, which might have introduced a bias in the analysis of the prevalence of this complication. Because embolisation has been widely used as a prophylactic treatment of AMLs since the 1990s, publications may be biased toward reporting of complications and alternative surgical treatment modalities.

Conclusions

The present analysis showed that the prevalence of major bleeding is significantly higher in AMLs larger than 6 cm. Therefore, conservative treatment can be considered for AMLs less than 6 cm in diameter, whereas a threshold for invasive treatment of 4 cm may not be appropriate. Among treatment methods, embolisation was associated with a significantly higher risk of re-intervention. Further studies are needed to define risk factors for bleeding and assess the relative benefits of different treatment modalities.

Abbreviations
AML: angiomyolipoma; HR: hazard ratio; CI: confidence interval.

Competing interests
Markku Vaarala is a consultant for Amgen, Astellas, and Janssen and received a speaker honorarium from Amgen, Astellas, and Novartis. Trial participation: Amgen, Aragon Pharmaceuticals, Astellas, AstraZeneca, Pfizer, Orexo, Millenium Pharmaceuticals, and Janssen. The other authors declare that they have no conflict of interest.

Authors' contributions
MHV and FB participated in the study design. TK and FB acquired the data. BL, CT, SC, and UR provided the patient cohort data. FB analysed and interpreted the data. MHV, FB, AM, and TK drafted the manuscript. FB, BL, CT, SC, UR, and VD'A critically revised the manuscript for important intellectual content. All authors read and approved the final manuscript.

Acknowledgements
We are grateful to the study nurses Katja Vaihoja and Tuula Kivimaa for their technical assistance.

Author details
[1]Department of Surgery and Medical Research Center Oulu, Oulu University Hospital and University of Oulu, PO Box 21, 90029 OYS Oulu, Finland. [2]Division of Urology, Michigan State University, Grand Rapids, Michigan, USA. [3]Department of Urology, Glickman Urological and Kidney Institute, Cleveland Clinic, Cleveland, Ohio, USA. [4]Sheba Medical Center, Tel-Hashomer, Sackler School of Medicine, Tel-Aviv University, Tel-Aviv, Israel.

References
1. Tamboli P, Ro JY, Amin MB, Ligato S, Ayala AG. Benign tumors and tumor-like lesions of the adult kidney. Part II: Benign mesenchymal and mixed neoplasms, and tumor-like lesions. Adv Anat Pathol. 2000;7:47–66.
2. Nelson CP, Sanda MG. Contemporary diagnosis and management of renal angiomyolipoma. J Urol. 2002;168:1315–25.
3. Bissler JJ, Kingswood JC. Renal angiomyolipomata. Kidney Int. 2004;66:924–34.
4. Martignoni G, Amin MB. Angiomyolipoma. World Health Organization Classification of Tumours. Pathology and Genetics of Tumours of the Urinary System and Male Genital Organs. In: Eble JN, Sauter G, Epstein JI, Sesterhenn IA (editors). Lyon:IARC Press; 2004. p. 65–67.
5. Fittschen A, Wendlik I, Oeztuerk S, Kratzer W, Akinli AS, Haenle MM, et al. Prevalence of sporadic renal angiomyolipoma: a retrospective analysis of 61,389 in- and out-patients. Abdom Imaging. 2014;39:1009–13.
6. Fujii Y, Komai Y, Saito K, Iimura Y, Yonese J, Kawakami S, et al. Incidence of benign pathologic lesions at partial nephrectomy for presumed RCC renal masses: Japanese dual-center experience with 176 consecutive patients. Urology. 2008;72:598–602.
7. Kutikov A, Fossett LK, Ramchandani P, Tomaszewski JE, Siegelman ES, Banner MP, et al. Incidence of benign pathologic findings at partial nephrectomy for solitary renal mass presumed to be renal cell carcinoma on preoperative imaging. Urology. 2006;68:737–40.
8. Oesterling JE, Fishman EK, Goldman SM, Marshall FF. The management of renal angiomyolipoma. J Urol. 1986;135:1121–4.
9. Steiner MS, Goldman SM, Fishman EK, Marshall FF. The natural history of renal angiomyolipoma. J Urol. 1993;150:1782–6.
10. Ljungberg B, Bensalah K, Bex A, Canfield S, Dabestani S, Hofmann F, et al. Guidelines on Renal Cell Carcinoma. 2015. http://uroweb.org/wp-content/uploads/EAU-Guidelines-Renal-Cell-Cancer-2015-v2.pdf. Accessed 28 Dec 2015.
11. Ouzaid I, Autorino R, Fatica R, Herts BR, McLennan G, Remer EM, et al. Active surveillance for renal angiomyolipoma: outcomes and factors predictive of delayed intervention. BJU Int. 2014;114:412–7.
12. Ramon J, Rimon U, Garniek A, Golan G, Bensaid P, Kitrey ND, et al. Renal angiomyolipoma: long-term results following selective arterial embolization. Eur Urol. 2009;55:1155–61.
13. Mues AC, Palacios JM, Haramis G, Casazza C, Badani K, Gupta M, et al. Contemporary experience in the management of angiomyolipoma. J Endourol. 2010;24:1883–6.
14. Dickinson M, Ruckle H, Beaghler M, Hadley HR. Renal angiomyolipoma: optimal treatment based on size and symptoms. Clin Nephrol. 1998;49:281–6.
15. Moher D, Liberati A, Tetzlaff J, Altman DG, PRISMA Group. Preferred reporting items for systematic reviews and meta-analyses: the PRISMA statement. BMJ. 2009;339:b2535.
16. Liberati A, Altman DG, Tetzlaff J, Mulrow C, Gotzsche PC, Ioannidis JP, et al. The PRISMA statement for reporting systematic reviews and meta-analyses of studies that evaluate healthcare interventions: explanation and elaboration. BMJ. 2009;339:b2700.
17. Lane BR, Aydin H, Danforth TL, Zhou M, Remer EM, Novick AC, et al. Clinical correlates of renal angiomyolipoma subtypes in 209 patients: classic, fat poor, tuberous sclerosis associated and epithelioid. J Urol. 2008;180:836–43.
18. Rimon U, Duvdevani M, Garniek A, Golan G, Bensaid P, Ramon J, et al. Ethanol and polyvinyl alcohol mixture for transcatheter embolization of renal angiomyolipoma. AJR Am J Roentgenol. 2006;187:762–8.
19. Sooriakumaran P, Gibbs P, Coughlin G, Attard V, Elmslie F, Kingswood C, et al. Angiomyolipomata: challenges, solutions, and future prospects based on over 100 cases treated. BJU Int. 2010;105:101–6.
20. De Luca S, Terrone C, Rossetti SR. Management of renal angiomyolipoma: a report of 53 cases. BJU Int. 1999;83:215–8.
21. Rimon U, Duvdevani M, Garniek A, Golan G, Bensaid P, Ramon J, et al. Large renal angiomyolipomas: digital subtraction angiographic grading and presentation with bleeding. Clin Radiol. 2006;61:520–6.
22. Yamakado K, Tanaka N, Nakagawa T, Kobayashi S, Yanagawa M, Takeda K. Renal angiomyolipoma: relationships between tumor size, aneurysm formation, and rupture. Radiology. 2002;225:78–82.
23. Koh KB, George J. Radiological parameters of bleeding renal angiomyolipoma. Scand J Urol Nephrol. 1996;30:265–8.
24. Kothary N, Soulen MC, Clark TW, Wein AJ, Shlansky-Goldberg RD, Crino PB, et al. Renal angiomyolipoma: long-term results after arterial embolization. J Vasc Interv Radiol. 2005;16:45–50.
25. Lenton J, Kessel D, Watkinson AF. Embolization of renal angiomyolipoma: immediate complications and long-term outcomes. Clin Radiol. 2008;63:864–70.
26. Han YM, Kim JK, Roh BS, Song HY, Lee JM, Lee YH, et al. Renal angiomyolipoma: selective arterial embolization—effectiveness and changes in angiomyogenic components in long-term follow-up. Radiology. 1997;204:65–70.
27. Ewalt DH, Diamond N, Rees C, Sparagana SP, Delgado M, Batchelor L, et al. Long-term outcome of transcatheter embolization of renal angiomyolipomas due to tuberous sclerosis complex. J Urol. 2005;174:1764–6.
28. Lee W, Kim TS, Chung JW, Han JK, Kim SH, Park JH. Renal angiomyolipoma: embolotherapy with a mixture of alcohol and iodized oil. J Vasc Interv Radiol. 1998;9:255–61.
29. Castle SM, Gorbatiy V, Ekwenna O, Young E, Leveillee RJ. Radiofrequency ablation (RFA) therapy for renal angiomyolipoma (AML): an alternative to angio-embolization and nephron-sparing surgery. BJU Int. 2012;109:384–7.
30. Gregory SM, Anderson CJ, Patel U. Radiofrequency ablation of large renal angiomyolipoma: median-term follow-up. Cardiovasc Intervent Radiol. 2013;36:682–9.
31. Atwell TD, Farrell MA, Callstrom MR, Charboneau JW, Leibovich BC, Frank I, et al. Percutaneous cryoablation of large renal masses: technical feasibility and short-term outcome. AJR Am J Roentgenol. 2007;188:1195–200.
32. Vricella GJ, Haaga JR, Adler BL, Dean N, Cherullo EE, Flick S, et al. Percutaneous cryoablation of renal masses: impact of patient selection and treatment parameters on outcomes. Urology. 2011;77:649–54.

33. Boorjian SA, Frank I, Inman B, Lohse CM, Cheville JC, Leibovich BC, et al. The role of partial nephrectomy for the management of sporadic renal angiomyolipoma. Urology. 2007;70:1064–8.

34. Heidenreich A, Hegele A, Varga Z, von Knobloch R, Hofmann R. Nephron-sparing surgery for renal angiomyolipoma. Eur Urol. 2002;41:267–73.

35. Mourikis D, Chatziioannou A, Antoniou A, Kehagias D, Gikas D, Vlahos L. Selective arterial embolization in the management of symptomatic renal angiomyolipomas. Eur J Radiol. 1999;32:153–9.

9

Feasibly of axitinib as first-line therapy for advanced or metastatic renal cell carcinoma

Takuya Koie, Chikara Ohyama*, Takahiro Yoneyama, Hayato Yamamoto, Atsushi Imai, Shingo Hatakeyama, Yasuhiro Hashimoto, Tohru Yoneyama, Yuki Tobisawa and Kazuyuki Mori

Abstract

Background: Clinical benefit of axitinib as a first line agent to treat patients with metastatic renal cell carcinoma (mRCC), or locally advanced renal cell carcinoma (RCC) have not been clearly demonstrated. The aim of this study was to evaluate the efficacy and safety of axitinib as first-line therapy in Japanese patients with locally advanced RCC or mRCC.

Methods: In this retrospective study, we focused on eighteen patients who underwent first-line therapy with axitinib between May 2012 and May 2014 at Hirosaki University. Axitinib was orally administered at a dose of 10 mg daily. Progression-free survival (PFS) was the primary endpoint, while secondary endpoints included overall response rate (ORR) and adverse events (AEs).

Results: All patients had histologically proven clear cell RCC. The median duration of the administration of axitinib was 10.8 months. According to the response evaluation criteria for solid tumors, five patients (27.8%) achieved a partial response and nine (50%) had stable disease. The 1-year PFS rate was 84.4%, and the median PFS was 20.4 months (95% confidence interval, 17.5 – 21.7). No serious AEs were reported during the study, and there were no toxicity-related deaths.

Conclusions: In the current study, axitinib showed acceptable oncological outcomes and favorable safety profile as first-line therapy for locally advanced RCC or mRCC in treatment-naïve Japanese patients. Thus, first-line therapy with axitinib may provide a feasible option for treatment of advanced RCC or mRCC patients.

Keywords: Axitinib renal cell carcinoma, First-line, Vascular endothelial growth factor receptor, Advanced renal cell carcinoma, Metastatic renal cell carcinoma

Background

Although the innate chemoresistance of renal cell carcinoma (RCC) is a limitation in the systemic treatment for metastatic renal cell carcinoma (mRCC) [1], the clinical benefits of using targeted agents to treat patients with mRCC or locally advanced RCC have become increasingly clear [2]. Currently, six targeted agents are approved for the treatment of mRCC in Japan, including the multi-targeted receptor tyrosine kinase inhibitors (TKIs): sunitinib, pazopanib, axitinib and sorafenib; and the mammalian target of rapamycin inhibitors (mTORs): everolimus and temsirolimus.

There is no doubt that initial treatment of low- or intermediate-risk mRCC patients [3] with a vascular endothelial growth factor (VEGF)-targeted agent significantly improves clinical outcomes compared with conventional immunotherapy [4]. Of these, sorafenib, sunitinib and pazopanib have been approved as first-line treatment for advanced RCC or mRCC based on several clinical trials conducted in Western countries [2-4]. Similarly, first-line therapy with temsirolimus has demonstrated efficacy in patients with poor-risk mRCC [3,5]. However, based on the incidence and severity of adverse events (AEs) in several clinical trials [6-9], Japanese

* Correspondence: coyama@cc.hirosaki-u.ac.jp
Department of Urology, Hirosaki University Graduate School of Medicine, 5 Zaifucho, Hirosaki 036-8562, Japan

patients with mRCC have been shown to exhibit greater AEs to TKIs compared with their Western counterparts.

Axitinib, an effective and selective second-generation inhibitor of VEGF receptors-1, 2, and 3 [10], has demonstrated clinical efficacy in patients with mRCC in phase II studies [11,12]. Single-agent axitinib is active and well tolerated as a second-line treatment for mRCC [11,12]. Conversely, no significant increase in progression-free survival (PFS) was found in treatment-naïve mRCC patients who were treated with axitinib, when compared with those treated with sorafenib [13]. However, it is possible that Japanese patients may exhibit a different response to axitinib, in terms of antitumor effects or profile of AEs, when compared with their Western counterparts [14]. In the National Comprehensive Cancer Network guideline 2015, axitinib is recommended as a treatment option for first-line therapy in patients with locally advanced or metastatic RCC.

This study, which was carried out at a single institution in Japan, aimed to evaluate the efficacy and safety of axitinib as first-line therapy in patients with advanced or mRCC.

Methods
Study population
In this retrospective study, we reviewed the clinical and pathological records of a total of 39 locally advanced RCC or mRCC patients who were administered VEGFR-TKIs or mTORs between May 2012 and May 2014 at Hirosaki University. We focused on 18 patients who underwent first-line therapy with axitinib. Eligible patients had histologically confirmed clear cell RCC, with local progression or distant metastases. Data on patient demographics and tumor characteristics were obtained from the patients' medical charts. Memorial Sloan-Kettering Cancer Center (MSKCC) criteria were evaluated based on the five risk factors: low Karnofsky performance status (<80), high LDH (>1.5 times the upper limit of normal), low serum hemoglobin, high corrected serum calcium (>10 mg/dL), and time from initial diagnosis to axitinib treatment of <1 year [3].

The study protocol and informed consent documents were reviewed and approved by the Hirosaki University institutional review board.

Treatment
Axitinib was administered orally at a dose of 10 mg daily. The axitinib dose was reduced in patients with grade 3 AEs based on the Common Terminology Criteria for Adverse Events (version 4) or two readings of systolic blood pressure at 150 mmHg or higher, or diastolic blood pressure at 100 mmHg or higher, while maintaining maximal antihypertensive therapy. In this study, none of the patients received axitinib dose titration.

Patient evaluation
Based on the results of percutaneous ultrasonography-guided biopsy, the diagnosis of RCC was confirmed by a single pathologist at our institution.

Baseline evaluations included complete history-taking and physical examinations, assessment of Eastern Cooperative Oncology Group performance status (ECOG PS), abdominal and pelvic computed tomography (CT) or magnetic resonance imaging (MRI), and chest radiography or CT. Tumors were measured at baseline before the administration of axitinib. The response to treatment was assessed using the Response Evaluation Criteria in Solid Tumors, version 1.1 [15]. Bone lesions were considered non-measurable.

All tumors were staged according to the cancer staging manual (7th edition), published by the American Joint Committee on Cancer [16].

Endpoints and statistical analysis
The primary endpoint was the PFS. The secondary endpoints were overall response rate (ORR) and AEs. The PFS was defined as the time between the initiation of axitinib treatment and the date on the CT scan that identified progressive disease (PD), or other records of clear clinical evidence of PD, or death.

Data were analyzed using IBM SPSS Statistics 20 (IBM Corp., Armonk, NY, USA). Survival after axitinib administration was estimated using the Kaplan–Meier method. All P values were 2-sided, and the significance level was set at a P value of < 0.05.

Results
Patient characteristics and treatment
The pretreatment characteristics of the patients are listed in Table 1. All patients had histologically proven clear cell RCC. The median duration of the administration of axitinib was 10.8 months. Seven patients received reduced axitinib dosing. Five patients received a continuous reduced dose of 3 mg twice daily; of these patients, four had exhibited systolic blood pressure of 150 mmHg or higher, one had suffered general malaise, and one had developed grade 3 proteinuria. Two patients received a continuous reduced dose of 1 mg twice daily due to general malaise.

Clinical response and PFS
According to the response evaluation criteria in solid tumors (RECIST) criteria, five patients achieved a partial response, nine had stable disease, and four had PD. Median duration of response was 10.8 months (interquartile range [IQR], 5.6-18.3). Tumor shrinkage was observed

Table 1 Patient characteristics

Variable	Value
Age (years), median (IQR)	73 (64–78)
Sex, number (%)	
Male	12 (67)
Female	6 (33)
ECOG PS, number (%)	
0	14 (77.8)
1	2 (11.1)
2	1 (5.6)
3	1 (5.6)
MSKCC risk group*, number (%)	
Favorable	10 (55.6)
Intermediate	5 (27.8)
Poor	3 (16.7)
Site of metastasis, number (%)	
None	5 (27.8)
Lung	5 (27.8)
Lymph node	4 (22.2)
IVC thrombus	4 (22.2)
Bone	2 (11.1)
Liver	1 (5.6)
Prior to nephrectomy, number (%)	4 (22.2)
Follow-up period (months), median (IQR)	11.5 (5.1–17.4)

* Risk groups are stratified in accordance with the Memorial Sloan-Kettering Cancer Center (MSKCC) criteria associated with shorter survival based on five risk factors: low Karnofsky performance status (<80%), high LDH (>1.5 times the upper limit of normal), low serum hemoglobin, high corrected serum calcium (>10 mg/dL), and interval of <1 year between initial diagnosis and axitinib treatment [3]
ECOG PS, Eastern Cooperative Oncology Group performance status; IVC, inferior vena cava

in 15 patients (primary renal tumor in 10 patients and metastatic site in 5 patients), with a median decrease of 20% in tumor size (IQR, 4.7–33.5; Figure 1).

Three patients underwent open radical nephrectomy after axitinib treatment. Median operative time was 100 minutes (range: 95–128); the median estimated blood loss was 225 mL (range: 50–380 mL). No intraoperative or postoperative complications, as defined by the Clavien-Dindo classification [17], were encountered. The kidney was noted to be adherent to surrounding tissues, including the peritoneum, in all three cases. Pathological examination on final nephrectomy specimens confirmed the presence of clear cell RCC in all three patients; pathological stages were further diagnosed as pT1b, pT3a, and pT3b.

At the end of the follow-up period, none of the patients had died of cancer or other causes. The 1-year PFS rate was 84.4% (Figure 2). The median PFS was 20.4 months (95% confidence interval, 15.8–21.5). The 1-year PFS rate was 55.6% in the patients with locally advanced RCC (locally advanced group) and 100% in the patients with metastasis (metastasis group) ($P = 0.373$). The median PFS was not reached in the locally advanced group, and it was 20.4 months in the metastasis group. According to the MSKCC risk stratification, the PFS did not differ significantly among all risk groups ($P = 0.985$). Two patients received sunitinib as a second-line treatment, and one patient underwent third-line therapy with pazopanib. One patient received best supportive care. The duration of effectiveness in the patients who were administered sunitinib or pazopanib as second-line treatment were 3 and 6 months, respectively.

Safety of axitinib treatment

The AEs are shown in Table 2. Hypertension was the most frequent AE. Grade 3 proteinuria was observed in two patients. Other toxicities were infrequent and mild. No serious grade 4 AEs were reported during the study, and there were no toxicity-related deaths.

Discussion

Till 2005, the standard of care was limited to cytokine therapy, including interferon-alpha (IFN-α) and/or interleukin-2, and these treatments were frequently associated with limited efficacy and high toxicity [18]. A better understanding of the molecular mechanisms that target angiogenesis by direct inhibition of VEGF or mTOR has led to improved treatment options for RCC. Clinical trials using novel targeted agents, including TKIs or mTORs, have been evaluated in large randomized controlled studies conducted in both the first- and second-line setting [19]. Of these, sunitinib demonstrated superior efficacy to IFN-α as first-line mRCC therapy, with a median PFS of 11 versus 5 months ($P < 0.001$), respectively, in a randomized phase III trial [4]. Sunitinib is currently regarded as the reference standard of care for the first-line treatment of mRCC.

Several studies have reported widely variable rates and grades of sunitinib-related AEs [6,8,9,20]. The rates of incidence for the most common grade 3/4 AEs that require dose discontinuation and/or reduction, including hand-foot syndrome (HFS), stomatitis, and hypertension were similar to the rates reported in previous trials [21,22]. However, differences in ethnicity-based treatment tolerance may have also played a role. Miyake et al. reported that the rates of incidence of AEs ≥ grade 3 in a phase III clinical trial and a phase II Japanese clinical trial were 61% and 95%, respectively [9]. Similarly, *ad hoc* analyses indicate that several AEs occur at a significantly higher rate in Asian patients relative to Caucasian patients; for example, HFS occurred in 70% of Asian patients compared with 28% of Caucasian patients ($P < 0.001$) [8]. Although the standard sunitinib schedule

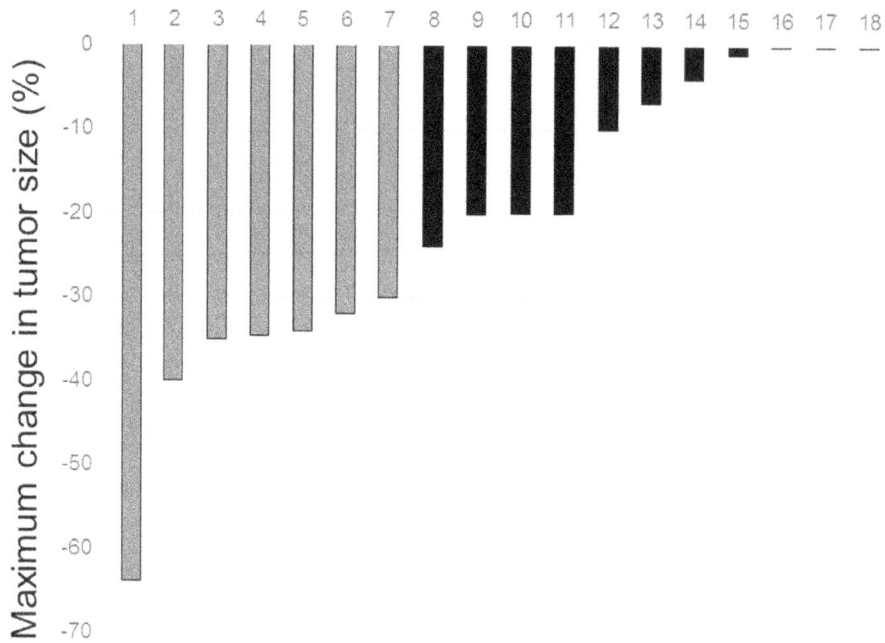

Figure 1 Waterfall plot showing tumor response to axitinib by RECIST. Bars represent individual evaluable patients. Gray, partial response; black, stable disease.

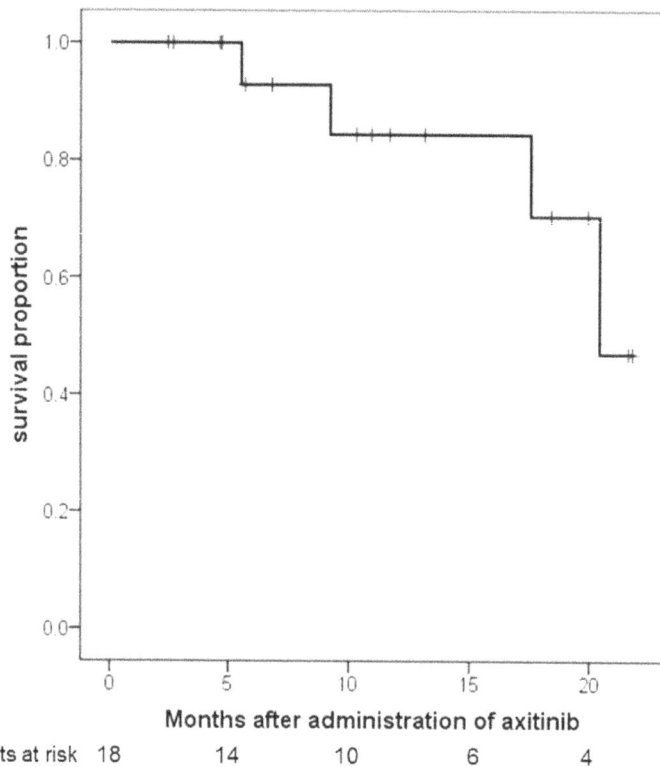

Figure 2 Kaplan-Meier analysis of progression-free survival. The 1-year progression-free survival rate was 84.4% (95% confidence interval, 15.8-21.5).

Table 2 Adverse events

Adverse events	Any grade, number (%)	Grade 3, number (%)
Hypertension	7 (38.9)	1 (5.6)
Proteinuria	5 (27.8)	2 (11.1)
Hypothyroidism	3 (16.7)	0
General malaise	3 (16.7)	0
Hand-foot syndrome	2 (11.1)	0
Anemia	1 (5.6)	0
Stomatitis	1 (5.6)	0
Renal impairment	1 (5.6)	0

involves four weeks of treatment and two weeks of rest, a modified schedule of sunitinib treatment, with two weeks of treatment and one week of rest, was associated with significantly decreased toxicity [23].

Common AEs of axitinib include diarrhea, hypertension, fatigue, anorexia and weight loss. The safety profile of axitinib is generally manageable with standard medical intervention [24]. In the AXIS study, discontinuation rates due to treatment-related AEs were 4% in the axitinib arm and 8% in the sorafenib arm, while dose interruptions and reductions were required in 77% and 31% of axitinib recipients [25]. The AXIS study protocol allowed for dose escalation in the absence of hypertension or grade 2 AEs, which may have been partially responsible for the subsequent increase in dose-reduction rate [26].

In this study, the treatment-naïve cRCC patients had a relatively longer PFS without axitinib dose titration, compared with other clinical trials. Rini et al. reported that in treatment-naïve mRCC patients who initially tolerated axitinib at a dose of 5 mg twice daily, a significantly higher proportion achieved an objective response with axitinib dose titration than with placebo titration [27]. Furthermore, based on the results from a phase 3 trial evaluating axitinib versus sorafenib in treatment-naïve patients with mRCC, the median PFS was 10.1 months with axitinib and 6.5 months with sorafenib ($P = 0.038$) [13]. In addition, median PFS was 13.7 months with axitinib and 6.6 months with sorafenib in patients with ECOG PS 0 ($P = 0.022$) [13]. In this study, the differences in PFS were not significant between all risk groups, according to the MSKCC risk stratification. Although brief exposure to higher axitinib doses may achieve immediate tumor shrinkage, a substantial proportion of patients may subsequently be forced to lower axitinib doses, which may lead to lower rates of long term disease control.

The current study has several limitations. First, it is a retrospective study, with an inherent potential for bias. Second, a relatively small number of patients were enrolled in this study, and the follow-up period was relatively short. In this study, the number of enrolled patients was relatively high age compared with other randomized trials [13,27]. AEs were also effectively managed with medications or axitinib dose reduction in this study. Although a large proportion of patients in other randomized control studies were recruited from North America and Western Europe, some patients were recruited from Asia, but the number was not large enough. Therefore, axitinib as first-line therapy may provide a treatment option for selected Japanese patients with locally advanced or mRCC.

Conclusions

In the current study, axitinib showed improved oncological outcomes and an acceptable safety profile as the first-line therapy for advanced RCC or mRCC in treatment-naïve patients. Thus, first-line therapy with axitinib may provide a promising treatment option for advanced RCC or mRCC patients. Further trials in the first-line setting are warranted.

Consent

Written informed consent was obtained from the patient for publication of this case report and the accompanying images. A copy of the written consent is available for review by the Editor-in-Chief of this journal.

Abbreviations

AEs: Adverse events; cRCC: clear cell renal cell carcinoma; CT: Computed tomography; ECOG PS: Eastern Cooperative Oncology Group performance status; IFN-α: Interferon-alpha; mRCC: metastatic renal cell carcinoma; mTORs: mammalian target of rapamycin inhibitors; MRI: Magnetic resonance imaging; MSKCC: Memorial Sloan-Kettering Cancer Center; ORR: Overall response rate; PD: Progressive disease; PFS: Progression-free survival; RCC: Renal cell carcinoma; RECIST: Response evaluation criteria in solid tumors; TKIs: Tyrosine kinase inhibitors; VEGF: Vascular endothelial growth factor.

Competing interests

The authors declare that they have no competing interests.

Authors' contributions

TK was involved in the drafting of the manuscript. TK, HY, AI, SH, TY and YH performed the clinical follow-up and contributed to the manuscript. TY, YT, and KM collected data and performed statistical analysis. YH reviewed the pathological specimen. CO and TK performed the operation. CO was responsible for the conception and design of this study, interpretation of the data, and critical revision of the manuscript. All authors read and approved the final manuscript.

Authors' information

TK: Associate professor. CO: Professor and Chairman. TY: Lecturer. HY: Assistant professor. AI: Assistant professor. SH: Lecturer. YH: Associate professor. TY: Assistant professor. YT: Assistant professor. KM: Assistant professor. Department of Urology, Hirosaki University Graduate School of Medicine, Hirosaki, Japan.

References

1. Motzer RJ, Russo P. Systemic therapy for renal cell carcinoma. J Urol. 2000;163:408–17.

2. Barrios CH, Hernandez-Barajas D, Brown MP, Lee SH, Fein L, Liu JH, et al. Phase II trial of continuous once-daily dosing of sunitinib as first-line treatment in patients with metastatic renal cell carcinoma. Cancer. 2012;118:1252–9.

3. Motzer RJ, Bacik J, Murphy BA, Russo P, Mazumdar M. Interferon-alfa as a comparative treatment for clinical trials of new therapies against advanced renal cell carcinoma. J Clin Oncol. 2002;20:289–96.

4. Motzer RJ, Hutson TE, Tomczak P, Michaelson MD, Bukowski RM, Oudard S, et al. Overall survival and update results for sunitinib compared with interferon alfa in patients with metastatic renal cell carcinoma. J Clin Oncol. 2009;27:3584–90.

5. Hudes G, Carducci M, Tomczak P, Dutcher J, Figlin R, Kapoor A, et al. Temsirolimus, interferon alfa, or both for advanced renal-cell carcinoma. N Eng J Med. 2007;356:227–81.

6. Tomita Y, Shinohara N, Yuasa T, Fujimoto H, Niwakawa M, Mugiya S, et al. Overall survival and updated results from a phase II study of sunitinib in Japanese patients with metastatic renal cell carcinoma. Jpn J Clin Oncol. 2010;40:1166–72.

7. Ueda T, Uemura H, Tomita Y, Tsukamoto T, Kanayama H, Shinohara N, et al. Efficacy and safety of axitinib versus sorafenib in metastatic renal cell carcinoma: subgroup analysis of Japanese patients from the global randomized Phase 3 AXIS trial. Jpn J Clin Oncol. 2013;43:616–28.

8. Motzer RJ, Escudier B, Bukowski R, Rini BI, Hutson TE, Barrios CH, et al. Prognostic factors for survival in 1059 patients treated with sunitinib for metastatic renal cell carcinoma. Br J Cancer. 2013;108:2470–7.

9. Miyake H, Miyazaki A, Harada K, Fijisawa M. Assessment of efficacy, safety and quality of life of 110 patients treated with sunitinib as first-line therapy for metastatic renal cell carcinoma: experience in real-world clinical practice in Japan. Med Oncol. 2014;31:978.

10. Hu-Lowe DD, Zou HY, Grazzini ML, Hallin ME, Wickman GR, Amundson K, et al. Nonclinical antiangiogenesis and antitumor activities of axitinib (AG-013736), an oral, potent, and selective inhibitor of vascular endothelial growth factor receptor tyrosine kinases 1, 2, 3. Clin Cancer Res. 2008;14:7272–83.

11. Rini BI, Wilding G, Hudes G, Stadler WM, Kim S, Tarazi J, et al. Phase II study of axitinib in sorafenib-refractory metastatic renal cell carcinoma. J Clin Oncol. 2009;27:4462–8.

12. Tomita Y, Uemura H, Fujimoto H, Kanayama HO, Shinohara N, Nakazawa H, et al. Key predictive factors of axitinib (AG-013736)-induced proteinuria and efficacy: a phase II study in Japanese patients with cytokine-refractory metastatic renal cell Carcinoma. Eur J Cancer. 2011;47:2592–602.

13. Hutson TE, Lesovoy V, Al-Shukri S, Stus VP, Lipatov ON, Bair AH, et al. Axitinib versus sorafenib as first-line therapy in patients with metastatic renal-cell carcinoma: a randomized open-label phase 3 trial. Lancet Oncol. 2013;14:1287–94.

14. Eisenhauer EA, Therasse P, Bogaerts J, Schwartz LH, Sargent D, Ford R, et al. New response evaluation criteria in solid tumours: revised RECIST guideline (version 1.1). Eur J Cancer. 2009;45:228–47.

15. Koie T, Ohyama C, Okamoto A, Yamamoto H, Imai A, Hatakeyama S, et al. Presurgical therapy with axitinib for advanced renal cell carcinoma: a case report. BMC Res Notes. 2013;6:484.

16. American Joint Committee on Cancer (AJC). Urinary Bladder. In: Edge SB, Byrd DR, Compton CC, et al., editors. AJCC Cancer Staging Manual, 7th edn. New York: Springer; 2010. p. 497–505.

17. Clavien PA, Barkun J, De Oliveira ML, Vauthey JN, Dindo D, Schulick RD, et al. The Clavien-Dindo classification of surgical complications. Ann Surg. 2009;250:187–96.

18. Negrier S, Escudier B, Lasset C, Douillard JY, Savary J, Chevreau C, et al. Recombinant human interleukin-2, recombinant human interferon alfa-2a, or both in metastatic renal-cell carcinoma. Groupe Français d'Immunothérapie. N Eng J Med. 1998;338:1272–8.

19. Patard JJ, Pignot G, Escudier B, Eisen T, Bex A, Sternberg C, et al. ICUD-EAU International Consultation on Kidney Cancer 2010: treatment of metastatic disease. Eur Urol. 2011;60:684–90.

20. Ibrahim EM, Kazkaz GA, Abouelkhair KM, Bayer AM, Elmasri OA. Sunitinib adverse events in metastatic renal cell carcinoma: a meta-analysis. Int J Clin Oncol. 2013;18:1060–9.

21. Motzer RJ, Michaelson MD, Redman BG, Hudes GR, Wilding G, Figlin RA, et al. Activity of SU11248, a multitargeted inhibitor of vascular endothelial growth factor receptor and platelet-derived growth factor receptor, in patients with metastatic renal cell carcinoma. J Clin Oncol. 2006;24:16–24.

22. Motzer RJ, Rini BI, Bukowski RM, Curti BD, George DJ, Hudes GR, et al. Sunitinib in patients with metastatic renal cell carcinoma. JAMA. 2006;295:2516–24.

23. Najjar YG, Mittal K, Elson P, Wood L, Garcia JA, Dreicer R, et al. A 2 weeks on and 1 week off schedule of sunitinib is associated with decreased toxicity in metastatic renal cell carcinoma. Eur J Cancer. 2014;50:1084–9.

24. Escudier B, Gore M. Axitinib for the management of metastatic renal cell carcinoma. Drugs R D. 2011;11:113–26.

25. Rini BI, Escudier B, Tomezak P, Kaprin A, Szczylik C, Hutson TE, et al. Comparative effectiveness of axitinib versus sorafenib in advanced renal cell carcinoma (AXIS): a randomised phase 3 trial. Lancet. 2011;378:1931–9.

26. Calvo E, Grünwald V, Bellmunt J. Controversies in renal cell carcinoma: treatment choice after progression on vascular endothelial growth factor-targeted therapy. Eur J Cancer. 2014;50:1321–9.

27. Rini BI, Melichar B, Ueda T, Grünwald V, Fishman MN, Arranz JA, et al. Axitinib with or without dose titration for first-line metastatic renal-cell carcinoma: a randomised double-blind phase 2 trial. Lancet Oncol. 2013;14:1233–42.

10

Sixteen years post radiotherapy of nasopharyngeal carcinoma elicited multi-dysfunction along PTX and chronic kidney disease with microcytic anemia

Yi-Ting Lin[1,2], Chia-Chun Huang[3], Charng-Cherng Chyau[2*], Kuan-Chou Chen[4,5*] and Robert Y Peng[2]

Abstract

Background: The hypothalamic–pituitary (h-p) unit is a particularly radiosensitive region in the central nervous system. As a consequence, radiation-induced irreversible, progressively chronic onset hypopituitarism (RIH) commonly develops after radiation treatments and can result in variably impaired pituitary function, which is frequently associated with increased morbidity and mortality.

Case presentation: A 38-year-old male subject, previously having received radiotherapy for treatment of nasopharygeal carcinoma (NPCA) 16 years ago, appeared at OPD complaining about his failure in penile erection, loss of pubic hair, atrophy of external genitalia: testicles reduced to 2×1.5 cm; penile size shrunk to only 4 cm long. Characteristically, he showed extremely lowered human growth hormone, (HGH, 0.115 ng/mL), testosterone (<0.1 ng/mL), total thyroxine (tT4: 4.740 g/mL), free T4 (fT4, 0.410 ng/mL), cortisol (2.34 g/dL); lowered LH (1.37 mIU/mL) and estradiol (22 pg/mL); highly elevated TSH (7.12 IU/mL). As contrast, he had low end normal ACTH, FSH, total T3, free T3, and estriol; high end normal prolactin (11.71 ng/mL), distinctly implicating hypopituitarism-induced hypothyroidism and hypogonadism. serologically, he showed severely lowered Hb (10.6 g/dL), HCT (32.7%), MCV (77.6 fL), MCH (25.3 pg), MCHC (32.6 g/dL), and platelet count (139×103/L) with extraordinarily elevated RDW (18.2%), together with severely lowered ferritin (23.6 ng/mL) and serum iron levels; highly elevated total iron binding capacity (TIBC, 509 g/dL) and transferrin (363.4 mg/dL), suggesting microcytic anemia. Severely reduced estimated glomerular filtration rate (e-GFR) (89 mL/mim/1.73 m2) pointed to CKD2. Hypocortisolemia with hyponatremia indicated secondary adrenal insufficiency. Replacement therapy using androgen, cortisol, and Ringer's solution has shown beneficial in improving life quality.

Conclusions: To our believe, we are the first group who report such complicate PTX dysfunction with adrenal cortisol insufficiency concomitantly occurring in a single patient.

Keywords: Radiotherapy, Hypopituitarism, Hypothyroidism, Hypogonadism, Adrenal insufficiency, Chronic kidney disease, Microcytic anemia

* Correspondence: ccchyau@sunrise.hk.edu.tw; kc.chen416@msa.hinet.net
[2]Research Institute of Biotechnology, Hungkuang University, 34 Chung-Chie Road, Shalu County, Taichung City 43302, Taiwan
[4]Department of Urology, Taipei Medical University-Shuang Ho Hospital, Taipei Medical University, 250, Wu-Xin St, Xin-Yi District 110 Taipei, Taiwan
Full list of author information is available at the end of the article

Background

The hypothalamic–pituitary (h-p) unit is a particularly radiosensitive region of the central nervous system. As a consequence, radiation-induced hypopituitarism (RIH) commonly develops after radiation treatments [1,2]. RIH, an irreversible and progressive chronic onset disorder, can result in a variable impairment of pituitary function [1,2], usually associated with increased morbidity and mortality [3].

Selective radiosensitivity of the neuroendocrine axes, with the human growth hormone (HGH) axis being the most vulnerable, accounts for the high frequency of HGH deficiency (GHD) following irradiation of the h–p axis with doses less than 30 Gy [2]. Life table analysis shows that the percent damages are dose- and time-dependent, and the frequency of GHD can substantially increase to reach as high as 50–100% [3]. At average, to lose 75% of the normal axis function of GHD may take 3.3 years, for LH/FSH, 7.8 years; and ACTH, 8.2 years [4]. Abnormalities in gonadotrophin secretion occurs dose-dependently but infrequently, and hyperprolactinemia is usually subclinical [2].

Thyroid hormones, directly or indirectly through erythropoietin, stimulate growth of erythroid colonies. Anemia is often the first sign of hypothyroidism diagnosed in 20-60% patients with hypothyroidism [5]. Numerous mechanisms are involved in the pathogenesis of these anemias which can be microcytic, macrocytic and normocytic [6]. Microcytic anemia is usually ascribed to malabsorption and failure in transport of iron. Macrocytosis is found in up to 55% patients with hypothyroidism and may result from the insufficiency of the thyroid hormones themselves without nutritive [5] like vitamin B_{12} and folic acid, and is frequently seen in pernicious anemia. Normocytic anemia is characterized by reticulopenia, hypoplasia of erythroid lineage, and decreased level of erythropoietin and mainly is associated with regular erythrocyte survival [6]. Worth note, pernicious anemia occurs 20 times more frequently in patients with hypothyroidism than generally [5].

We report a male patient who showed apparently shrunken penis and reduced testicular size, erectile dysfunction and loss of libido 16 years post radiotherapy of his nasopharyngeal carcinoma (NPCA).

Case presentation

A 38 years old male patient visited the Urological Outpatient Department and complained mainly about complete loss of penile erection already for half a year. The fact was soon recognized that he had been diagnosed to be with NPC, epidermoid carcinoma, nonkeratinizing in July 2, 1997, Stage cT3N2bM0 (previous AJCC staging system, 4th edition, not AJCC 7th staging system). The overall cumulative radiotherapy dose was 7140 cGy/42 fractions. The fraction dose was 170 cGy. The irradiation was delivered with conventional 2-dimensional radiotherapy using the linear accelerator equipped with 6 MV energy. Complete tumor response was achieved. The physical examination revealed shrunken external genitalia with penile size severely reduced to only 4 cm long accompanied with complete loss of pubic hair (Figure 1). His testicles are apparently with atrophy, size severely reduced to approximately 2×1.5 cm (not shown). Tracing back to the past history, the patient was diagnosed with nasopharyngeal carcinoma (NPCA) and as in the above mentioned he had received cumulative radiotherapy dose 7140 cGy/42 fractions (170 cGy/per fraction) sixteen years ago and didn't receive any extra surgery or

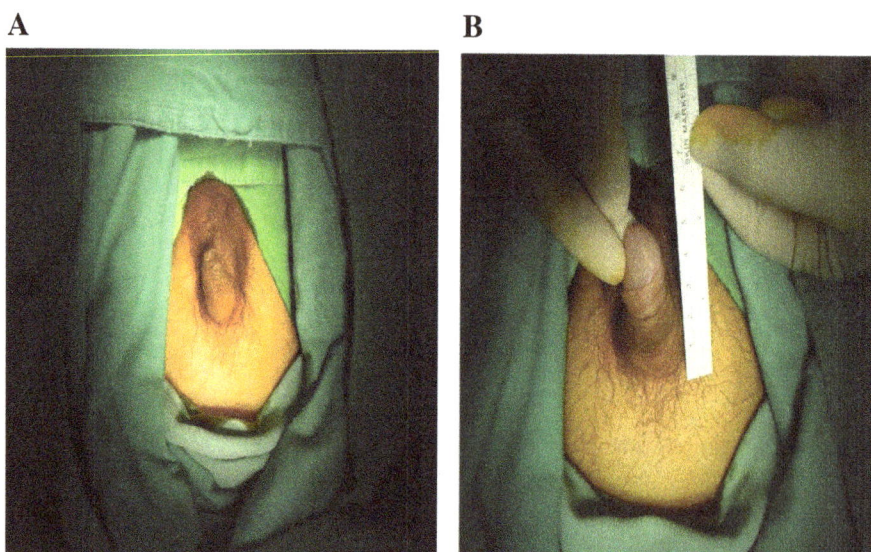

Figure 1 Appearance of this genital organ-penis. Shrunken penis is apparently with size reduced to only 4 cm long post radiotherapy for treating nasopharyngeal carcinoma (NPCA) 16 years ago. (**A**: Penis regularly appearing, **B**: Measuring size of penis)(patient: male, age 38).

chemotherapy for this NPCA. The NPCA was successfully treated and didn't recur up to present. In the same duration, he successfully went on to father three healthy children, age 16, 15 and 10 respectively.

The sagittal views reveal his hypophysis has been injured severely. The nasal pharyngeal area is severely deformed. (Figure 2). After testis biopsy, the pathological report showed pictures of mature testis with spermatogenesis, well developed seminiferous tubules and Leydig cells, yet the number of mature spermatozoa is fair per cross section of seminiferous tubules. The thickening of tubular wall indicates early stage testicular atrophy (Figure 3).

The laboratory data revealed extremely lowered HGH, lower levels of LH, testosterone, E2, total thyroxine and free T4, accompanied with severely lowered cortisol, low end level ACTH, FSH, total T3, and free T3; highly elevated TSH, high end normal prolactin, and normal estriol were also noticed (Table 1). Complete blood count revealed low RBC, severely lowered Hb, HCT, MCV, MCH, MCHC, PLT, MPV, elevated RDW (Table 2); severely lowered ferritin, low serum iron levels, highly elevated serum total iron binding capacity, elevated transferrin and the low end marginal e-GFR (Table 3). This patient was commenced on replacement therapy with cortisone injections, Ringer's solution (3%), thyroxine (T4), and testosterone replacement were immediately prescribed.

Discussion

Concomitant occurrence of low end normal ACTH, extremely lowered HGH, and highly elevated TSH level with significantly lowered tT4 and fT4 (Table 1) implicated the second stage hypothyroidism (Figure 4). Buchanan et al. indicated that hypothyroidism also can

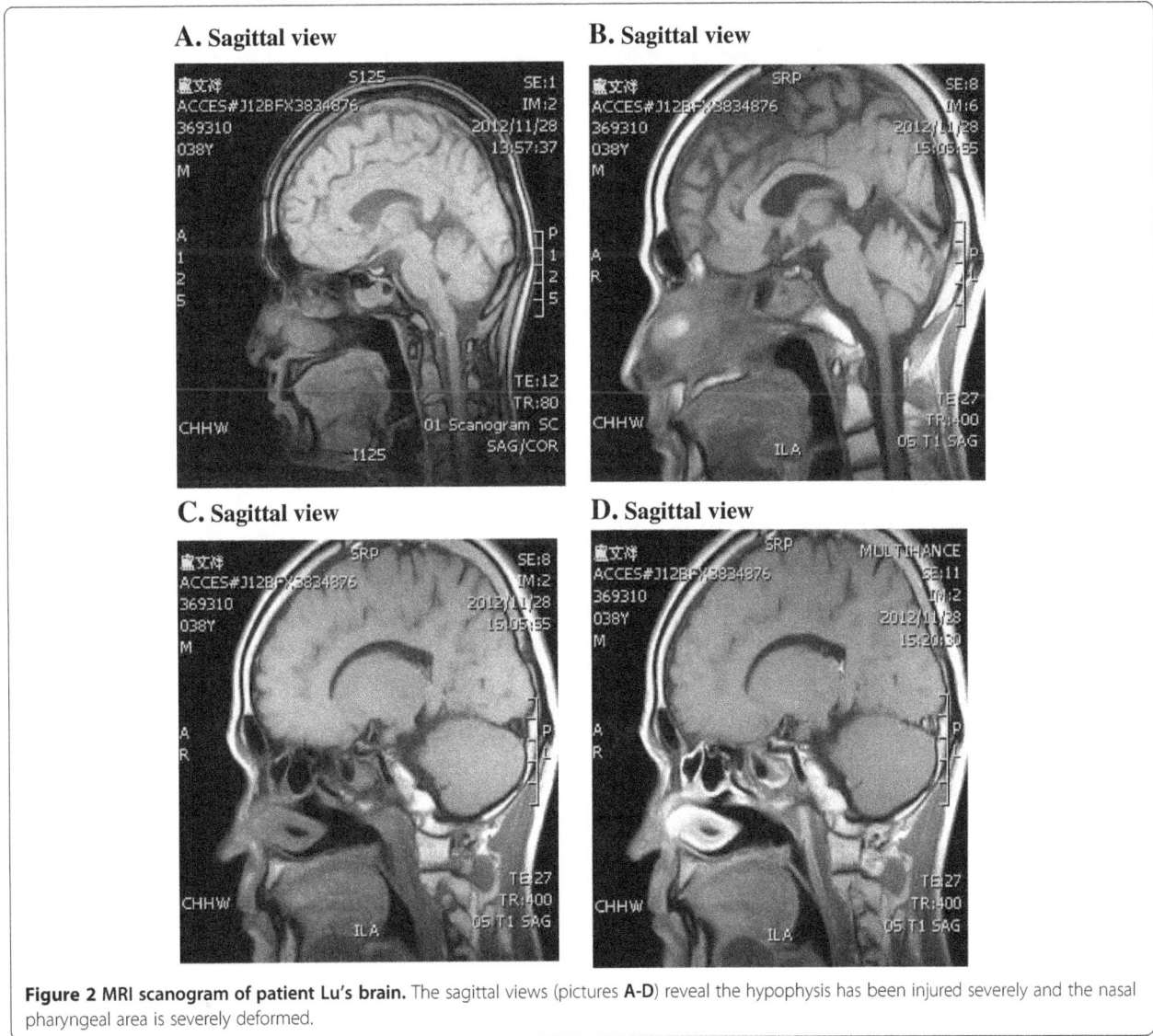

Figure 2 MRI scanogram of patient Lu's brain. The sagittal views (pictures **A-D**) reveal the hypophysis has been injured severely and the nasal pharyngeal area is severely deformed.

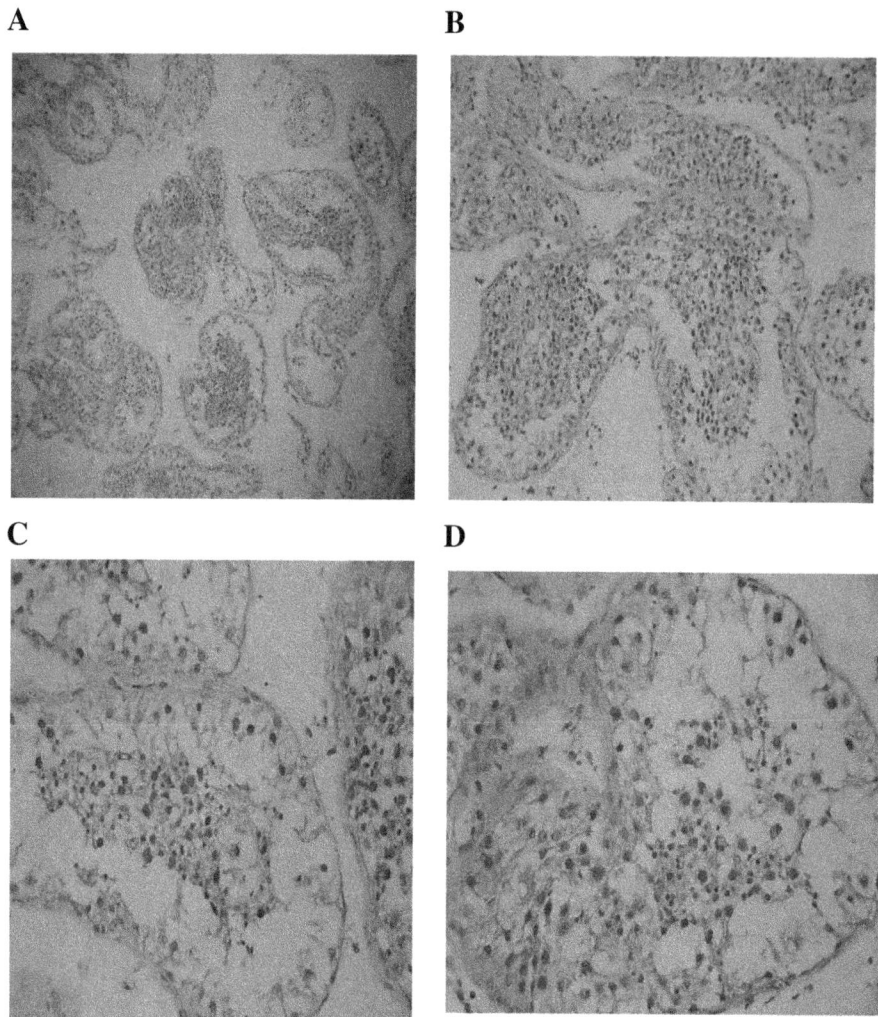

Figure 3 Hematoxylin-Eosin stain of testicualr tissues. **A**: 100×; **B**: 200×; **C**: 300×; and **D**: 400× (date: December 20, 2012). The thickening of seminiferous tubular walls is a typical symptom of early testicular atrophy. The Leydig cells and Sertoli cells appear normal with mature spermatogenesis, however with reduced density and lack of compact cell linings as usually seen in normal subjects.

be associated with increased FSH secretion [7]. However such a manifestation did not occur in this male victim (Table 1).

The HE stain of the patient's seminiferous tubule revealed normal maturation of spermatozoa, but much less in population, implying infertility (Figure 3). Diminished secretion of LH can result in hypogonadism [8] (refer to Table 1 and Figure 4).

Secondary hypocortisolemia associated with hyponatremia (Table 3, Figure 4) occurred because of lacking adrenocorticotropin that is responsible for triggering the adrenal gland to produce the adrenal cortisol [9,10].

An e-GFR 89 mL/min/1.73 m^2 implied stage 2 chronic kidney disease (CKD2) (Table 3). Hypocortisolemia (Table 1) can cause reduced e-GFR.

This patient was affiliated with microcytic anemia as evidenced by hypothyroidism (Table 1), low Hb, MCV (Table 2) and severely lowered ferritin (Table 3). Pituitary gland has an influence on erythropoiesis. Anaemia is thought to be due to loss of thyrotrophic and adrenotrophic hormones [11]. Testosterone enhances erythropoiesis by increasing renal erythropoietin production [11-13]. Severely lowered ferritin (Table 3) implies poor iron absorption by the duodenal lumen (Figure 5) [14].

This patient was commenced on replacement therapy with cortisone injection, Ringer's solution (3%), thyroxine (T4), and testosterone replacement were immediately prescribed. Muscle strength was rapidly restored after replacement. Unlike primary hypogonadism, secondary hypogonadism often has a cause that is amenable to specific treatment. For that reason, finding the cause carries particular importance [18]. If the hypogonadism occurred postpubertally, usually only LH need to be replaced. In hypogonadism secondary to hypothalamic disease,

Table 1 Endocrine analysis

Hormone	Value	Normal range	Comment
ACTH, pg/mL	12.2	9.0–52.0 (website 1)	Low end normal
GH, ng/mL	0.115	1.000–9.000 (website 2)	Severely lower
Prolactin, ng/mL (EIA)	11.71	male: 2.64–13.13; 4–23 (website 3); (3–15, website 4)	High end normal
FSH, mIU/mL (EIA/LIA)	4.91	males: 1.27–19.26; 1.4–18.1 (male) (website 5)	Low end normal
LH, mIU/mL	1.37	males: 1.50–9.30 (website 5)	Lower
Estradiol, E2 (EIA/LIA), pg/mL	22	males: 25–70 (website: 4)	Lower
Estriol (E3) (EIA), pg/mL	<0.017	0–3 (website: 6)	Normal
Testosterone (EIA/LIA), ng/mL	<0.1	Blood: 3.0–12.0 (website 5)	Trace only
T4 total (biochem), µg/dL	4.740	6.09–12.23	Extremely lower
Free T4 (EIA/LIA), ng/dL	0.41	0.54–1.40	Extremely lower
T3 total, (EIA/LIA), ng/dL	92.88	87.00–178.00	Low end normal
Free T3 (EIA/LIA), pg/mL	2.780	2.500–3.900; 2.300–6.190 (website 7)	Low end normal
TSH (EIA/LIA), µIU/mL	7.12	0.34–5.60	Highly elevated
Cortisol, µg/dL	-		-
At 8 am	2.34	6.7–22.6	Severely lowered;
At 16 pm	3.74	0–10	Low end

Websites: 1. http://www.nlm.nih.gov/medlineplus/ency/article/003695.htm.
2. Medline Plus. 3. Selleckchem.com. 4-30 ng/ml in females and 4-23 ng/mL in males. 4. MedHelp. 5. Health Board. 6. High-Pro.com. 7. Men's Health Message Board. 7. About.Com. Thyroid disease. Practice Notebook. Updated July 31, 2003; by Kenneth N. Woliner, M.D., A.B.F.P. Website: Nova Tech ImmunodiagnosticaGmbH.

spermatogenesis can also be stimulated by pulsatile administration of GnRH. Testosterone can be replaced whether the hypogonadism is primary or secondary. Unlike estrogen, testosterone itself is not suitable for oral replacement, because it is catabolized rapidly during its first pass through the liver. Derivatives of testosterone that are alkylated in the 17α position do not undergo this rapid hepatic catabolism; however, these agents appear to lack

Table 2 Complete blood count*

	Value obtained	Normal range	Comment
WBC, 10^3/µL	5.2	3.5–9.6	Normal
RBC, 10^6/µL	4.21	4.20–6.23	Low end margin
Hb, g/dL	10.6	13–18	Severely lower
HCT, %	32.7	38.8–53.1	Severely lower
MCV, fL	77.6	80.0–100.0	Severely lower
MCH, pg	25.3	27.0–32.0	Severely lower
MCHC, g/dL	32.6	33.3–36.0	Lower
PLT, 10^3/µL	139	150–450	Severely lower
PDW, %	17.6	15.5–18.0	Normal
MPV, fL	6.6	6.8–13.5	Lower
RDW, %	18.2	12.1–15.2	Highly elevated

*WBC: white blood cells. RBC: red blood cells. Hb: hemoglobin. HCT: hematocrit. MCV: mean corpuscular volume. MCH: mean corpusulr hemoglobin. MCHC: mean corpusular hemoglobin concentration. PLT: platelet count. PDW: platelet distribution width. MPV: mean platelet volume. RDW: red blood cell distribution width.

the full virilizing effect of testosterone, and they may cause hepatic toxicity, including cholestatic jaundice, a cystic condition of the liver called peliosis, and, possibly, hepatocellular carcinoma. Consequently, the 17α-alkylated androgens should not be used to treat testosterone deficiency [18].

During replacement therapy, clinicians should monitor patients for the efficacy and side effects of testosterone. Serum testosterone concentrations can vary with any of these preparations, so testosterone should be measured more than once to determine whether the initial dose is optimal. Serum testosterone should be measured again after a dose is changed and then once or twice a year. If the serum testosterone concentration is maintained within the normal range, the patient should experience reversal of the consequences of testosterone deficiency. Specifically, energy, libido, hemoglobin concentration, muscle mass, and bone density will increase [18]. Noteworthy, hypogonadism has been associated with several risk factors of atherosclerosis including obesity, Type II DM, dyslipidemia and hypertension.

Hypogonadism having low testosterone levels with increased carotid intima-media thickness (IMT) may evidence early atherosclerosis. In addition, low testosterone increases the susceptibility to myocardial ischemia. Erectile dysfunction is a symptom of hypogonadism, but also an end result of atherosclerosis and a predictor of coronary artery atherosclerosis (CAD) [19].

Table 3 Biochemical tests of serum

Parameters	Value obtained	Normal range	Comment
Serum BUN, mg/dL	16	8–20	Normal
s-GOT (AST), IU/L	28	15–41	Normal
s-GPT (ALT), IU/L	14	10–40	Normal
TIBC, µg/dL	509	255–450	Highly elevated
Ferritin (EIA), ng/mL	23.6	30.0–336.2	Severely lower
Transferrin (Nephelometry), mg/dL	363.4	180–329	Highly elevated
Serum Iron (Fe), µg/dL	55	Adult male: 45–182	Lower margin
Creatinine (bood), mg/dL	0.95	0.70–1.20	Normal
e-GFR, mL/min/1.73 m^2	89	90–120	Low end margin
Na$^+$, mEq/L or mmol/L	124	135–146	Severely lower
Cu^{2+} (blood), µg/dL	129.75	70-140	Normal

TIBC: Total iron binding capacity. e-GFR: estimated glomerular filtration rate.
s-GOT: serum glutamate-oxaloacetate transaminase. s-GPT: serum glutamate-pyruvate transaminase.

The replacement therapy was subsequently associated with rise in haemoglobin to 12.3 g/dL after 3 months and 13.5 g/dL, MCV 86 after 7 months. It is important to remember the role of pituitary hormones in erythropoiesis and consider hypopituitarism in the differential diagnosis of iron deficiency anaemia. Steroid and testosterone replacement corrected anaemia in this patient however it is not clear which hormone played a major role.

Hypopituitarism associated secondary adrenal insufficiency must be frequently noted to avoid the occurrence of severe hyponatremia. Replacement therapy with testosterone, thyroid hormone, coritsol and saline

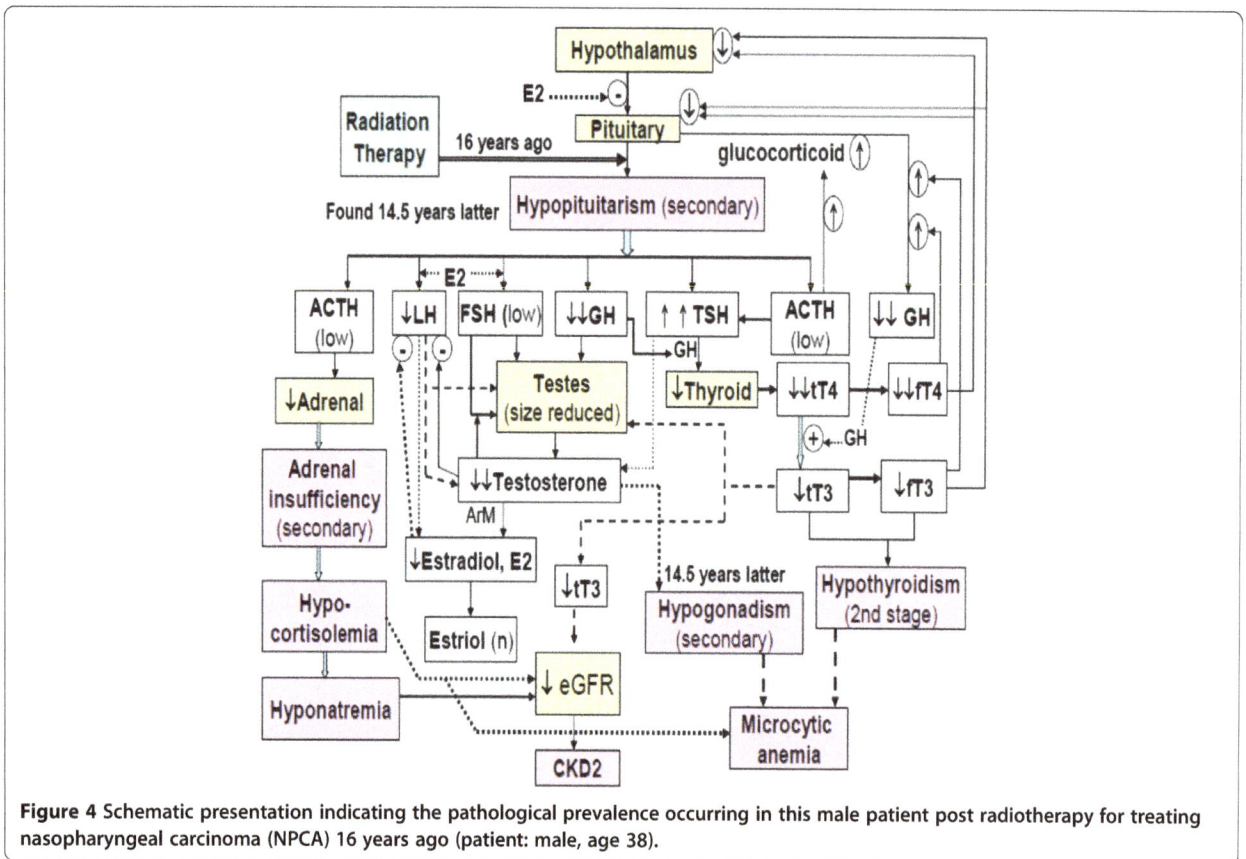

Figure 4 Schematic presentation indicating the pathological prevalence occurring in this male patient post radiotherapy for treating nasopharyngeal carcinoma (NPCA) 16 years ago (patient: male, age 38).

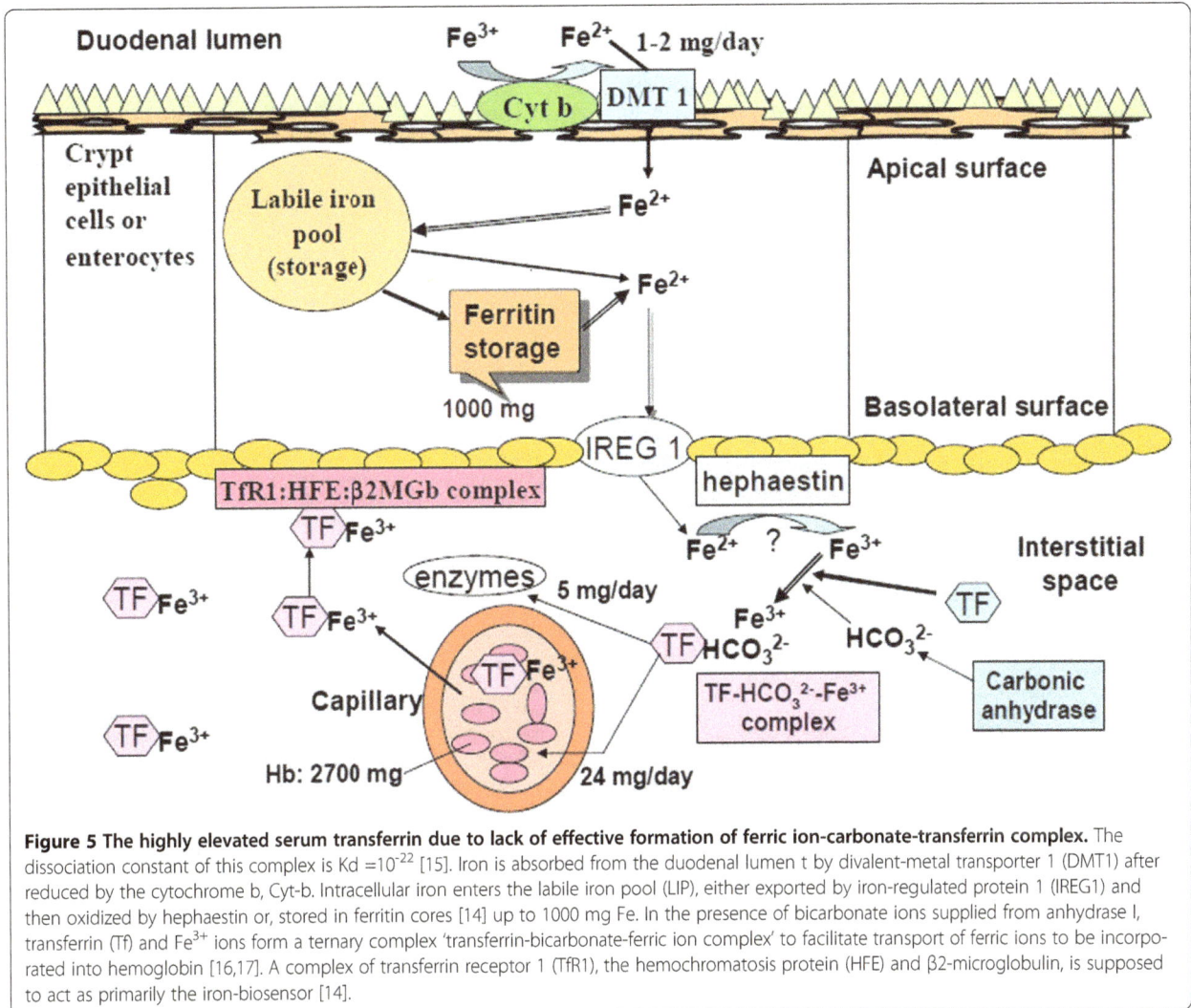

Figure 5 The highly elevated serum transferrin due to lack of effective formation of ferric ion-carbonate-transferrin complex. The dissociation constant of this complex is Kd =10^{-22} [15]. Iron is absorbed from the duodenal lumen t by divalent-metal transporter 1 (DMT1) after reduced by the cytochrome b, Cyt-b. Intracellular iron enters the labile iron pool (LIP), either exported by iron-regulated protein 1 (IREG1) and then oxidized by hephaestin or, stored in ferritin cores [14] up to 1000 mg Fe. In the presence of bicarbonate ions supplied from anhydrase I, transferrin (Tf) and Fe^{3+} ions form a ternary complex 'transferrin-bicarbonate-ferric ion complex' to facilitate transport of ferric ions to be incorporated into hemoglobin [16,17]. A complex of transferrin receptor 1 (TfR1), the hemochromatosis protein (HFE) and β2-microglobulin, is supposed to act as primarily the iron-biosensor [14].

infusion are effective strategies. Cortisol inhibits sodium loss through the small intestine of mammals. Sodium depletion, however, does not affect cortisol levels. So cortisol cannot be used to regulate serum sodium [20]. The original task of cortisol may have been sodium transport [21].

Radiation-induced GHD may progressively and frequently develop in the first 10 years after radiation delivery [22]. Radiation induced anterior pituitary hormone deficiencies are irreversible and progressive; a recognized complication of cranial irradiation in cancer survivors– in particular, a very sensitivity and high incidence of GH deficiency (GHD) is observed [2], some cases may reach a prevalence of GHD between 50 and 100%. Replacement not only could improve the life quality, but also sustain the life expectancy.

Regular assessments of anterior-pituitary function are imperative in such patients, to achieve a timely diagnosis and to enable introduction of appropriate hormone-replacement therapy [2,23,24]. To increase tumour-related survival rates, a long-term monitoring tailored to the individual risk profile is required to avoid the sequelae of untreated pituitary hormonal deficiencies and resultant decrease in the quality of life [1].

Conclusions

Damage resulting from radiotherapy is a progressive, chronic, and irreversible process. This case has taken 16 years to elicit PTX axis and adrenal dysfunction and concomitantly, secondary hypopituitarism complicated with second stage hypothyroidism, microcytic anemia, secondary hypocortisolemia with hyponatremia, secondary hypogonadism, and CKD2. Replacement therapy using T4, testosterone, cortisol, and 3% Ringer's solution infusion has shown rather beneficial to his life quality.

To our believe, we are the first group who report such a complicate PTX dysfunction which also involves adrenal cortisol insufficiency, chronic kidney disease and microcytic anemia concomitantly in a single patient.

Consent

Written informed consent was obtained from the patient for publication of this Case report and any accompanying images. A copy of the written consent is available for review by the Editor of this journal.

Abbreviations

ACTH: Adrenocorticotropic hormone; LH: Leutenizing hormone; TSH: Thyroid stimulating hormone; HGH or GH: Human growth hormone; FSH: Follicular stimulating hormone; tT4: Total thyroxine; fT4: Free T4; tT3: Total T3; fT3: Free T3; E2: Estradiol; ArM: Aromatase; N: Normal.

Competing interests

The authors declare that they have no competing interests.

Authors' contributions

YTL was responsible for concept, design, acquisition and interpretation of data. CCC and RYP contributed to design and critical revision of the manuscript and KCC was responsible for the critical revision of the manuscript. All authors have read and approved the final manuscript.

Acknowledgement

The authors are grateful for financial support offered by the National Science Council, NSC-103-2320-B-038-025. We also thank Professor Robert Y. Peng for providing medical writing services.

Author details

[1]Department of Urology, St. Joseph's Hospital, 74, Sinsheng Road, Huwei County, Yunlin Hsien 632, Taiwan. [2]Research Institute of Biotechnology, Hungkuang University, 34 Chung-Chie Road, Shalu County, Taichung City 43302, Taiwan. [3]Department of Radiation Oncology, Changhua Christian Hospital, No.135 Nan Shiau Street, Changhua 500, Taiwan. [4]Department of Urology, Taipei Medical University-Shuang Ho Hospital, Taipei Medical University, 250, Wu-Xin St, Xin-Yi District 110 Taipei, Taiwan. [5]Department of Urology, School of Medicine, Taipei Medical University, 250, Wu-Xin St, Xin-Yi District 110 Taipei, Taiwan.

References

1. Fernandez A, Brada M, Zabuliene L, Karavitaki N, Wass JA: Radiation-induced hypopituitarism. Endocr Relat Cancer 2009, 16:733.
2. Darzy KH, Shalet SM: Hypopituitarism following radiotherapy. Pituitary 2009, 12:40.
3. Tomlinson JW, Holden N, Hills RK, Wheatley K, Clayton RN, Bates AS, Sheppard MC, Stewart PM: Association between premature mortality and hypopituitarism. West Midlands prospective hypopituitary study group. Lancet 2001, 357:425.
4. Littley MD, Shalet SM, Beardwell CG, Ahmed SR, Applegate G, Sutton ML: Hypopituitarism following external radiotherapy for pituitary tumors in adults. Q J Med 1989, 70:145.
5. Antonijević N, Nesović M, Trbojević B, Milosević R: Anemia in hypothyroidism. Med Pregl 1999, 52:136.
6. Kosenli A, Erdogan M, Ganidagli S, Kulaksizoglu M, Solmaz S, Kosenli O, Unsal C, Canataroglu A: Anemia frequency and etiology in primary hypothyroidism. European Congress of Endocrinology, Istanbul, Turkey, 25 April 2009 - 29 April 2009. Eur Soc Endocrinol Endocr Abst 2009, 20:140.
7. Buchanan CR, Stanhope R, Adlard P: Gonadotrophin, growth hormone and prolactin secretion in children with primary hypothyroidism. Clin Endocrinol (Oxf) 1988, 29:427.
8. Pitteloud N, Dwyer AA, DeCruz S: Inhibition of luteinizing hormone secretion by testosterone in men requires aromatization for its pituitary but not its hypothalamic effects: evidence from the Tandem Study of Normal and Gonadotropin-Releasing Hormone-Deficient Men. J Clin Endocrinol Metab 2008, 93:784.
9. Diederich S, Franzen NF, Bahr V, Oelkers W: Severe hyponatremia due to hypopituitarism with adrenal insufficiency: report on 28 cases. Eur J Endocrinol 2003, 148:609.
10. Waikar SS, Mount DB, Curhan GC: Mortality after hospitalization with mild, moderate, and severe hyponatremia. Am J Med 2009, 122:857.
11. King R, Mizban N, Rajeswaran C: Iron deficiency anaemia due to hypopituitarism. Endocr Abst 2009, 19:P278.
12. Malgor LA, Valsecia M, Vergés E, De Markowsky EE: Blockade of the in vitro effects of testosterone and erythropoietin on Cfu-E and Bfu-E proliferation by pretreatment of the donor rats with cyproterone and flutamide. Acta Physiol Pharmacol Ther Latinoam 1998, 48:99.
13. Angelin-Duclos C, Domenget C, Kolbus A: Thyroid hormone T3 acting through the thyroid hormone α receptor is necessary for implementation of erythropoiesis in the neonatal spleen environment in the mouse. Development 2005, 132:925.
14. Chorney MJ, Yoshida Y, Meyer PN: The enigmatic role of the hemochromatosis protein (HFE) in iron absorption. Trends Mol Med 2003, 9:118.
15. Aisen P, Listowsky I: Iron transport and storage proteins. Ann Rev Biochem 1980, 49:357.
16. Supuran CT: Carbonic anhydrase inhibition with natural products: novel chemotypes and inhibition mechanisms. Mol Diver 2011, 15:305.
17. Sarikaya SB, Gülçin I, Supuran CT: Carbonic anhydrase inhibitors: Inhibition of human erythrocyte isozymes I and II with a series of phenolic acids. Chem Biol Drug Des 2010, 75:515.
18. Snyder PJ: Testes and testicular disorders: male hypogonadism, Endocrinology. University of Pennsylvania Medical School: From ACP Medicine Online Posted 06/07/2006 Peter J. Snyder, M.D. Etiology. ACP Medicine Online. 2002; ©2002 WebMD Inc. (Synder, P.J.: Professor of Endocrinology, Diabetes, and Metabolism; 2006.
19. Fahed AC, Gholmieh JM, Azar ST: Connecting the lines between hypogonadism and atherosclerosis. Int J Endocrinol 2012, 2012:793953.
20. Mason PA, Fraser R, Morton JJ, Semple PF, Wilson A: The effect of sodium deprivation and of angiotensin II infusion on the peripheral plasma concentrations of 18-hydroxycorticosterone, aldosterone and other corticosteroids in man. J Steroid Biochem 1977, 8:799.
21. Gorbman A, Dickhoff WW, Vigna SR, Clark NB, Muller AF: Comparative Endocrinol. New York: Wiley; 1983. ISBN ISBN 0-471-06266-9.
22. Toogood AA, Ryder WD, Beardwell CG, Shalet SM: The evolution of radiation-induced growth hormone deficiency in adults is determined by the baseline growth hormone status. Clin Endocrinol 1995, 43:97.
23. Agha A, Walker D, Perry L, Drake WM, Chew SL, Jenkins PJ, Grossman AB, Monson JP: Unmasking of central hypothyroidism following growth hormone replacement in adult hypopituitary patients. Clinical Endocrinol (Oxf) 2007, 66:72.
24. Appelman-Dijkstra NM, Kokshoorn NE, Dekkers OM, Neelis KJ, Biermasz NR, Romijn JA, Smith JWA, Pereira AM: Pituitary dysfunction in adult patients after cranial radiotherapy: systematic review and meta-analysis. J Clinical Endocrinol Metab 2011, 96:2330.

11

Effects of stimulating interleukin -2/anti-interleukin -2 antibody complexes on renal cell carcinoma

Kyu-Hyun Han[1†], Ki Won Kim[2†], Ji-Jing Yan[1], Jae-Ghi Lee[1], Eun Mi Lee[1], Miyeon Han[3], Eun Jin Cho[3], Seong Sik Kang[4], Hye Jin Lim[4], Tai Yeon Koo[4], Curie Ahn[1,3,4] and Jaeseok Yang[1,4*]

Abstract

Background: Current therapies for advanced renal cell carcinoma (RCC) have low cure rates or significant side effects. It has been reported that complexes composed of interleukin (IL)-2 and stimulating anti-IL-2 antibody (IL-2C) suppress malignant melanoma growth. We investigated whether it could have similar effects on RCC.

Methods: A syngeneic RCC model was established by subcutaneously injecting RENCA cells into BALB/c mice, which were administered IL-2C or phosphate-buffered saline every other day for 4 weeks. RCC size was measured serially, and its weight was assessed 4 weeks after RENCA injection. Immune cell infiltration into RCC lesions and spleen was assessed by flow cytometry and immunohistochemistry.

Results: IL-2C treatment increased the numbers of CD8[+] memory T and natural killer (NK) cells in healthy BALB/c mice ($P < 0.01$). In the spleen of RCC mice, IL-2C treatment also increased the number of CD8[+] memory T, NK cells, and macrophages as compared to PBS-treated controls ($P < 0.01$). The number of interferon-γ- and IL-10-producing splenocytes increased and decreased, respectively after 4 weeks in the IL-2C-treated mice ($P < 0.01$). Tumor-infiltrating immune cells including CD4[+] T, CD8[+] T, NK cells as well as macrophages were increased in IL-2C-treated mice than controls ($P < 0.05$). Pulmonary edema, the most serious side effect of IL-2 therapy, was not exacerbated by IL-2C treatment. However, IL-2C had insignificant inhibitory effect on RCC growth ($P = 0.1756$).

Conclusions: IL-2C enhanced immune response without significant side effects; however, this activity was not sufficient to inhibit RCC growth in a syngeneic, murine model.

Keywords: CD8[+] T cell, Immune complex, Interleukin-2, NK cell, Renal cell carcinoma, Tumor

Background

Renal cell carcinoma (RCC) is the most common primary malignancy of the renal parenchyma, comprising 3 % of all adult malignancies, and its incidence has been increasing [1, 2]. Although early RCC can be cured by surgery, one-third of RCC patients exhibit metastasis at diagnosis. Metastatic RCC has poor prognosis, with a 5-year survival rate of only 10 % [3], and approximately 20-25 % of patients with metastatic RCC do not respond to treatment and symptoms progress rapidly [4]. Sorafenib is one of target drugs against RCC that prolongs patient survival, but rarely leads to complete remission [5–7]; moreover, long-term sorafenib treatment can exacerbate RCC by creating ischemic conditions [8, 9].

RCC is considered as an immunogenic tumor owing to its spontaneous regression, variable growth, late metastasis, high degree of T cell infiltration, and high incidence in immunosuppressed patients. However, RCC can also suppress the anti-tumor immunity of naïve and memory CD4[+] T, natural killer (NK), and dendritic cells [10], and evade the cytotoxic effect of NK cells [11, 12]. Therefore, a drug that potentiates immune response may be effective in the treatment of

* Correspondence: jcyjs@dreamwiz.com
†Equal contributors
[1]Transplantation Research Institute, Seoul National University College of Medicine, Seoul, Republic of Korea
[4]Transplantation Center, Seoul National University Hospital, 101 Daehak-ro, Jongno-gu, Seoul 110-744, Republic of Korea
Full list of author information is available at the end of the article

RCC. Indeed, high doses of interleukin (IL)-2 have been shown to suppress RCC progression without inducing tumor ischemia, leading to complete remission in 10–20 % of patients [13, 14]. Blockade of CTLA4, a T-cell inhibitory receptor with ipilimumab, and increasing T-cell proliferation and cytotoxic effects with PD-1/PD-L1 axis inhibition also induced regression of renal cell carcinoma in some patients [15, 16]. However, high-dose IL-2 therapy also induces systemic inflammatory responses, including capillary leak syndrome, heart failure, and pulmonary edema, thereby hindering the broad application of high-dose IL-2 therapy in the treatment of advanced RCC [17, 18].

Recently, immune complexes (IL-2C) composed of with low-dose IL-2 and stimulating anti-IL-2 antibody (S4B6) have been shown to enhance immune responses via selective structural interactions [19–23]. Stimulating IL-2C can preferentially expand memory $CD8^+$ T and NK cells—while more weakly affecting regulatory T cells—via the interaction of anti-IL-2 antibodies (S4B6) and CD25 binding region of IL-2, leading to inhibition of both leukemia and melanoma [19, 23]. Interestingly, the half-life of IL-2 is increased in IL-2C; as such, low-dose IL-2C has immune enhancing effects that are comparable to those of high-dose IL-2 therapy without

accompanying serious side effects such as capillary leak syndrome [19, 23]. Low-dose IL-2C therapy is therefore expected to be an effective and safe treatment for immunogenic tumors.

Here, we investigated the efficacy and safety of low-dose IL-2C treatment for RCC in a syngeneic murine model. We found that IL-2C treatment enhanced anti-tumor immunity against RCC without causing pulmonary edema, although it did not have sufficient potency to suppress tumor growth.

Methods
Cells and mice
The RENCA, a murine RCC cell line from a BALB/c mouse background was purchased from Korean Cell line Bank (Seoul, Korea), and cultured in Eagle's Minimum Essential Medium (Gibco/Invitrogen, Grand Island, NY, USA) containing 10 % fetal bovine serum (Gibco/Invitrogen) at 37 °C and 5 % CO_2. BALB/c mice were purchased from Orient Bio Inc. (Seongnam, Korea) and maintained at the Biomedical Research Institute of Seoul National University Hospital. Mouse experimental protocols were approved by the Animal Ethics Committee of Seoul National University College of Medicine.

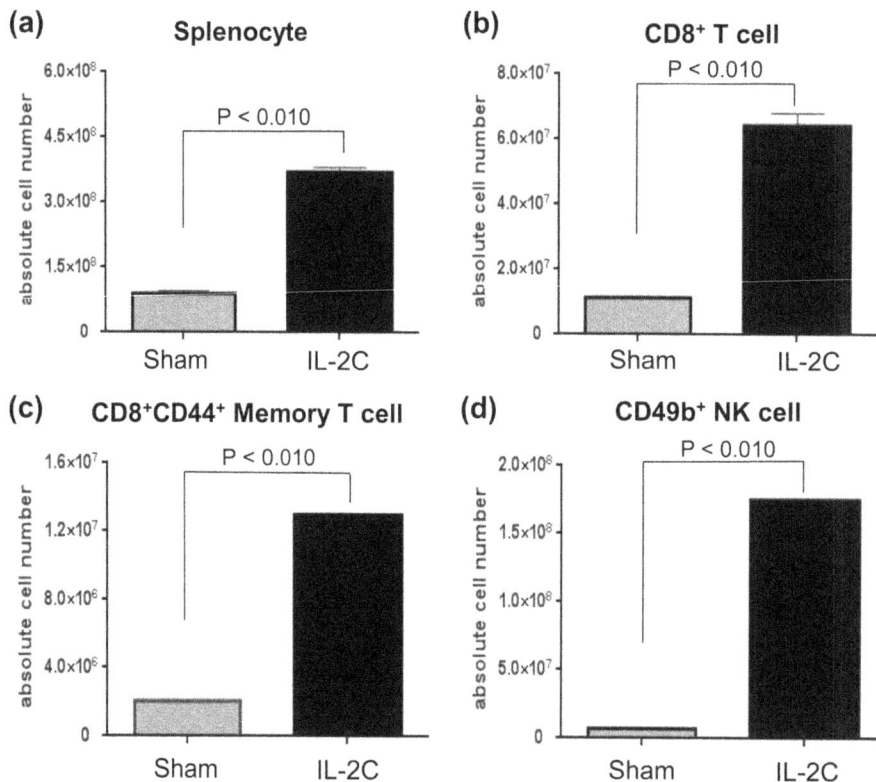

Fig. 1 IL-2C treatment induces the expansion of $CD8^+$ memory T and NK cells in the spleen. Mice were treated with IL-2C by intraperitoneal injection for 5 days. The total numbers of (**a**) splenocytes, (**b**) $CD8^+$ T cells, (**c**) $CD8^+$ memory T cells, (**d**) and NK cells were higher in IL-2C-treated than in PBS-treated mice ($P < 0.010$)

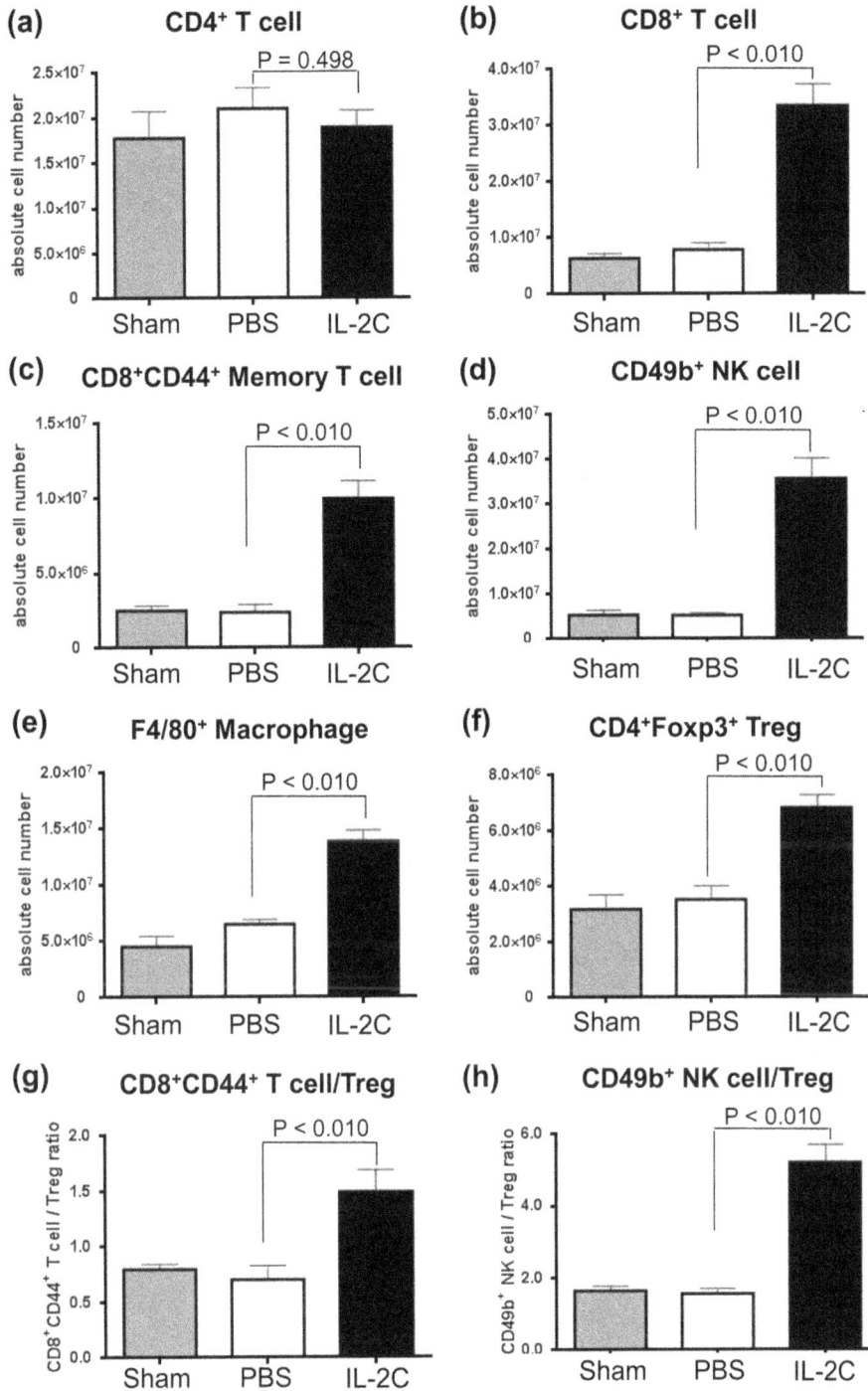

Fig. 2 IL-2C treatment induces the expansion of immune cells in the spleen of mice with RCC. Syngeneic RENCA cells were implanted subcutaneously in mice, and IL-2C or PBS was administered every other day for 4 weeks. (a) The number of CD4[+] T cells was similar between the two groups (P = 0.498), while the numbers of (b) CD8[+] T cells, (c) CD8[+] memory T cells, (d) NK cells, (e) macrophages, and (f) Tregs were higher in the IL-2C group than in the PBS group (P < 0.010). (g, h) CD8[+] memory T cell/Treg and NK cell/Treg ratios were higher in the IL-2C group than the PBS group (P < 0.010 in both cases). Treg, regulatory T cell

Preparation of IL-2/anti-IL-2 antibody complex

Recombinant murine IL-2 was purchased from eBioscience (San Diego, CA, USA) and the S4B6 anti-mouse IL-2 monoclonal antibodies was provided by Dr. Charles D. Surh (La Jolla Institute for Allergy and Immunology, La Jolla, CA, USA). S4B6 (7.5 µg) was mixed with IL-2 (1.5 µg, equivalent to 8555 IU) and incubated at 37 °C for 30 min before use. To evaluate the immune-enhancing effects of

IL-2 under normal conditions, IL-2C or phosphate-buffered saline (PBS) was administered daily to mice by intraperitoneal injection for 5 days, before the spleen was harvested for immune cell analysis.

In vivo tumor model

Eight-week old BALB/c mice were subcutaneously injected with RENCA cells (1×10^5) in 0.1 ml of 1× PBS to induce syngeneic RCC formation. IL-2C (treatment group) or PBS (control group) was intraperitoneally administered to mice every other day from day 0 to 28. Tumor size (length × width) was measured every other day using calipers. IL-2C with S4B6 (7.5 µg) and IL-2 (1.5 µg) or phosphate-buffered saline (PBS) was administered every 2 days to mice by intraperitoneal injection until 28 days. In high-dose IL-2 group, higher dose of IL-2 (35 µg, 200,000 IU) was administered to mice with the same schedule. Spleen, lung and tumor tissues were harvested 28 days after injection of RENCA cells. Tumor weight was measured after harvest. Pulmonary edema was assessed by lung weight, which was calculated by subtracting the dry weight from the wet weight.

Flow cytometry

Splenocytes were labeled with the following antibodies: anti-CD4-allophycocyanin (APC), anti-CD8-fluorescein isothiocyanate (FITC), anti-CD44-APC, anti-CD45-FITC, anti-CD49-phycoerythrin (PE), and anti-F4/80-PE and the vital dye 7-aminoactinomycin D (7-AAD) (BD Biosciences, San Jose, CA, USA). Forkhead homeobox protein 3 (Foxp3) was labeled using the anti-mouse Foxp3-FITC staining kit (eBioscience) according to the manufacturer's instructions. For analysis of tumor-infiltrating cells, tumors were dissociated with 200U/ml collagenase IV at 37 °C for 30 min. Flow cytometric analysis was carried out on a Canto II Instrument (BD Biosciences).

Enzyme-linked immunoSPOT (ELISPOT) assay

Interferon (IFN)-γ- or IL-10-producing T cells were detected with the ELISPOT assay. Spleens were harvested 28 days after mice were injected with RENCA cells. A 96-well plate was coated with anti-IFN-γ or -IL-10 capture antibodies using ELISPOT mouse IFN-γ or mouse IL-10 kits (BD biosciences). For IFN-γ ELISPOT, splenocytes (1×10^5/well) were incubated with 5 ng/ml phorbol 12-myristate 13-acetate (Sigma, St. Louis, MO, USA) and 500 ng/ml of inomycin (Sigma) at 37 °C for 8 h. For IL-10 ELISPOT, splenocytes (5×10^5/well) were incubated with 1 µg/ml of lipopolysaccharide (Sigma) for 24 h. Detection antibodies were then added, along with horseradish peroxidase (HRP)-streptavidin (BD Biosciences). After adding 3'-amino-9-ethylcarbazole substrate (BD Biosciences) for development, colored spots were measured with an ELSPOT reader (Cellular- Technology, Cleveland, OH, USA).

Immunohistochemistry

Tumor tissue with overlying skin was harvested on day 28. Anti-CD4, anti-CD8, anti-CD49b and anti-F4/80 antibodies (eBioscience) were incubated with tissue sections at 4 °C overnight. Sections were then treated sequentially with secondary antibody (ZytoChem Plus HRP One-Step Polymer anti-mouse; Zytomed, Berlin, Germany) and substrate solution (ImmPACT NovaRED Peroxidase Substrate Kit; Vector, Burlingame, CA, USA). Pulmonary edema was assessed by hematoxylin and eosin staining.

Statistical analysis

Continuous variables were compared between the IL-2C and the PBS groups using the Student's t-test. RCC growth over 4 weeks was compared between the two groups with the linear mixed model. A P value < 0.050 was considered statistically significant. Analyses were carried out using SPSS v.22.0 software (SPSS Inc., Chicago, IL, USA).

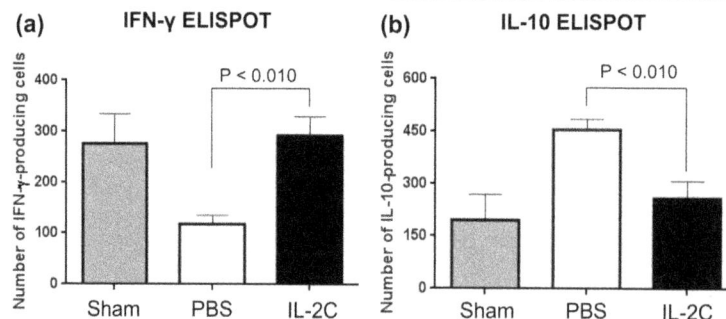

Fig. 3 IL-2C treatment increases the number of IFN-γ⁺ splenocytes, but decreased the number of IL-10⁺ splenocytes. After syngeneic RENCA cells were implanted in mice, splenocytes were harvested on day 28 and analyzed for IFN-γ and IL-10 production by ELISPOT. **a, b** The number of IFN-γ-producing splenocytes was higher (**a**) but the number of IL-10-producing splenocytes were lower (**b**) in IL-2C-treated mice than in PBS-treated mice (P < 0.010 in both cases)

Results

IL-2/anti-IL-2 antibody complex treatment induces the expansion of CD8⁺ memory T and NK cells in the spleen

IL-2C were injected into healthy mice for 5 consecutive days to evaluate its immune-enhancing effects. The total numbers of splenocytes (Fig. 1a; $P < 0.010$) and CD8$^+$ T cells (Fig. 1b; $P < 0.010$) were increased in the IL-2C group as compared to the PBS group. IL-2C treatment also increased the numbers of CD44$^+$CD8$^+$ memory T (Fig. 1c; $P < 0.010$) and CD49b$^+$ NK (Fig. 1d; $P < 0.010$) cells. These results suggest that IL-2C treatment can enhance anti-tumor immunity.

IL-2/anti-IL-2 antibody complex treatment induces the expansion of CD8$^+$ memory T and NK cells in the spleen of RCC mice

Mice were subcutaneously injected with syngeneic RENCA cells, followed by IL-2C or PBS administration every other day for 4 weeks. A sham group received PBS without RENCA cell implantation. Among RCC mice, there was no difference in the number of CD4$^+$ T cells between the IL-2C and PBS groups (Fig. 2a; $P = 0.498$). However, IL-2C treatment induced the expansion of CD8$^+$ T, CD8$^+$ memory T, and NK cells as well as macrophages (Fig. 2b–e; $P < 0.010$), and increased the number of splenic

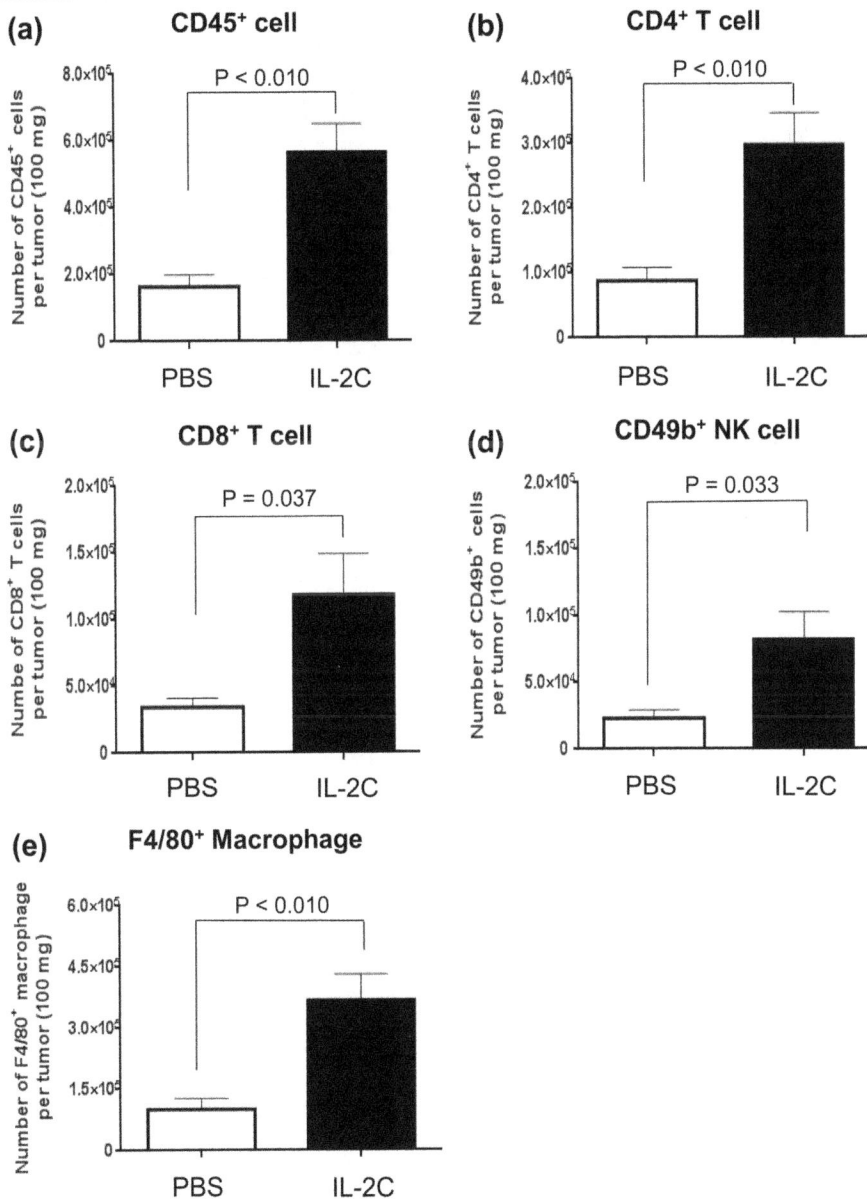

Fig. 4 Flow cytometric analysis of immune cell infiltration into RCC lesions. Tumors were harvested on day 28 after mice were implanted with RENCA cells and immune cells were detected by flow cytometry. IL-2C treatment increased infiltration of (**a**) CD45$^+$ cells ($P < 0.010$), (**b**) CD4$^+$ T cells ($P < 0.010$), (**c**) CD8$^+$ T cells ($P = 0.037$), (**d**) NK cells ($P = 0.033$) (**e**) and macrophages ($P < 0.010$) into tumors

CD4$^+$Foxp3$^+$ regulatory T cells (Fig. 2f; P = 0.040), albeit to a lesser degree than for CD8$^+$ memory T or NK cells. As a result, CD8$^+$ memory T cell/regulatory T cell (Fig. 2g; $P < 0.010$) and NK cell/regulatory T cell (Fig. 2h; $P < 0.010$) ratios were increased in the IL-2C relative to the PBS group. These data indicate that IL-2C treatment enhances anti-tumor immunity against RCC.

IL-2/anti-IL-2 antibody complex treatment increases IFN-γ$^+$ and decreases IL-10$^+$ splenocyte populations

We analyzed Th1 and Th2 cytokine responses in the spleen of RCC mice (Fig. 3). The number of IFN-γ-producing splenocytes was lower in RCC mice treated with PBS than in the sham group. Meanwhile, IL-2C-treated mice had a higher number of IFN-γ$^+$ splenocytes than those in the PBS group (Fig. 3a; $P < 0.010$). The number of IL-10-producing

splenocytes was higher in RCC mice treated with PBS than in the sham group ($P < 0.010$), but this was decreased by IL-2C treatment (Fig. 3b; $P < 0.01$). These results indicate that IL-2C can shift the immune response from Th2 to Th1 in the RCC environment.

IL-2/anti-IL-2 antibody complex treatment increases immune cell infiltration into RCC lesions

Given the immune-stimulating effects of IL-2C on the spleen in RCC, we investigated whether immune cell infiltration of immune cells into RCC lesions was induced by IL-2C treatment. Flow cytometric analysis showed higher numbers of infiltrating CD45$^+$ (Fig. 4a; $P < 0.010$), CD4$^+$ T (Fig. 4b; $P < 0.010$), CD8$^+$ T (Fig. 4c; P = 0.037), and NK (Fig. 4d; P = 0.033) cells as well as macrophages (Fig. 4e; $P < 0.010$) in the IL-2C group than in the PBS

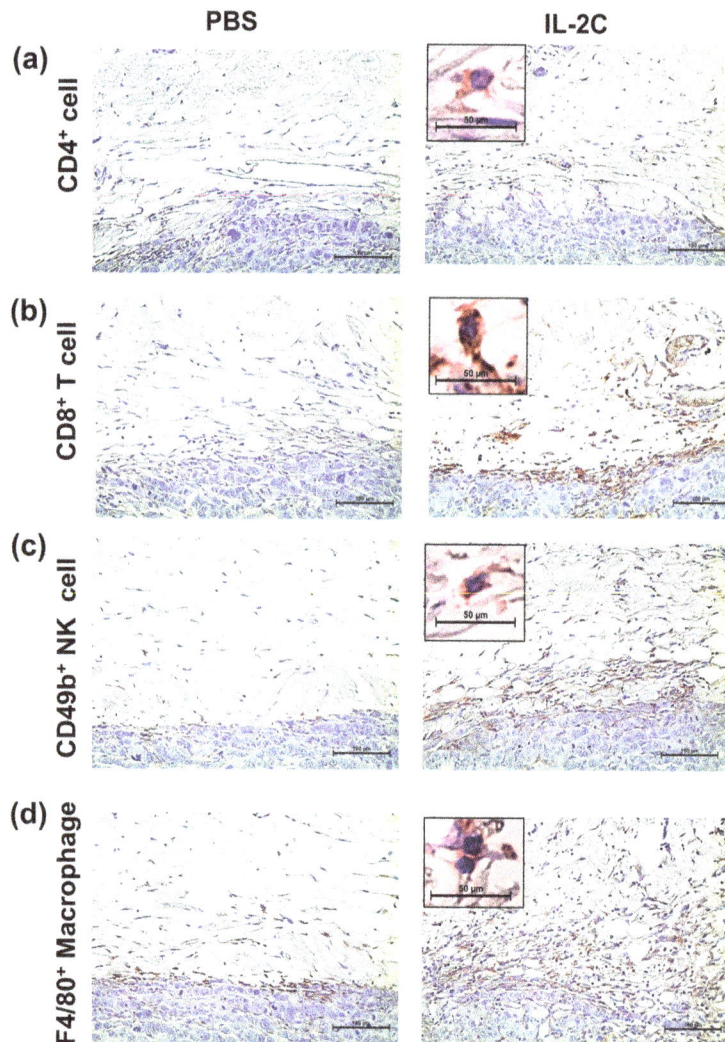

Fig. 5 Immunohistochemical analysis of immune cell infiltration into RCC lesions. Tumors were harvested on day 28 after mice were implanted with RENCA cells and immune cells were detected by immunohistochemistry. The size of immune cell populations, including (**a**) CD4$^+$ T cells, (**b**) CD8$^+$ T cells, (**c**) NK cells and (**d**) macrophages along tumor margins was increased by IL-2C treatment. Images are shown at 200× magnification. Insets show immunoreactive cells at 1000× magnification

group. In addition, an immunohistochemical analysis found that IL-2C treatment increased CD4$^+$ T, CD8$^+$ T, and NK cells as well as macrophages recruitment to RCC lesions (Fig. 5). However, there was no perigraft infiltration of regulatory T cells (data not shown). Taken together, these data demonstrate that IL-2C stimulates the infiltration of immune cells into RCC lesions.

Anti-tumorigenic effects of IL-2/anti-IL-2 antibody complex were not sufficient to suppress RCC growth

The size of RCC lesions increased progressively over time in both PBS-treated and IL-2C-treated mice (Fig. 6a; $P < 0.010$); however, the rate of growth was higher in the former group (Fig. 6a; $P = 0.036$), although the difference was slight. However, tumor weights on day 28 did not differ significantly between the two groups (Fig. 6b; $P = 0.176$). These data suggest that the potentiation of anti-tumor immunity by IL-2C was not sufficient to suppress RCC growth significantly.

IL-2/anti-IL-2 antibody complex treatment does not induce pulmonary edema

Pulmonary edema is a manifestation of capillary leak syndrome and is the most serious side effect of high-dose of IL-2 therapy [23]. On day 28, there was no significant difference in lung weights between IL-2C- and PBS-treated mice (Fig. 7a; $P = 0.184$). A histologic examination revealed no evidence of increased pulmonary edema by IL-2C treatment (Fig. 7b). These results demonstrate that IL-2C is safe for use, as it does not carry a significant risk of pulmonary edema development.

Comparison between IL-2/anti-IL-2 antibody complex treatment and high-dose IL-2 therapy

When immune potentiating effects of IL-2C were compared with those of high-dose IL-2 therapy, the IL-2C therapy increased total leukocytes, CD8$^+$ T cells, NK cells, and macrophages in both spleen (Fig. 8) and peritumor tissues (data not shown) to greater extent than the high-dose IL-2 therapy. The ratio of either splenic CD8$^+$CD44$^+$ T cells/Tregs or CD49b + NK cell/Tregs were not significantly increased in the high-dose IL-2 group (Fig. 8d-e). There was no difference in RCC weight between the IL-2C group and the high-dose IL-2 group (Fig. 8f). Pulmonary edema looked more severe in the high-dose IL-2 group than IL-2 complex group (Fig. 8g); however there was no significant difference in lung weight between the two groups ($P > 0.05$). Taken together, IL-2C induced more immune potentiating effects with lesser dose than high-dose IL-2 therapy; however IL-2C did not show significant benefits in either tumor reduction or pulmonary edema in the present dose.

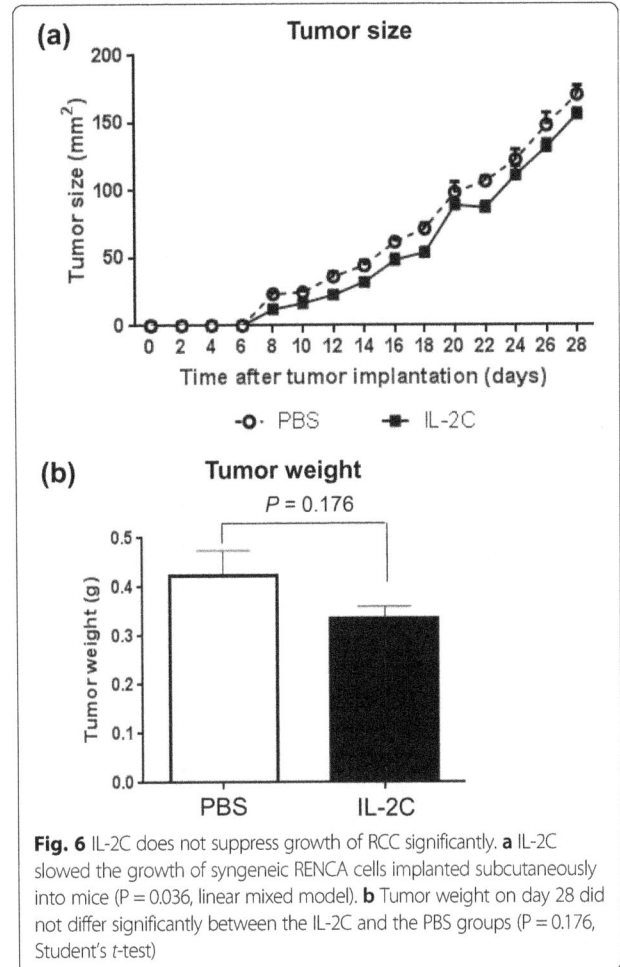

Fig. 6 IL-2C does not suppress growth of RCC significantly. **a** IL-2C slowed the growth of syngeneic RENCA cells implanted subcutaneously into mice (P = 0.036, linear mixed model). **b** Tumor weight on day 28 did not differ significantly between the IL-2C and the PBS groups (P = 0.176, Student's *t*-test)

Discussion

The present study investigated for the first time the anti-tumorigenic effects of IL-2C against RCC in vivo. We found that stimulating IL-2C induced the expansion of CD8$^+$ memory T and NK cell populations, shifted the Th1/Th2 balance in favor of Th1, and increased immune cell infiltration into tumor tissue in mice with RCC, all without inducing serious side effects such as pulmonary edema. However, the enhancement of anti-tumor immunity by IL-2C was not sufficient to inhibit RCC growth significantly.

IL-2C can enhance or suppress immunity depending on the type of anti-IL-2 monoclonal antibody. For example, the monoclonal antibody JES6-1 binds to the IL-2 epitope, and hinders binding to IL-2 receptor (R)-β while enabling binding to IL-2R-α. Since both CD8$^+$ memory T and NK cells constitutively express IL-2R-β, and regulatory T cells constitutively express both IL-2R-β and IL-2R-α, an IL-2C comprising JES6-1 preferentially induced the expansion of regulatory T cells [24]. In contrast, S4B6 binds to an epitope of IL-2 such that binding to IL-2R-α is blocked in favor of IL-2R-β

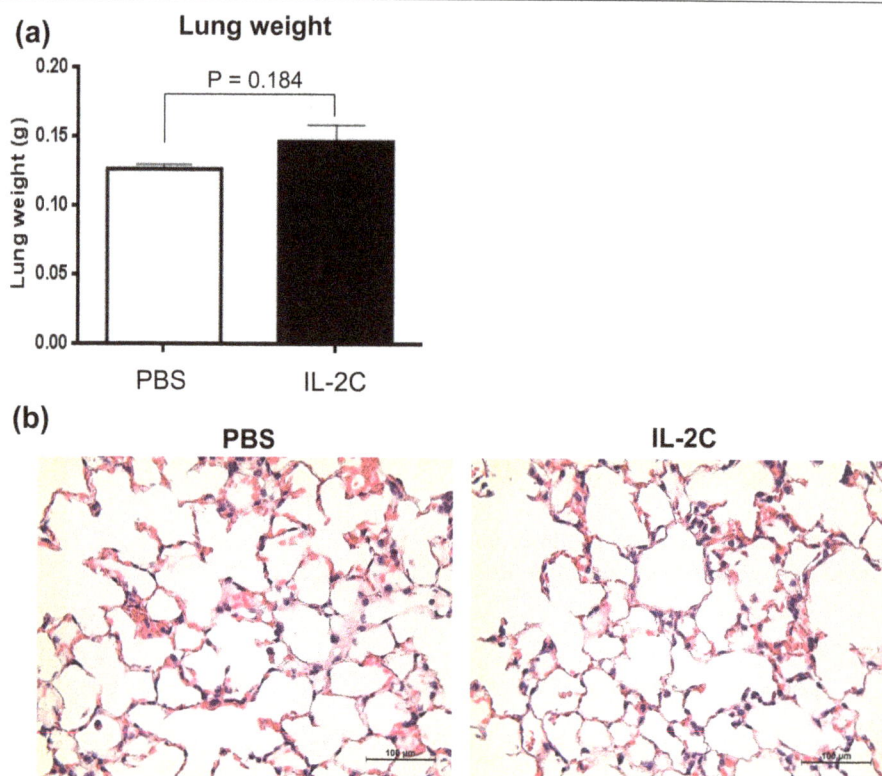

Fig. 7 IL-2C does not exacerbate pulmonary edema in mice with RCC. Lung weight was measured by subtracting dry from wet weight immediately after harvesting on day 28. **a** Lung weight did not differ significantly between IL-2C-treated mice and PBS-treated mice (P = 0.184). **b** IL-2C treatment did not increase pulmonary edema, as visualized by hematoxylin and eosin staining. Images are shown at 400× magnification

binding [23]. Therefore, IL-2C comprising S4B6 induces the expansion of CD8[+] memory T and NK cells over regulatory T cells.

Immune complexes consisting of low-dose IL-2 and the S4B6 clone of the anti-IL-2 antibody was found to inhibit metastasis of melanoma and leukemia in a mouse model by inducing the expansion of CD8[+] T and NK cell populations [19, 23]. In accordance with these findings, we also found that S4B6-containing IL-2C increased CD8[+] T and NK cell number as well as their infiltration into RCC lesion, although the growth of RCC was not significantly affected in a syngeneic RCC mice model.

There are a few possible explanations for the insufficient effects of IL-2C on RCC growth. Firstly, immunosuppression by RCC is strong enough to counter immune-potentiating effects of IL-2C, which promotes RCC proliferation and survival [10–12]. For instance, RCC exhibits resistance to NK cell-mediated lysis, despite IL-2C-induced NK cell expansion and infiltration into RCC lesions [11, 12]. Secondly, the immunogenicity of RCC may be lower than that of malignant melanoma. Tumor-associated antigens are required for immune cell infiltration into tumors [25, 26]; however, there are fewer RCC-associated antigens than tumor-associated antigens

that have been found in melanoma [27]. Therefore, a relative lack of targeting antigens may be a reason why adoptive therapy with CD8[+] tumor-infiltrating lymphocytes has not been clinically effective for RCC treatment [28]. Third, lack of kidney-specific microenvironment might have influenced the results. However, when we injected RENCA cells into the renal subcapsular space, the results were the same as those in the subcutaneous RCC model (data not shown).

The amount of IL-2 that was used in IL-2C therapy was 23 times lower than the amount of IL-2 in high-dose IL-2 therapy [23]. Based on a previous report [23] and our results, low-doses of IL-2C do not cause significant adverse reactions such as pulmonary edema, and is therefore safe for clinical application. However, because even high-dose IL-2 therapy in the present study did not increase lung weight significantly, further studies using higher dose of IL-2C and IL-2 are needed to confirm safety as well as insufficient efficacy of IL-2C in comparison to high-dose IL-2.

Since IL-2C alone cannot suppress RCC growth, additional studies are needed to determine the impacts of other therapies used in combination with IL-2C on RCC. For example, IL-15 can also induce the expansion

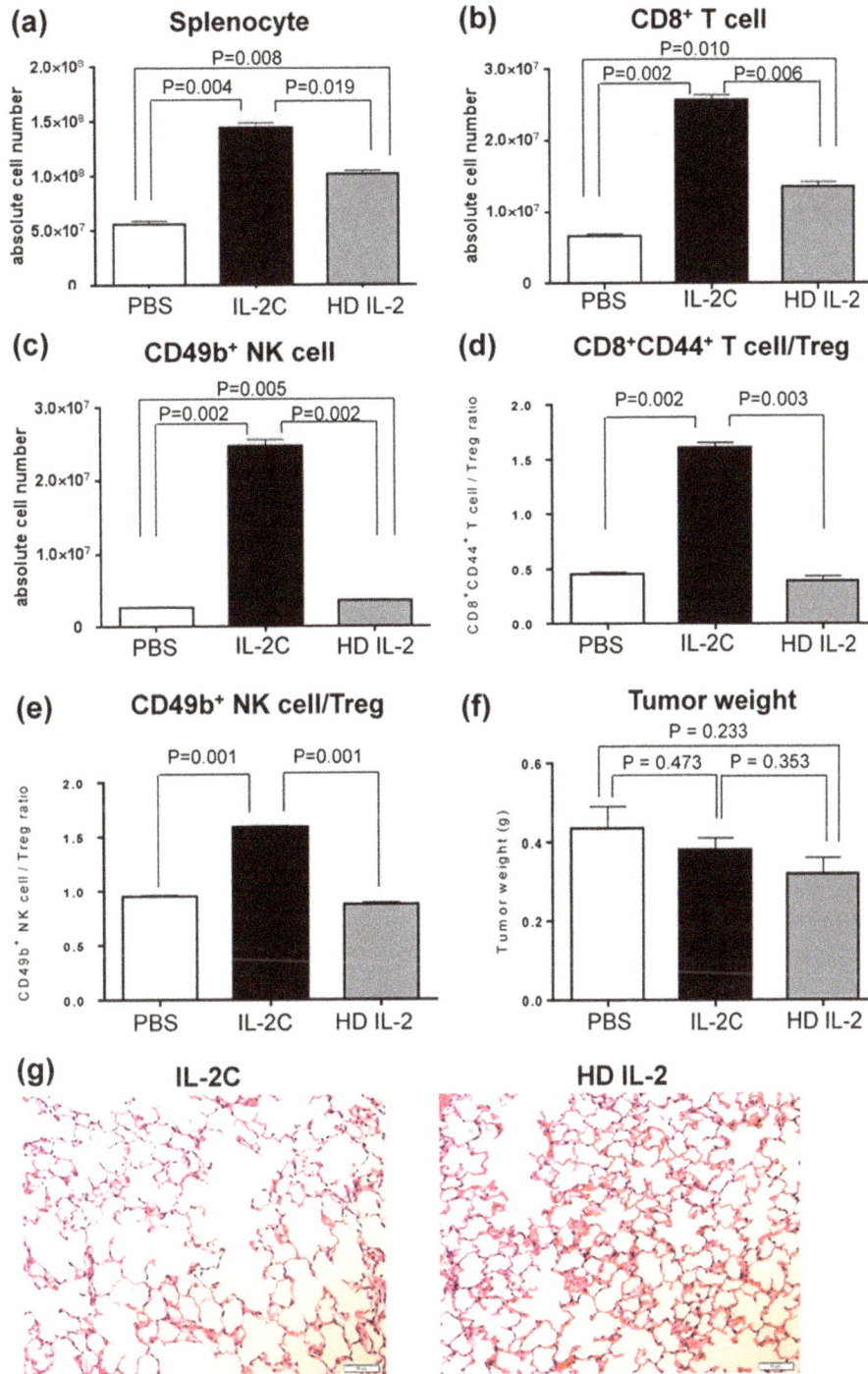

Fig. 8 Comparison between IL-2C therapy and high-dose IL-2 therapy. IL-2C treatment induces more expansion of splenic immune cells than high-dose IL-2 therapy (**a-e**). **a** Both IL-2C (P = 0.004) and high-dose IL-2 (P = 0.008) increased the number of splenocytes; however, the effect of IL-2C was greater than that of high-dose IL-2 (P = 0.019). **b** CD8+ T cells were also increased more by IL-2C than high-dose IL-2 (P = 0.006). **c** Only IL-2C increased the number of NK cells (P = 0.002). **d-e** IL-2C increased both ratio of CD8+CD44+ T cells/Tregs (P = 0.002, **d**), and ratio of CD49b+ NK cells/Tregs (P = 0.001, **e**), whereas high-dose IL-2 did not. **f** Either IL-2C or high-dose IL-2 did not suppress growth of RCC significantly. Tumor weight on day 28 did not differ significantly between the IL-2C and the high-dose IL-2 groups (P = 0.353). **g** Pulmonary edema looked more severe in the high-dose IL-2 group than IL-2 complex group; however difference was not significant. Images are shown at 200× magnification. IL-2C, interleukin-2/anti-interleukin-2 antibody complex; HD, high dose; Treg, regulatory T cell

of NK and CD8$^+$ T cell populations and thereby suppress the growth of malignant melanoma [29], and a complex of IL-15 and soluble IL-15Rα has even more potent effects [30]. Therefore, it is worth investigating whether IL-2C used in conjunction with an IL-15 complex has greater effectiveness in suppressing RCC growth. We may also try to combine IL-2C with the current target agents such as sorafenib to obtain additive effects.

Conclusions

Stimulating IL-2C treatment potentiated anti-tumor immunity without causing significant side effects; however, given that the immune-enhancing effects of IL-2C were not sufficiently strong to suppress RCC growth, its use in combination with other therapy should be considered.

Abbreviations

7-AAD: 7-aminoactinomycin D; APC: Allophycocyanin; FITC: Fluorescein isothiocyanate; Foxp3: Forkhead homeobox protein 3; IFN: Interferon; IL: Interleukin; IL-2C: Complex of interleukin (IL)-2 and stimulating anti-IL-2 antibody; NK cell: Natural killer cell; PBS: Phosphate-buffered saline; PE: Phycoerythrin; RCC: Renal cell carcinoma; RENCA: Murine renal cell carcinoma..

Competing interests

The authors declare that they have no competing interests.

Authors' contributions

KHH and KWK performed the design of the study, experiments, data analysis, and drafted the manuscript. JJY and JGL contributed to the design of study, experiments and data analysis. EML and MH helped the experiments and data analysis. EJC, SSK, HJL and TYK contributed the experiments. CA provided intellectual advice to the study. JY conceived of and designed the study and supervised the work. All authors read and approved the final manuscript.

Acknowledgements

This work was supported by a grant from the Korean Health Technology R&D Project, Ministry of Health & Welfare, Republic of Korea (A111355), and by a grant (0320140430, 2014-1033) from the SNUH Research Fund. We thank Charles D Surh for providing anti-IL-2 antibody.

Author details

[1]Transplantation Research Institute, Seoul National University College of Medicine, Seoul, Republic of Korea. [2]Nephrology clinic, Center for Clinical Specialty, National Cancer Center, Seoul, Republic of Korea. [3]Department of Internal Medicine, Seoul National University College of Medicine, Seoul, Republic of Korea. [4]Transplantation Center, Seoul National University Hospital, 101 Daehak-ro, Jongno-gu, Seoul 110-744, Republic of Korea.

References

1. Symbas NP, Townsend MF, El-Galley R, Keane TE, Graham SD, Petros JA. Poor prognosis associated with thrombocytosis in patients with renal cell carcinoma. BJU Int. 2000;86(3):203–7.
2. Sun M, Thuret R, Abdollah F, Lughezzani G, Schmitges J, Tian Z, et al. Age-adjusted incidence, mortality, and survival rates of stage-specific renal cell carcinoma in North America: a trend analysis. Eur Urol. 2011; 59(1):135–41.
3. Patil S, Manola J, Elson P, Negrier S, Escudier B, Eisen T, et al. Improvement in overall survival of patients with advanced renal cell carcinoma: prognostic factor trend analysis from an international data set of clinical trials. J Urol. 2012;188(6):2095–100.
4. Buti S, Bersanelli M, Sikokis A, Maines F, Facchinetti F, Bria E, et al. Chemotherapy in metastatic renal cell carcinoma today? A systematic review. Anticancer Drugs. 2013;24(6):535–54.
5. Haas N, Manola J, Ky B, Flaherty KT, Uzzo RG, Kane C, et al. Effects of adjuvant sorafenib and sunitinib on cardiac function in renal cell carcinoma patients without overt metastases:results from ASSURE, ECOG2805. Clin Cancer Res. 2015;21(18):4048–54.
6. Fishman MN, Tomshine J, Fulp WJ, Foreman PK. A systematic review of the efficacy and safety experience reported for sorafenib in advanced renal cell carcinoma (RCC) in the post-approval setting. PLoS One. 2015;10(4): e0120877.
7. Eichelberg C, Vervenne WL, De Santis M, Fischer von Weikersthal L, Goebell PJ, Lerchenmuller C, et al. SWITCH: a randomised, sequential, open-label study to evaluate the efficacy and safety of sorafenib-sunitinib versus sunitinib-sorafenib in the treatment of metastatic renal cell cancer. Eur Urol. 2015;68(5):837–47.
8. Pantaleo MA, Mandrioli A, Saponara M, Nannini M, Erente G, Lolli C, et al. Development of coronary artery stenosis in a patient with metastatic renal cell carcinoma treated with sorafenib. BMC Cancer. 2012;12:231.
9. Escudier B, Eisen T, Stadler WM, Szczylik C, Oudard S, Staehler M, et al. Sorafenib for treatment of renal cell carcinoma: Final efficacy and safety results of the phase III treatment approaches in renal cancer global evaluation trial. J Clin Oncol. 2009;27(20):3312–18.
10. Porta C, Bonomi L, Lillaz B, Paglino C, Rovati B, Imarisio I, et al. Renal cell carcinoma-induced immunosuppression: an immunophenotypic study of lymphocyte subpopulations and circulating dendritic cells. Anticancer Res. 2007;27(1A):165–73.
11. Messai Y, Noman MZ, Janji B, Hasmim M, Escudier B, Chouaib S. The autophagy sensor ITPR1 protects renal carcinoma cells from NK-mediated killing. Autophagy. 2015;0. doi:10.1080/15548627.2015.1017194.
12. Messai Y, Noman MZ, Hasmim M, Janji B, Tittarelli A, Boutet M, et al. ITPR1 protects renal cancer cells against natural killer cells by inducing autophagy. Cancer Res. 2014;74(23):6820–32.
13. Atkins MB. Cytokine-based therapy and biochemotherapy for advanced melanoma. Clin Cancer Res. 2006;12(7 Pt 2):2353s–8s.
14. Leibovich BC, Han KR, Bui MH, Pantuck AJ, Dorey FJ, Figlin RA, et al. Scoring algorithm to predict survival after nephrectomy and immunotherapy in patients with metastatic renal cell carcinoma: a stratification tool for prospective clinical trials. Cancer. 2003;98(12):2566–75.
15. Yang JC, Hughes M, Kammula U, Royal R, Sherry RM, Topalian SL, et al. Ipilimumab (anti-CTLA4 antibody) causes regression of metastatic renal cell cancer associated with enteritis and hypophysitis. J Immunother. 2007;30(8):825–30.
16. Topalian SL, Hodi FS, Brahmer JR, Gettinger SN, Smith DC, McDermott DF, et al. Safety, activity, and immune correlates of anti-PD-1 antibody in cancer. N Engl J Med. 2012;366(26):2443–54.
17. Pautier P, Locher C, Robert C, Deroussent A, Flament C, Le Cesne A, et al. Phase I clinical trial combining imatinib mesylate and IL-2 in refractory cancer patients: IL-2 interferes with the pharmacokinetics of imatinib mesylate. Oncoimmunology. 2013;2(2):e23079.
18. Lam ET, Wong MK, Agarwal N, Redman BG, Logan T, Gao D, et al. Retrospective analysis of the safety and efficacy of high-dose interleukin-2 after prior tyrosine kinase inhibitor therapy in patients with advanced renal cell carcinoma. J Immunother. 2014;37(7):360–5.
19. Tomala J, Chmelova H, Mrkvan T, Rihova B, Kovar M. In vivo expansion of activated naive CD8+ T cells and NK cells driven by complexes of IL-2 and anti-IL-2 monoclonal antibody as novel approach of cancer immunotherapy. J Immunol. 2009;183(8):4904–12.
20. Smith C, Martinez M, Peet J, Khanna R. Differential outcome of IL-2/anti-IL-2 complex therapy on effector and memory CD8+ T cells following vaccination with an adenoviral vector encoding EBV epitopes. J Immunol. 2011;186(10):5784–90.
21. Mostbock S, Lutsiak ME, Milenic DE, Baidoo K, Schlom J, Sabzevari H. IL-2/ anti-IL-2 antibody complex enhances vaccine-mediated antigen-specific CD8+ T cell responses and increases the ratio of effector/memory CD8+ T cells to regulatory T cells. J Immunol. 2008;180(7):5118–29.
22. Lin GH, Stone JC, Surh CD, Watts TH. In vivo accumulation of T cells in response to IL-2/anti-IL-2 mAb complexes is dependent in part on the TNF family ligand 4-1BBL. Immunol Cell Biol. 2012;90(7):743–7.
23. Krieg C, Letourneau S, Pantaleo G, Boyman O. Improved IL-2 immunotherapy by selective stimulation of IL-2 receptors on

lymphocytes and endothelial cells. Proc Natl Acad Sci U S A. 2010; 107(26):11906–11.

24. Boyman O, Kovar M, Rubinstein MP, Surh CD, Sprent J. Selective stimulation of T cell subsets with antibody-cytokine immune complexes. Science. 2006; 311(5769):1924–7.

25. Reinherz EL. Alphabeta TCR-mediated recognition: relevance to tumor-antigen discovery and cancer immunotherapy. Cancer Immunol Res. 2015; 3(4):305–12.

26. Osada T, Nagaoka K, Takahara M, Yang XY, Liu CX, Guo H, et al. Precision cancer immunotherapy: optimizing dendritic cell-based strategies to induce tumor antigen-specific T-cell responses against individual patient tumors. J Immunother. 2015;38(4):155–64.

27. Vissers JL, De Vries IJ, Schreurs MW, Engelen LP, Oosterwijk E, Figdor CG. The renal cell carcinoma-associated antigen G250 encodes a human leukocyte antigen (HLA)-A2.1-restricted epitope recognized by cytotoxic T lymphocytes. Cancer Res. 1999;59(21):5554–9.

28. Figlin RA, Thompson JA, Bukowski RM, Vogelzang NJ, Novick AC, Lange P, et al. Multicenter, randomized, phase III trial of CD8(+) tumor-infiltrating lymphocytes in combination with recombinant interleukin-2 in metastatic renal cell carcinoma. J Clin Oncol. 1999;17(8):2521–9.

29. Klebanoff CA, Finkelstein SE, Surman DR, Lichtman MK, Gattinoni L, Theoret MR, et al. IL-15 enhances the in vivo antitumor activity of tumor-reactive CD8+ T cells. Proc Natl Acad Sci U S A. 2004;101(7):1969–74.

30. Rubinstein MP, Kovar M, Purton JF, Cho JH, Boyman O, Surh CD, et al. Converting IL-15 to a superagonist by binding to soluble IL-15R{alpha}. Proc Natl Acad Sci U S A. 2006;103(24):9166–71.

12

IgG4-related kidney disease from the renal pelvis that mimicked urothelial carcinoma

Hui Zhang[1†], Xinyu Ren[1†], Wen Zhang[2], Di Yang[1] and Ruie Feng[1*]

Abstract

Background: IgG4-related kidney disease is a comprehensive term for renal lesions associated with IgG4-related disease, which mainly manifests as plasma cell-rich tubulointerstitial nephritis with increased IgG4+ plasma cells and fibrosis. IgG4-related kidney disease in the renal pelvis is rare.

Case presentation: We describe a 53-year-old Asian woman who was referred to our hospital with a space-occupying renal lesion discovered by medical examination. A physical examination and laboratory evaluation revealed no significant abnormalities. Computed tomography scans showed a soft-tissue mass with an irregular border and mild homogeneous enhancement in the right renal pelvis and calyces. A positron emission tomography/computed tomography scan revealed soft-tissue density shadows with increased radionuclide uptake. To investigate a suspected pelvic carcinoma, a right ureteronephrectomy was performed. A pathologic examination of the renal sections showed a dense lymphoplasmacytic infiltrate rich in IgG4+ plasma cells, with fibrosis beneath the urothelial epithelium of the renal pelvis. Postoperatively, the serum IgG4 level was significantly elevated. The patient was diagnosed with IgG4-related kidney disease.

Conclusion: We present a case of IgG4-related kidney disease mimicking urothelial carcinoma in the renal pelvis. When a buried and solitary hypovascular tumor is detected in the kidney, we must consider IgG4-related kidney disease as a differential diagnosis. Accordingly, elevated serum IgG4, radiologic findings, and pathologic examination may improve the diagnosis.

Keywords: IgG4-related disease, IgG4-related kidney disease, Renal pelvis, Urothelial carcinoma

Background

IgG4-related disease (IgG4-RD) has recently been proposed and is considered to involve conditions of systemic inflammatory fibrosis, including autoimmune pancreatitis, retroperitoneal fibrosis, chronic sclerosing cholangitis, and inflammatory pseudotumor. IgG4-RD has now been reported in nearly every organ, though it was first identified in the pancreas and salivary glands [1–6]. This disease manifests as organ enlargement or nodular/hyperplastic lesions in various organs concurrently or metachronously as a result of marked infiltration of lymphocytes and IgG4-positive plasma cells as well as fibrosis.

IgG4-related kidney disease (IgG4-RKD) is a comprehensive term for renal lesions associated with IgG4-RD, which mainly manifests as plasma cell-rich tubulointerstitial nephritis (TIN) with increased IgG4+ plasma cells and fibrosis (IgG4-related TIN, IgG4-TIN) [6, 7]. Few data exist on the epidemiological and clinical features of large series of patients. The mean age at diagnosis of the reviewed cases is 65 years, and 73–87 % are men [8]. IgG4-RKD is common and predominantly involves the cortex of the kidney; however, we report a rare case of IgG4-RKD involving a renal pelvic lesion that mimicked urothelial carcinoma.

Case presentation

A 53-year-old woman was referred to our hospital with a space-occupying renal lesion that was discovered incidentally by an ultrasound scan. The patient's past medical history was positive for a gastric ulcer.

* Correspondence: fengruie1@163.com
†Equal contributors
[1]Department of Pathology, Peking Union Medical College Hospital, Chinese Academy of Medical Sciences and Peking Union Medical College, 1 Shuaifu Yuan, Beijing 100730, PR China
Full list of author information is available at the end of the article

A physical examination revealed no significant abnormalities. Laboratory evaluations, including urinalysis, were within normal limits, and urinary cytology was negative. Computed tomography (CT) scans showed a soft-tissue density mass with an irregular border and mild homogeneous enhancement in the right renal pelvis and calyces (Fig. 1). A positron emission tomography/CT scan revealed soft-tissue density shadows with increased radionuclide uptake, which suggested a malignant lesion.

Because pelvic carcinoma was suspected, a right ureteronephrectomy was performed. Gross examination revealed only thickened mucosa of the renal pelvis but no obvious abnormalities in the renal cortex or medulla (Fig. 2). A pathologic examination of the renal sections showed numerous lymphoid follicles and prominent fibrosis beneath the urothelial epithelium of the thickened mucosa (Fig. 3a). Additionally, numerous plasma cells and scattered eosinophils were identified in the interfollicular area (Fig. 3b). The infiltrating lymphocytes and plasma cells did not show significant cytological atypia. Immunohistochemistry demonstrated that more than 40 % of the plasma cells were IgG4+ (Fig. 3c, 3d). All of these histologic changes were confined to the renal pelvis and did not involve the renal parenchyma. The postoperative serum IgG4 level was 3250 mg/L (80–1400 mg/L). The patient was diagnosed with IgG4-RKD and no specific therapy was administered. The postoperative serum IgG4 level decreased from 3250 mg/L to 2450 mg/L at 2 months.

Discussion

IgG4-RKD is a comprehensive term for renal lesions, including renal parenchymal lesions and renal pelvic lesions, related to IgG4-RD, which is a recently recognized and proposed clinical entity characterized by a dense lymphoplasmacytic infiltrate rich in IgG4+ plasma cells with fibrosis that affects several organs [6, 9]. TIN involving tubules and/or the interstitium of the kidney is the most dominant feature of IgG4-RKD [9]; however, IgG4-RKD in the renal pelvis is rare [7–10]. Here, we report a rare case of IgG4-RKD that mimicked renal pelvic carcinoma.

A comprehensive English and non-English search for all articles pertinent to IgG4-RD of the renal pelvis was conducted using PubMed. Since Naoto Kuroda [11] first reported a case of IgG4-RD arising in the renal pelvis in 2009, six cases of IgG4-RD of the renal pelvis have been reported previously in the world literature (Table 1) [12–16]. The mean age at diagnosis was 59.8 years (range: 49 to 80 years), with a male: female ratio of 1:1. Most patients presented with renal lesions in the left kidney, with a left-to-right presentation ratio of 2:1. Patients visited the hospital with or without complaints of non-characteristic presentations (i.e., flank pain), and none of the patients had hematuria. Hypocomplementemia and elevated serum IgG are characteristic features of IgG4-RD. Elevated serum IgG and IgG4 were found in all patients, but no hypocomplementemia was found in these seven cases, including our case (Table 1). Although hypocomplementemia is a distinct feature of IgG4-RD, a relatively low proportion of patients actually have it.

Patients with IgG4-RD often have lesions in several organs, either synchronously or metachronously, although others may show the involvement of only a single organ. Renal lesions are recognized as extra-pancreatic manifestations of IgG4-RD; the condition can develop as IgG4-RKD singly or associated with the lesions of other organs.

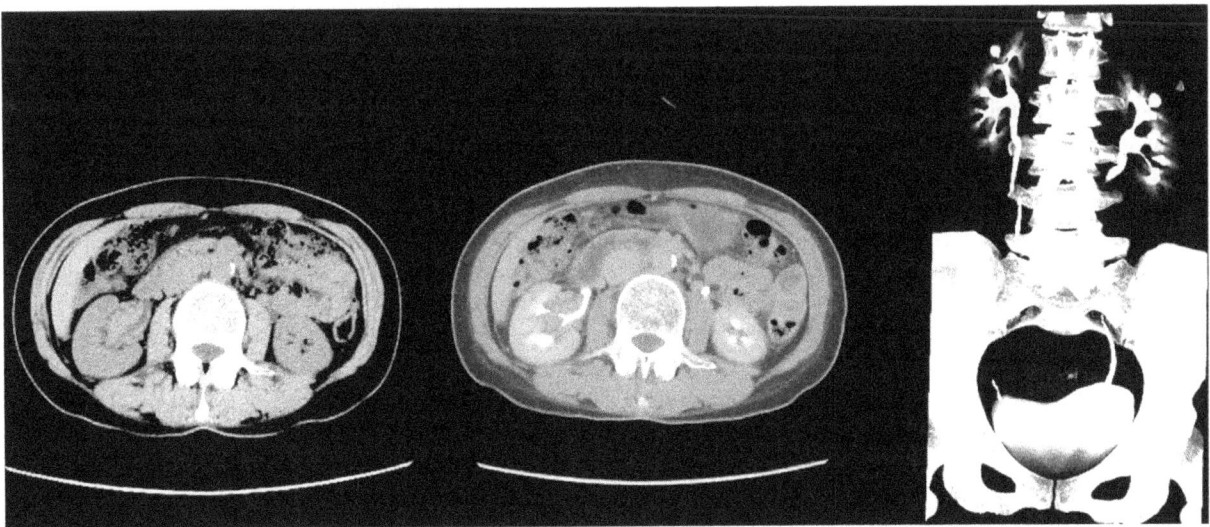

Fig. 1 Abdominal computed tomography scans. These scans showed a soft-tissue density mass with an irregular border and mild homogeneous enhancement in the right renal pelvis and calyces

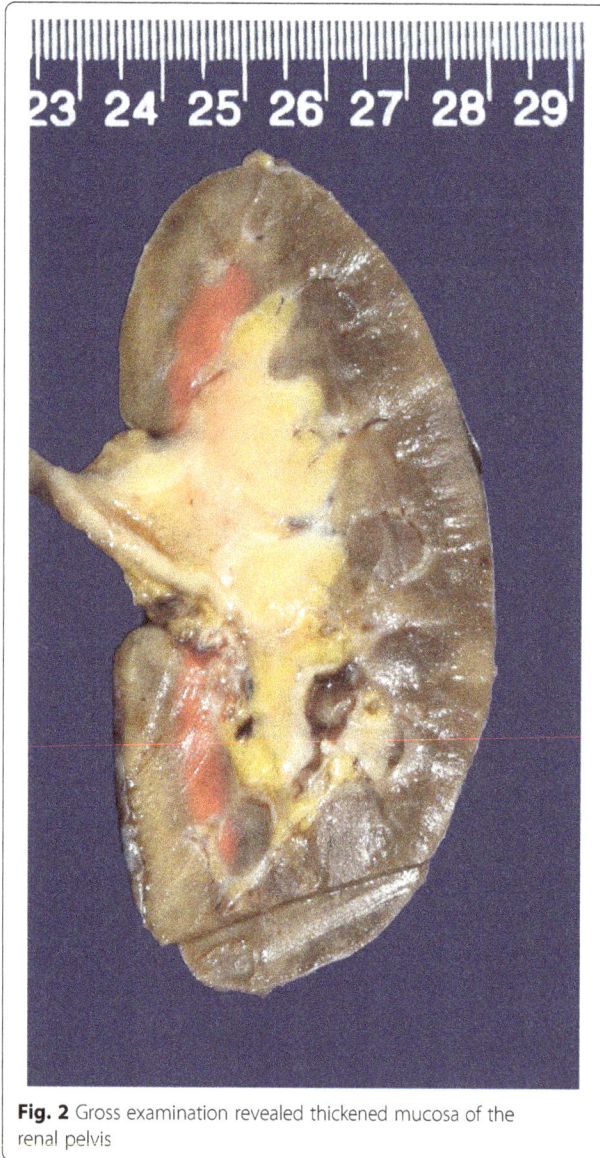

Fig. 2 Gross examination revealed thickened mucosa of the renal pelvis

infiltrating IgG4+ plasma cells and fibrosis; and (5) extra-renal histology showing prominent lymphoplasmacytic infiltration with infiltrating IgG4+ plasma cells. The diagnosis is classified into three stages—definite, probable, and possible—according to the combinations of the above conditions. In their diagnostic criteria, abnormal renal imaging findings were essential for making a definitive diagnosis. In the present case, all of these conditions, including imaging studies that identified low-density lesions, pathologic examinations that revealed characteristic changes, and elevated serum IgG4, prompted the definitive diagnosis of IgG4-RKD.

A rapid response to corticosteroid therapy is a characteristic feature of IgG4-RD, and corticosteroids are typically the first line of therapy, although no controlled trial has been performed. Moreover, the protocol used for corticosteroid therapy varies among countries and institutions [1]. Because of the decreased level of serum IgG4 after ureteronephrectomy, our patient received a close follow-up without corticosteroid therapy. In the reported cases, patients with IgG4-RKD arising from the renal pelvis were treated according to different strategies, including surgical treatment alone for two patients, corticosteroid therapy alone for two patients, and surgical and corticosteroid treatment for the remaining two patients. The renal lesions improved or resolved after the corticosteroid treatment in three patients who received corticosteroid treatment (Table 1). Takahashi and colleagues [17] also found that lesions progressed in three IgG4-TIN patients receiving no corticosteroid treatment or surgical resection and that lesions regressed in all IgG4-TIN patients who underwent corticosteroid treatment. These observations indicate that effective interventions should begin as soon as possible for irreversible fibrosis in IgG4-RKD. Because corticosteroid treatment has a remarkable effect in this type of disease, at least in the short term, this treatment is vital to avoid unnecessary surgery. CT-guided biopsy or laparoscopic biopsy of the original tumor might help to rule out malignancy.

Recent studies have revealed several characteristic clinical features of IgG4-RKD, including predominance in middle-aged to older men, frequent association with IgG4-RD in other organs, high levels of serum IgG and IgG4, and a good initial response to corticosteroids. However, longer follow-up data for IgG4-RKD, including relapse information, are still sparse. Takako Saeki and his colleagues [18] retrospectively analyzed the longer-term clinical course of 43 patients with IgG4-TIN in detail in a larger cohort. This analysis included the largest series on the long-term outcomes of corticosteroid treatment of IgG4-RKD. Saeki et al. showed that 1 month after the start of treatment, most of the abnormal serology and radiology parameters had improved, and relapse of IgG4-related lesions occurred in 8 of 40 treated patients. These studies

In previous cases, renal and extra-renal (salivary gland) involvements in IgG4-RD have presented simultaneously in two patients [11, 12]. In the current case, a systemic examination showed no other abnormal findings, inclusive of the salivary glands, lacrimal glands, and pancreas. Thus, the condition was diagnosed as IgG4-RD isolated in the renal pelvis without the involvement of other organs.

On the basis of the results of a diagnostic algorithm procedure and with references to several diagnostic criteria for AIP, Mitsuhiro Kawano [6] proposed diagnostic criteria for IgG4-RKD: (1) presence of some kidney damage, as manifested by laboratory examination; (2) kidney imaging studies showing abnormal renal findings, i.e., multiple low-density lesions on enhanced CT; (3) elevated serum IgG4 levels exceeding 135 mg/dL; (4) renal histology showing dense lymphoplasmacytic infiltration with

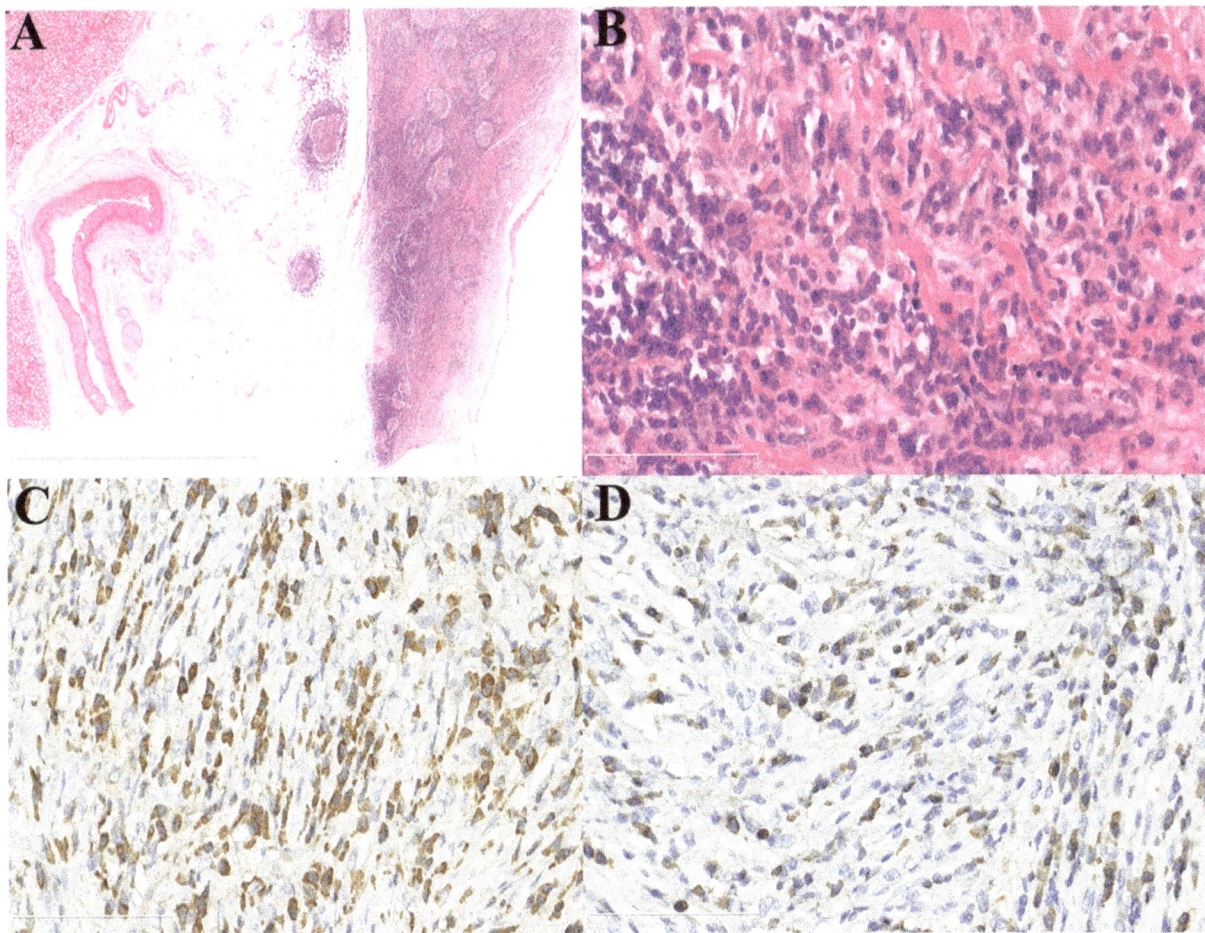

Fig. 3 Pathologic examination of the renal sections. (**a**). Numerous lymphoid follicles and prominent fibrosis beneath the urothelial epithelium of the renal pelvis; (**b**). Numerous plasma cells and scattered eosinophils were identified in the interfollicular area. Immunohistochemistry showed numerous IgG+ (**c**) and IgG4+ (**d**) plasma cells

indicate that the response of IgG4-RKD to corticosteroids is rapid and partial, and that irreversible lesions may remain, especially in patients with advanced renal damage. Patients with renal dysfunction should receive corticosteroid therapy, although spontaneous improvement of lesions can also occur in IgG4-TIN and the indications for corticosteroid therapy in IgG4-RKD have not been established. Careful attention should be paid to renal function during follow-up without therapy [18, 19]. A large-scale prospective

Table 1 Previous reports of IgG4-related kidney disease arising in the renal pelvis

Ref.	Age (years)	Sex	Manifestations	Hypocomplementemia	Extra-renal lesions	Location	Serum IgG4	Therapy	Findings at follow-up
12	58	M	None	NA	IgG4-related MD	Left	Elevated	Surgery + corticosteroid	Dead
13	80	M	NA	NA	None	Right	NA	Surgery	NA
14	69	M	NA	NA	None	Right	Elevated	Surgery + corticosteroid	Regression of the manifestations
11	49	F	None	None	IgG4-related MD	Left	Elevated	Surgery	NA
15	49	F	Bilateral lumbago	NA	None	Left	Elevated	Corticosteroid	Regression of the manifestations
16	54	F	Left flank discomfort and palpebral edema	None	None	Left	Elevated	Corticosteroid	Regression of the manifestations

F, female; M, male; MD, mikulicz's disease; NA, unavailable

study is necessary to determine a more useful treatment strategy for IgG4-RKD.

Conclusions

We present a case of IgG4-RKD that mimicked urothelial carcinoma in the renal pelvis. When a deep and solitary hypovascular tumor is detected in the kidney, we must consider IgG4-RKD as a differential diagnosis. Accordingly, elevated serum IgG4, radiologic findings, and pathologic examination may be helpful for the diagnosis.

Consent

Written informed consent was obtained from the patient for publication of this case report and any accompanying images.

Abbreviations

IgG-RD: IgG-related disease; IgG-RKD: IgG-related kidney disease; TIN: Tubulointerstitial nephritis; CT: Computed tomography.

Competing interests

The authors declare that they have no competing interests.

Authors' contributions

HZ and XYR drafted the manuscript and participated in the final diagnosis. WZ, DY, and REF critically revised the manuscript for important intellectual content and gave final approval of the version to be published. The final manuscript was read and approved by all authors.

Acknowledgments

The authors thank Yufeng Luo, Department of Pathology, for her technical assistance with immunohistochemistry staining. We also thank Shuo Li, Department of Radiology, for help with the preparation of the radiological materials.

Author details

[1]Department of Pathology, Peking Union Medical College Hospital, Chinese Academy of Medical Sciences and Peking Union Medical College, 1 Shuaifu Yuan, Beijing 100730, PR China. [2]Department of Rheumatology, Peking Union Medical College Hospital, Chinese Academy of Medical Sciences and Peking Union Medical College, Beijing 100730, PR China.

References

1. Hamano H, Kawa S, Horiuchi A, Unno H, Furuya N, Akamatsu T, et al. High serum IgG4 concentrations in patients with sclerosing pancreatitis. N Engl J Med. 2001;344:732–8.
2. Brito-Zerón P, Ramos-Casals M, Bosch X, Stone JH. The clinical spectrum of IgG4-related disease. Autoimmun Rev. 2014;13(12):1203–10.
3. Abraham SC, Cruz-Correa M, Argani P, Furth EE, Hruban RH, Boitnott JK. Lymphoplasmacytic chronic cholecystitis and biliary tract disease in patients with lymphoplasmacytic sclerosing pancreatitis. Am J Surg Pathol. 2003;27:441–51.
4. Zen Y, Harada K, Sasaki M, Sato Y, Tsuneyama K, Haratake J, et al. IgG4-related sclerosing cholangitis with and without hepatic inflammatory pseudotumor, and sclerosing pancreatitis-associated sclerosing cholangitis: do they belong to a spectrum of sclerosing pancreatitis? Am J Surg Pathol. 2004;28:1193–203.
5. Zen Y, Fujii T, Sato Y, Masuda S, Nakanuma Y. Pathological classification of hepatic inflammatory pseudotumor with respect to IgG4-related disease. Mod Pathol. 2007;20:884–94.
6. Kawano M, Saeki T, Nakashima H, Nishi S, Yamaguchi Y, Hisano S, et al. Proposal for diagnostic criteria for IgG4-related kidney disease. Clin Exp Nephrol. 2011;15:615–26.
7. Yamaguchi Y, Kanetsuna Y, Honda K, Yamanaka N, Kawano M, Nagata M. Japanese study group on IgG4-related nephropathy. Characteristic tubulointerstitial nephritis in IgG4-related disease. Hum Pathol. 2012;43:536–49.
8. Kawano M, Saeki T. IgG4-related kidney disease - an update. Curr Opin Nephrol Hypertens. 2015;24(2):193–201.
9. Saeki T, Kawano M. IgG4-related kidney disease. Kidney Int. 2014;85:251–7.
10. Lee LY, Yap H, Sampson S, Ford B, Hayman G, Marsh J, et al. IgG4- related disease as a rare cause of tubulointerstitial nephritis. J Clin Immunol. 2014;34:548–50.
11. Kuroda N, Nakamura S, Miyazaki K, Inoue K, Ohara M, Mizuno K, et al. Chronic sclerosing pyelitis with an increased number of IgG4-positive plasma cells. Med Mol Morphol. 2009;42:236–8.
12. Uehara T, Ikeda S, Hamano H, Kawa S, Moteki H, Matsuda K, et al. A case of Mikulicz's disease complicated by malignant lymphoma: a postmortem histopathological finding. Intern Med. 2012;51:419–23.
13. Takata M, Miyoshi M, Kohno M, Ito M, Komatsu K, Tsukahara K. Two cases of IgG4-related systemic disease arising from urinary tract. Hinyokika Kiyo. 2012;58:613–6.
14. Tsuzaka Y, Ookubo K, Sugiyama K, Morimoto H, Amano H, Oota N, et al. IgG4-related kidney disease: a long-term follow up case of pseudotumor of the renal pelvis. Nihon Hinyokika Gakkai Zasshi. 2014;105:51–5.
15. Inoue S, Takahashi C, Hikita K. A case of IgG4-related retroperitoneal fibrosis from the renal pelvis mimicking bilateral hydronephrosis. Urol Int. 2014 Apr;8.
16. Yiwei W, Xing C, Rongkui L, Hang W, Guomin W, Yingyong H, et al. IgG4-related systemic disease mimicking renal pelvic cancer: a rare case. World J Surg Oncol. 2014;12:395.
17. Takahashi N, Kawashima A, Fletcher JG, Chari ST. Renal involvement in patients with autoimmune pancreatitis: CT and MR imaging findings. Radiology. 2007;242(3):791–801.
18. Saeki T, Kawano M, Mizushima I, Yamamoto M, Wada Y, Nakashima H, et al. The clinical course of patients with IgG4-related kidney disease. Kidney Int. 2013;84(4):826–33.
19. Kawano M, Yamada K. Treatment of IgG4-related disease. Curr Immunol Rev. 2011;7:246–51.

13

Renal cell carcinoma with intramyocardial metastases

Anna M Czarnecka[1,4*], Pawel Sobczuk[1,2], Fei Lian[3] and Cezary Szczylik[1]

Abstract

Background: Cardiac metastases from renal cell carcinoma without vena caval involvement are extremely rare with a limited number of cases reported in the worldwide literature until now. Nevertheless, this rare location of metastasis may significantly influence patient treatment and prognosis. Cooperation between oncology, cardiology, and urology teams are indispensable in cases of patients suffering from intramyocardial tumors. For these individuals, treatment guidelines based on large-scale studies are unavailable and only case/case series analysis may provide clinicians with decision assistance.

Case presentation: In this paper, we report a case of a 50-year-old Caucasian male diagnosed with a 10.2 × 10.3 × 10.0 cm lower pole left renal mass in January 2002. He was subsequently treated with immunochemotherapy, tyrosine kinase inhibitors (TKIs), and mTOR inhibitors (mTORIs) - that is sunitinib, everolimus, and sorafenib. In March 2012, contrast-enhancing tumors in the left myocardium (⌀22 mm) and in the interventricular septum (⌀26 mm) were seen on CT. Cardiology testing was conducted and the patient was treated with pazopanib with a profound response. Overall survival since the clear cell renal cell carcinoma (ccRCC) diagnosis was 11 years 2 months and since diagnosis of multiple heart metastases was 1 year.

Conclusions: Cardiac metastases present a unique disease course in renal cell carcinoma. Cardiac metastases may remain asymptomatic, as in the case of this patient at the time of diagnosis. The most common cardiac presentation of renal cell carcinoma is hypertension, but other cardiac presentations include shortness of breath, cough, and arrhythmias. Targeted systemic therapy with tyrosine kinase inhibitors may be useful for this group of patients, but necrosis in the myocardium can result in tamponade and death. Regular cardiac magnetic resonance imaging scans are required for treatment monitoring.

Keywords: Renal cell carcinoma, Myocardium, Metastasis, Pazopanib, Axitinib

Background

Rare locations of metastasis may significantly influence patient treatment and prognosis. For these individuals, treatment guidelines based on large-scale studies are unavailable, and only case/case series analysis may provide clinicians with decision assistance. The incidence of primary and secondary heart tumors in unselected pathology necropsy reports is about 0.17% with secondary tumors more common. Secondary cardiac tumors are often found incidentally in even up to 20% of patients with metastatic cancer, sarcoma, or lymphoma [1]. Metastases spread to the pericardium, myocardium, and endocardium in descending order of frequency [2].

In general, cardiac metastases are 20 to 40 times more common than primary cardiac malignancies, and have been reported in different studies in approximately 2% to 18% of cases at autopsies. Intramyocardial metastases arise most often in the course of malignant melanoma, leukemia, lymphoma, and lung, esophageal and breast cancers [3,4]. At the same time, heart involvement *via* the inferior vena cava (IVC) is a well-known phenomenon in clear cell renal cell carcinoma (ccRCC) cases. Renal cell carcinoma (RCC) is known for invading the renal vein and further promoting tumor thrombosis of the vena cava and even the right atrium [1]. For these patients, long-term outcome after radical surgical treatment with RCC and tumor thrombus extension reaching

* Correspondence: anna.czarnecka@gmail.com
[1]Department of Oncology, Military Institute of Medicine, Warsaw, Poland
[4]Department of Oncology, Military Institute of Medicine, Laboratory of Molecular Oncology, Szaserow 128, 04-141 Warsaw, Poland
Full list of author information is available at the end of the article

up to the right atrium justifies an extensive procedure with median survival (including in-hospital mortality) of 25 months. Cardiopulmonary bypass with deep hypothermic circulatory arrest allows safe and precise extirpation of all intracaval and intracardiac tumor mass [5]. Manual repositioning of the tumor thrombus out of the right atrium into the inferior vena cava on the beating heart is also a safe and feasible approach with low risk of tumor thrombembolization [6].

In the absence of IVC involvement, cardiac metastases are exceptional in ccRCC with a limited number of cases reported in the worldwide literature (Table 1) [3]. No cases of well-documented cardiology diagnostics or oncological follow-ups with noted progression-free survival (PFS) and overall survival (OS) have been described in the literature before (Tables 1 and 2). No such cases have been reported in clinical trial of recently widely used sunitinib, sorafenib, pazopanib or axitinib [7-10]. In this report, we present the first case of a patient with intramyocardial metastases treated with tyrosine kinase inhibitors (TKI), who was carefully monitored.

Case presentation

We report a case of a 50-year-old Caucasian male who was diagnosed with a 10.2 × 10.3 × 10.0 cm lower pole left renal mass in January 2002. Subsequently, he underwent radical left nephrectomy in that same month. Pathology of the resected tumor was ccRCC, Fuhrman Grade 2. In the following year, metastasis in the right adrenal gland was diagnosed and the patient was referred for a metastasectomy, which was performed in September 2003, when a 6.1 × 5.5 × 4.9 cm metastatic tumor was removed. Subsequently, he was enrolled in immunochemotherapy treatment.

Between September 2003 and January 2004, the patient received two courses of immunochemotherapy with

a regimen of vinblastine, interleukin-2, and interferon alpha-2a (IFN-α-2a) in a single dosage of 4 mg intravenous vinblastine per m^2 of body surface, 4.5 MU/m^2 subcutaneous interleukin-2 q12h, qw1,3,5 and 3 MU/m^2 subcutaneous interferon alpha-2a qd, qw 2,4,6 [27]. The immunochemotherapy was terminated due to stenocardial chest pain without myocardial ischemia signs. After metastasectomy and immunochemotherapy, the patient remained disease free until 2006 when multiple right lung and right femoral bone metastases were diagnosed at a routine check-up. In September 2006, bi-lobectomy of the right lung was performed, and in November 2006, the patient underwent a total right hip replacement. Total rib replacement with subsequent rehabilitation enabled the patient to walk without walking aid (cane, crutches or walker) until final deterioration (see below). All surgical specimens were confirmed as ccRCC.

In March 2007, new lung lesions were detected, and in April 2007 the patient was started on immunotherapy of 9 MU subcutaneous interferon alpha-2a qd, qw 1,3,5 with moderate tolerance of body temperature elevation up to 100.0°F, grade 3 neutropenia, myalgia, arthralgia and bone pain. The lung disease progressed after seven months from the beginning of the immunotherapy and he was transferred to sunitinib treatment beginning in November 2007 at a standard dose and schedule (50 mg, 4/2 weeks). After six cycles, the dose was reduced to 37.5 mg due to hand-foot syndrome and mucositis grade 3. The patient continued sunitinib treatment with the best response of stable disease (SD) and received a total of 15 cycles. Pamindronate disodium 90 mg administered monthly was prescribed in parallel due to bone lesions with concurrent hypercalcemia. In October 2009, the patient underwent a femoral bone intramedullary locking ChM nail placement in order to prevent pathologic fracture.

Table 1 Blood test results on diagnosis and treatment of presented case

Blood test	16.04. 2012	01.08. 2012	02.08. 2012	08.01. 2013	30.01. 2013	15.02. 2013
CK (N = 55-70) [U/l]	47	49	58	20	16	16
CKMB (N = 0-16) [U/l]	39	11	13	13	11	23
Troponin I (N <0.035, MI > 0.12) [ng/ml]	0.070	0.055	0.066	0.097	0.076	0.076
NT-proBNP N < 125 [pg/ml]	799.4	-	-	-	1875.0	1879.3
LDH (135–232) [U/l]	243	-	178	-	134	196
Treatment	Pazopanib	IFN	IFN	Axitinib	BSC	BSC

Table 2 Summary of all reported cardiac intramyocardial metastases in clear cell renal cancer and the course of disease in those patients

Case no	Localization	Reference	Years from nephrectomy	Signs or symptoms	Diagnostic method	Treatment; treatment efficacy
1	LV	[11]	23	Weight loss	CT, TTE, MRI, CA	ND
2	LV	[12]	18	Dyspnea	CT, CA	Surgery - successful, 6 years follow-up
3	LV	[13]	7	Chest pain	TTE, TEE, CT, B	Chemotherapy - no response
4	LV	[4]	0	ND	PET-CT	ND
5	LV	[14]	ND	Dyspnea	CT, TTE	ND
6	LV, PE	[3]	8/12	Dyspnea, asthenia, and inferior limb edema, peripheral cyanosis	TTE	No
7	LV, PE	[15]	ND	ND	ND	Surgery - successful
8	RA	[16]	ND	Asymptomatic	TTE, CT	Surgery - successful
9	RA, LA, LV, PE	[13]	7	Endocarditis	TTE, CT, CA	Chemotherapy - no response
10	RV	[17]	19	ND	ND	Surgery - successful
11	RV	[18]	18	Asymptomatic	PET-CT	Sunitinib, everolimus - successful PR 6 months
12	RV	[1]	4.5	Arrhythmia, tachycardia	MRI, EBCT, CA, ECG, TEECG	Immunotherapy - no response
13	RV	[19]	5	Congestive heart failure (NYHA class III)	MRI, CT, CA, TEE	Echo-guided coil embolization - successful, 19 months follow-up
14	RV	[20]	0	Pansystolic murmur	TTE, MRI	ND
15	RV	[21]	0	Syncope, T wave abnormality, prolonged QT interval	ECG, TTE	Surgery - successful
16	RV	[22]	ND	Presyncope	TTE, B	ND
17	RV	[23]	ND	Asymptomatic	ND	ND
18	RV	[24]	ND	ND	X-ray	Surgery – died
19	RV	[25]	ND	Dyspnea	Post-mortem diagnosis	ND
20	RV, SE	[26]	4	cardiac murmur, monomorphic ventricular tachycardia	TTE	Sunitinib, ICD
21	SE	[2]	20	Raynaud's-like phenomena, systolic ejection murmur	TTE, MRI, TEE, B	Surgery -successful

Legend: TTE - Transthoracic echocardiography; TEE – transesophageal echocardiography, PA – pulmonary arteries, RA – right atrium, RV – right ventricle, SE- septum, CA - Coronary angiography, B- biopsy; ICD - implantable cardioverter-defibrillator, ND – no data available; EBCT - electron-beam CT; TEECG – trans -esophageal ECG; S-S; M-M; PE - pericardial effusion.

Due to further disease progression in the skeletal system, the patient was rescheduled on everolimus 10 mg/day. This treatment was continued with the best response of SD for the next 23 months (2009–2011), and was accompanied by zoledronic acid injections. As a result of a solitary new metastasis in the right kidney, the patient was referred for nephron-sparing surgery (NSS), which was performed in August 2010. In April 2011, multiple new skin metastases developed and the patient was referred for surgical consultation. In May 2011, scalp metastases were removed. After four weeks' recovery in July 2011, the patient started sorafenib (2 × 200 mg b.i.d.) treatment. From 2011 to2012, sorafenib treatment was continued with SD for 7 cycles on standard dose. The patient tolerated the treatment well with reported neuropathies grade 2. Standard follow-up

contrast-enhanced-CT scan was performed after 9 sorafenib cycles (March 2012). Metastases in the thoracic and abdominal lymph nodes, liver, right kidney, pancreas and skeleton were stable, but new lesions in the right lung (33 × 17 mm), in the right lumbar retroperitoneal region (27 × 20 mm), and in the psoas major muscle (∅10 mm) were described.

Moreover, contrast-enhancing tumors in the left myocardium (∅22 mm) and in the interventricular septum (∅26 mm) were described (Figure 1). This was defined as disease progression and the patient was transferred to pazopanib treatment in April 2012. In parallel, further laboratory tests and medical imaging were carried out (Table 2, Figure 2). In order to specify the diagnosis, we referred the patient for an echocardiogram that confirmed a 16 × 19 mm tumor localized between the

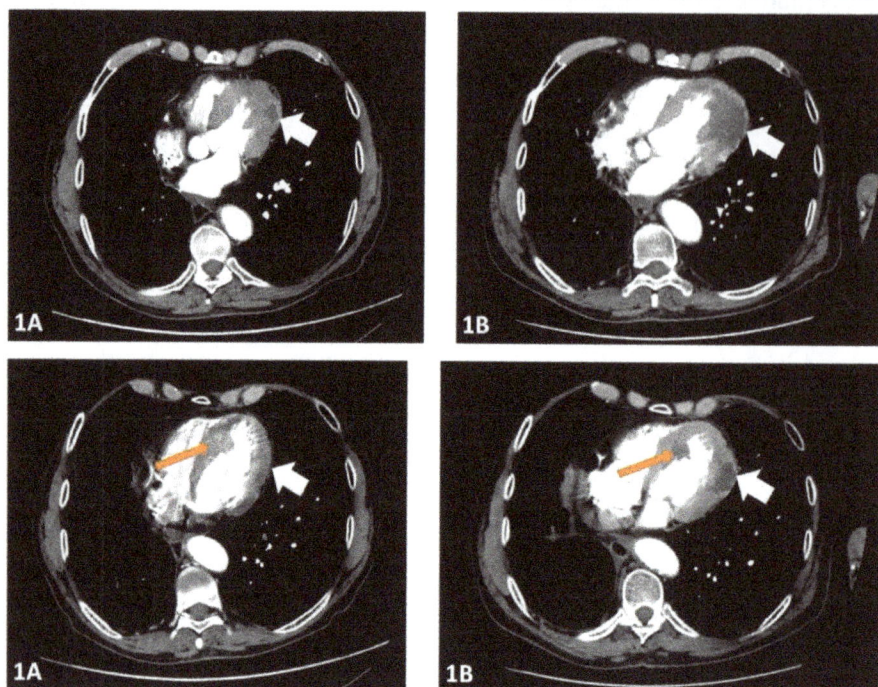

Figure 1 First CTimaging showing intramyocardial tumor in the LV in the left myocardium (white arrow 1A and 1B) and in the interventricular septum (red arrow 1A and 1B).

inferoseptal and apical septal segments with an estimated ejection fraction (EF) of 60%.

A subsequent cardiac MRI performed in April 2012 revealed multiple intramyocardial metastases (Figure 2), including tumors localized in segments: 1) apical inferior and apical lateral (∅13 × 7 mm); 2) apical septal and mid-inferoseptal (3 tumors: ∅10 mm, 11 mm, and 14 mm); 3) basal anterior (∅13 mm); 4) basal anteroseptal (∅18 mm); 5) mid-anteroseptal with pericardium infiltration (44 × 31 × 26 mm); and also in 6) anterior (∅14 mm) and posterior papillary (∅13 mm) muscles of the left ventricle (LV). On cardiac MRI, the EF was measured at 49.6% and hypokinetic muscles were described in the septum and anterolateral mid-ventricular segment. Cardiac single-photon emission computed tomography (SPECT) confirmed impaired myocardial perfusion in the inferolateral wall of the LV and anterior apex. Although the patient developed no signs or symptoms of cardiac dysrhythmia, a 24-hr Holter electrocardiogram (ECG) was performed and revealed ST-segment elevation, atrial extrasystoles, premature ventricular complexes, and a single episode of atrial fibrillation.

After five months of standard pazopanib treatment, a cardiac MRI in July 2012 (Figure 2) revealed SD with massive necrosis in the tumor localized in septal segments and an EF of 45%. At this point, the 24-h Holter ECG revealed no rhythm abnormalities. Due to massive necrosis – a typical TKI treatment effect – the patient

was referred for IFN-alpha treatment and received IFN-α-2a 3 million U, three times weekly for two months. This treatment was terminated due to poor tolerance with significant myalgia, arthralgia, and severe bone pain. In August 2012, a follow-up CT revealed progression according to RECIST-1.1 criteria with new lung and peritoneal tumors. In November 2012, axitinib treatment in a reduced dose (5 mg) was initiated. After two cycles of treatment, the patient's condition deteriorated and the patient passed in March 2013. OS since ccRCC diagnosis was 11 years 2 months, since first TKI treatment was 5 years 3 months, and since diagnosis of multiple heart metastases was 1 year.

Conclusions

Metastatic ccRCC involving the heart is well-recognized but a rare phenomenon, mostly arising as an intravascular protruding tumor. According to literature since 2000, right atrial in-growth of RCC was recently diagnosed in no more than 1% of cases at the time of nephrectomy. In post-mortem studies, cardiac metastasis was shown to be present in 11% of patients who died of RCC [3].

There are two mechanisms of cardiac involvement. Tumor extension through the renal vein and IVC is the main mechanism for the spread of cardiac ccRCC. On the other hand, metastases may also arise by diffuse systemic blood-borne spread or through the intrathoracic lymphatic system, especially in the presence of

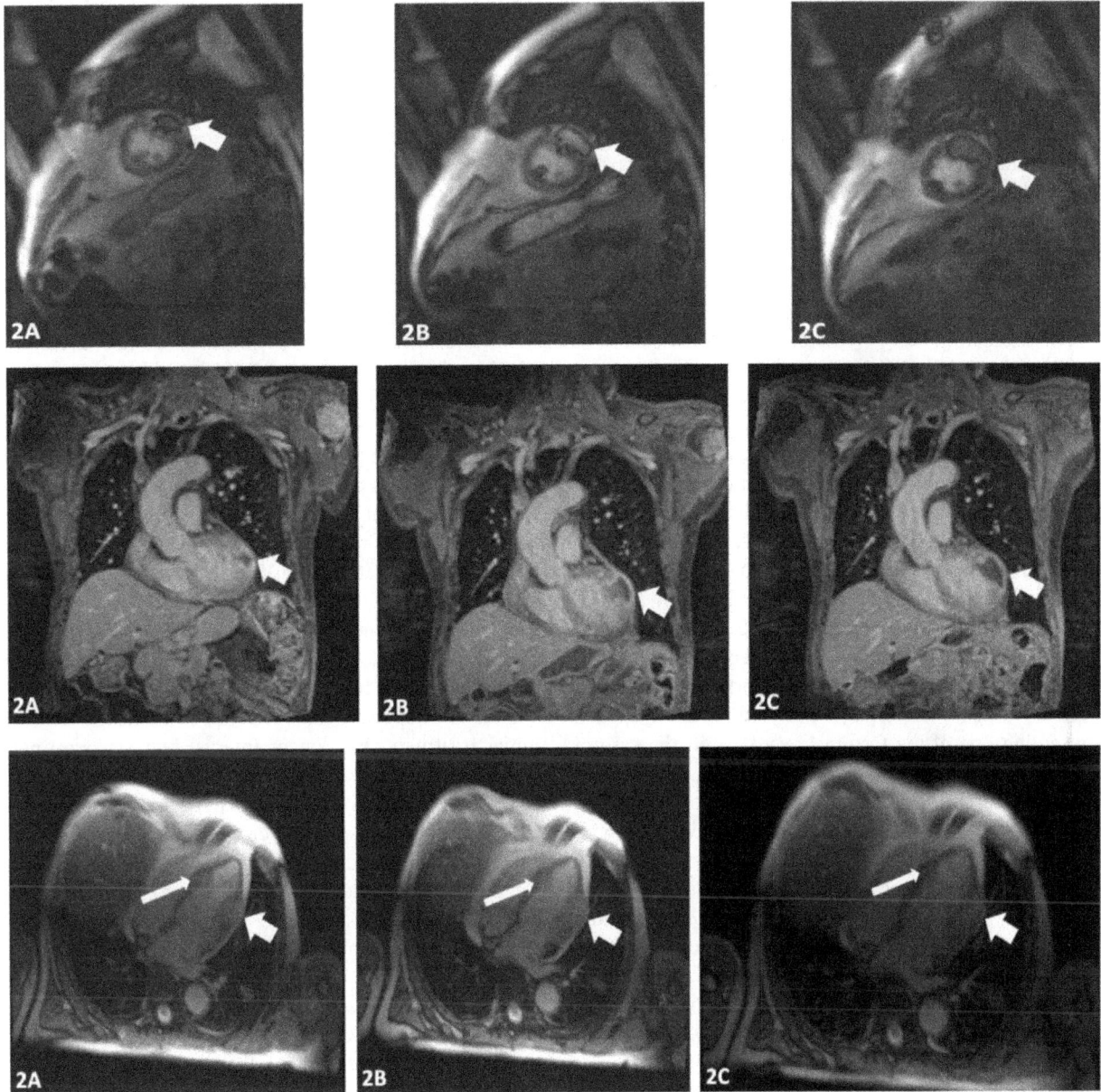

Figure 2 Cardiac-MRI performed on treatment onset and follow-up showing multiple (2A, 2B, and 2C) intramyocardial tumors and large necrosis on TKI treatment - coronal, horizontal and sagittal sections.

disseminated disease and pulmonary metastases [3]. It is clear that left ventricular metastases from ccRCC without vena caval or right atrial involvement are casuistic (Table 1). In the absence of either direct vena caval extension or systemic disease, involvement of the heart is extremely rare with only two cases known [12]. This specific pattern of metastasis should be considered a Stage 4 disease, with an expected five-year survival of less than 10% [20]. Up until now, only 21 cases of intramyocardial tumors of ccRCC have been described in the literature (Table 1). Majority of these cases were single tumors.

Only reports by two groups have shown multiple cardiac metastases from ccRCC [3,13]. Moreover only in two cases, the patients were treated with TKI, but in both cases, cardiac tumors were single, and no cardiac tests were reported nor was functional testing evaluation performed. In one of the cases the tumor actually developed on sorafenib treatment [14]. Other disease course and treatment is required if is a tumor thrombus that protrude to the heart, but not develop as intramyocarial metastases. In particular it was shown that tumor thrombus level does not predict recurrence or mortality in this group of ccRCC patients who present with IVC involvement in the renal vein (Group 1) or subdiaphragmatic IVC tumor thrombus (Group 2), in comparison to involvement of IVC above diaphragm or atrial extension (Group 3). Survival is determined by inherent aggressiveness of the cancer manifested by tumor size, grade and distant metastasis at presentation [28]. Pre-surgical treatment with sunitinib is able to ease surgery for ccRCC tumor thrombi and surgery after sunitinib treatment may be possible without additional morbidity. In this setting, two courses of pre-surgical therapy with sunitinib may be appropriate treatment [29].

Most ccRCC cardiac metastases remain asymptomatic, as in the case of this patient at the time of diagnosis. The most common cardiac presentation of renal cell carcinoma is hypertension, but other cardiac presentations include shortness of breath, cough, arrhythmias, chest pain, important hemodynamic impairment, and peripheral edema [21]. Tachyarrhythmia is also found often in this patients and may lead to syncope [21]. Coronary occlusion or compression from tumor masses can lead to myocardial infarction, heart failure, and death [12]. A typical clinical pattern of cardiac ccRCC disease progression is characterized by a worsening performance status, exacerbation of cardiac symptoms, including tamponade, arrhythmia, obstruction, or dilated cardiomyopathy, representing one of the terminal events as in the case of the reported patient [30]. Coronary occlusion or compression from tumor masses may also lead to myocardial infarction and death [12]. Pericardial involvement with effusion and cardiac tamponade is the most commonly recognized cause of hemodynamic compromise [24].

A variety of diagnostic imaging and hemodynamic techniques have been applied in the diagnostic process of all cases published, including echocardiography, CT, MRI, and even right heart catheterization and right ventriculography [24]. In our opinion cardiac MRI could be the diagnostic tool of choice in the assessment of patients with RCC when cardiac metastasis is suspected (Figure 2). Although there is overlap of the MRI characteristics of several cardiac masses, MRI is reliable tool to exclude lipomas, fibromas, and hemangiomas as well as thrombus or lipomatous hypertrophy. Also necrosis, extra-cardiac spread, and pericardial effusion may be identified with cardiac MRI [31]. Transthoracic echocardiography, transesophageal echocardiography, and PET-CT may also be used to diagnose cardiac metastases [20,30]. The capability of PET for absolute quantification in general and for blood flow quantification in particular is a substantial advantage. As we have shown in this case with SPECT, cardiac lesions visualized by functional imaging are correlated with anatomic data and provides sensitivity as well as the specificity of scintigraphic findings. Myocardium perfusion and coronary morphology

can be evaluated with SPECT/CT systems. For assessing absolute flow and coronary flow reserve imaging with SPECT also appears to be reliable [32]. Targeted systemic therapy may be useful for this group of patients [11], but profound necrosis in the heart wall may evoke tamponade, therefore follow-up cardiac MRI scans are required. Resection or embolization of ccRCC cardiac metastasis is dependent on the location and relationship of the tumor to the important local structures [11,19]. Finally, based on experience with this patient and literature data, we propose regular cardiac magnetic resonance imaging (MRI) evaluation in ccRCC patients receiving TKI treatment when intramyocardial ccRCC metastases are found. We believe that MRI combines noninvasive multiplanar imaging and the ability to acquire functional information with excellent contrast resolution [31].

Finally this case presents prolonged treatment with multiple lines of TKIs and mTOR inhibitor after immunotherapy. At this point of time third line therapy - following first-line TKI and mTOR inhibitors remains undefined, although sunitinib and other VEGF inhibitors have demonstrated activity in this setting [33]. Re-challenge with TKIs may provide clinical benefit in terms of PSF/OS after everolimus in patients with mRCC [34], as in this case. Recent data analysis has proven that globally PFS durations is shorter and response rate lower on re-challenge following initial treatment, but longer interval between treatments was shown to increase response to sunitinib re-challenge [35]. In a wide retrospective analysis in the sorafenib – mTOR inhibitor – sunitinib group subsequent PFS was of 11.7, 5.1 and 9.1 months, respectively, while in the sunitinib – mTOR inhibitor – sorafenib group PFS was 14.4, 4.3, and 3.9 months, respectively. This has led to conclusion that there is no significant difference between the two sequence modalities [36]. After failure of everolimus, re-exposure to TKIs was recently reported as a common clinical practice. It was demonstrates that patients obtain clinical benefit of therapies beyond immunotherapy – sunitinib/sorafenib – everolimus sequence. Drugs administered beyond was sunitinib (in 28.6% cases), sorafenib (in 28.6%) and other therapies (in 42.8%) in a recent report [37]. It was also shown that sunitinib and sorafenib re-challenge may be considered as it has had potential benefits in terms of PFS and may be tolerated in select mRCC patients [38,39]. This treatment modality may be effective due to a transient nature of sunitinib resistance [40,41] and in primarily sunitinib-responsive patients, re-challenge with sunitinib may be successfully introduced after mTOR inhibitor - refractory disease [42]. This case also confirms that sequential therapy enables to obtain prolong combined PSF as result of multiple lines of treatment. Although this patient obtained benefit from presented sequence immunotherapy – sunitinib – everolimus – sorafenib – pazopanib – axitinib, but for further cases 'ideal sequence' is still unknown. It should be hoped that TKIs, mTORIs with novel therapies (anti-PDL1, anti-PD1 anti-CTLA4) used in combination or sequentially have potential to provide best treatment and favorable outcomes in ccRCC. Results from ongoing and planned trials are expected to help shape future therapy [43].

Consent

The patient gave consent for all treatment procedures used and future scientific publications. Informed consent for this publication was obtained from relative of the patient. The patient passed prior to manuscript preparation.

Competing interests

CS has received honoraria for lectures from Pfizer, Roche, GSK, Novartis and Astellas. AMC has received honoraria for lectures from Pfizer, GSK, and Novartis. PS and FL indicate no potential conflict of interest.

Authors' contributions

Treatment: AMC, CS; Manuscript writing: All authors; Final approval of manuscript: All authors. Conception and design: CS, AMC; Collection and assembly of data: PS, AMC; Data interpretation: AMC, CS; Administrative support: PS, FL.

Authors' information

CS is a clinical oncology specialist since 1986, and has worked at Temple University School of Medicine, Jefferson Cancer Institute at Thomas Jefferson University, and in the last 10 years has participated in major renal cancer treatment clinical trials including AXIS, EU-ARCCS or TARGET and is an expert in renal cancer treatment; AMC specializes in clinical oncology and biotechnology, and has trained at the Universite degli Studi di Palermo, Paracelsus Medizinische Privatuniversität, and Emory University School of Medicine.

Acknowledgments

The authors thank Dr. Jerzy Czarnecki for fruitful discussions and manuscript proofreading. This work was supported by statutory funding from the Military Institute of Medicine. Proofreading services (Scribendi Inc.) fee was covered by CS.

Author details

[1]Department of Oncology, Military Institute of Medicine, Warsaw, Poland. [2]The Second Faculty of Medicine with the English Division and the Physiotherapy Division, Medical University of Warsaw, Warsaw, Poland. [3]Emory University School of Medicine, Atlanta, GA, USA. [4]Department of Oncology, Military Institute of Medicine, Laboratory of Molecular Oncology, Szaserow 128, 04-141 Warsaw, Poland.

References

1. Roigas J, Schroeder J, Rudolph B, Schnorr D: Renal cell cancer with a symptomatic heart metastasis. BJU Int 2002, 90(6):622–623.
2. Bradley SM, Bolling SF: Late renal cell carcinoma metastasis to the left ventricular outflow tract. Ann Thorac Surg 1995, 60(1):204–206.
3. Zustovich F, Gottardo F, De Zorzi L, Cecchetto A, Dal Bianco M, Mauro E, Cartei G: Cardiac metastasis from renal cell carcinoma without inferior vena involvement: a review of the literature based on a case report: two different patterns of spread? Int J Clin Oncol 2008, 13(3):271–274.
4. Pinnamaneni N, Muthukrishnan A: Left ventricular myocardium metastasis in a patient with primary renal cell carcinoma detected by 18 F-FDG PET/CT. Clin Nucl Med 2012, 37(7):e181–183.
5. Dominik J, Moravek P, Zacek P, Vojacek J, Brtko M, Podhola M, Pacovsky J, Harrer J: Long-term survival after radical surgery for renal cell carcinoma with tumour thrombus extension into the right atrium. BJU Int 2013, 111(3 Pt B):E59–64.
6. Schneider M, Hadaschik B, Hallscheidt P, Jakobi H, Fritz M, Motsch J, Pahernik S, Hohenfellner M: Manual repositioning of intra-atrial kidney cancer tumor thrombus: a technique reducing the need for cardiopulmonary bypass. Urology 2013, 81(4):909–914.
7. Motzer RJ, Hutson TE, Tomczak P, Michaelson MD, Bukowski RM, Rixe O, Oudard S, Negrier S, Szczylik C, Kim ST, Chen I, Bycott PW, Baum CM, Figlin RA: Sunitinib versus interferon alfa in metastatic renal-cell carcinoma. N Engl J Med 2007, 356(2):115–124.
8. Escudier B, Eisen T, Stadler WM, Szczylik C, Oudard S, Siebels M, Negrier S, Chevreau C, Solska E, Desai AA, Rolland F, Demkow T, Hutson TE, Gore M, Freeman S, Schwartz B, Shan M: Sorafenib in advanced clear-cell renal-cell carcinoma. N Engl J Med 2007, 356(2):125–134.
9. Rini BI, Escudier B, Tomczak P, Kaprin A, Szczylik C, Hutson TE, Michaelson MD, Gorbunova VA, Gore ME, Rusakov IG, Negrier S, Ou YC, Castellano D, Lim HY, Uemura H, Tarazi J: Comparative effectiveness of axitinib versus sorafenib in advanced renal cell carcinoma (AXIS): a randomised phase 3 trial. Lancet 2011, 378(9807):1931–1939.
10. Sternberg CN, Davis ID, Mardiak J, Szczylik C, Lee E, Wagstaff J, Barrios CH, Salman P, Gladkov OA, Kavina A, Zarba JJ, Chen M, McCann L, Pandite L, Roychowdhury DF, Hawkins RE: Pazopanib in locally advanced or metastatic renal cell carcinoma: results of a randomized phase III trial. J Clin Oncol 2011, 28(6):1061–1068.
11. Talukder MQ, Deo SV, Maleszewski JJ, Park SJ: Late isolated metastasis of renal cell carcinoma in the left ventricular myocardium. Interact Cardiovasc Thorac Surg 2010, 11(6):814–816.
12. Aburto J, Bruckner BA, Blackmon SH, Beyer EA, Reardon MJ: Renal cell carcinoma, metastatic to the left ventricle. Tex Heart Inst J 2009, 36(1):48–49.
13. Rohani M, Roumina S, Saha SK: Renal adenocarcinoma with intramyopericardial and right atrial metastasis, latter via coronary sinus: report of a case. Echocardiography 2005, 22(4):345–348.
14. Tokuyama Y, Iwamura M, Fujita T, Sugita A, Maeyama R, Bessho H, Ishikawa W, Tabata K, Yoshida K, Baba S: Myocardial metastasis from renal cell carcinoma treated with sorafenib. Hinyokika Kiyo 2011, 57(10):555–558.
15. Safi AM, Rachko M, Sadeghinia S, Zineldin A, Dong J, Stein RA: Left ventricular intracavitary mass and pericarditis secondary to metastatic renal cell carcinoma–a case report. Angiology 2003, 54(4):495–498.
16. Ishida N, Takemura H, Shimabukuro K, Matsuno Y: Complete resection of asymptomatic solitary right atrial metastasis from renal cell carcinoma without inferior vena cava involvement. J Thorac Cardiovasc Surg 2011, 142(3):e142–144.
17. Minale C, Ulbricht LJ, Holer H, Kobberling J, Cramer BM, Schubert GE: A rare form of heart metastasis: hypernephroma: successful surgical treatment. Z Kardiol 1995, 84(8):643–647.
18. Tatenuma T, Yao M, Sakata R, Sano F, Makiyama K, Nakaigawa N, Nakayama T, Inayama Y, Kubota Y: A case of myocardiac metastasis of clear cell renal cell carcinoma successfully treated with sunitinib. Hinyokika Kiyo 2013, 59(2):97–101.
19. Butz T, Schmidt HK, Fassbender D, Esdorn H, Wiemer M, Horstkotte D, Faber L: Echo-guided percutaneous coil embolization of a symptomatic massive metastasis of a renal cell carcinoma in the right ventricular outflow tract. Eur J Echocardiogr 2008, 9(5):725–727.
20. Otahbachi M, Cevik C, Sutthiwan P: Right ventricle and tricuspid valve metastasis in a patient with renal cell carcinoma. Anadolu Kardiyol Derg 2009, 9(4):E11–12.
21. Alghamdi A, Tam J: Cardiac metastasis from a renal cell carcinoma. Can J Cardiol 2006, 22(14):1231–1232.
22. Masaki M, Kuroda T, Hosen N, Hirota H, Terai K, Oshima Y, Nakaoka Y, Sugiyama S, Kimura R, Yoshihara S, Kawakami M, Iizuka N, Tomita Y, Ogawa H, Kawase I, Yamauchi-Takihara K: Solitary right ventricle metastasis by renal cell carcinoma. J Am Soc Echocardiogr 2004, 17(4):397–398.
23. Cheng AS: Cardiac metastasis from a renal cell carcinoma. Int J Clin Pract 2003, 57(5):437–438.
24. Labib SB, Schick EC Jr, Isner JM: Obstruction of right ventricular outflow tract caused by intracavitary metastatic disease: analysis of 14 cases. J Am Coll Cardiol 1992, 19(7):1664–1668.
25. Carroll JC, Quinn CC, Weitzel J, Sant GR: Metastatic renal cell carcinoma to the right cardiac ventricle without contiguous vena caval involvement. J Urol 1994, 151(1):133–134.

26. Zhang B, Malouf J, Young P, Kohli M, Dronca R: **Cardiac metastasis in renal cell carcinoma without vena cava or atrial involvement: an unusual presentation of metastatic disease.** *Rare Tumors* 2013, **5**(3):e29.

27. Pectasides D, Varthalitis J, Kostopoulou M, Mylonakis A, Triantaphyllis D, Papadopoulou M, Dimitriadis M, Athanassiou A: **An outpatient phase II study of subcutaneous interleukin-2 and interferon-alpha-2b in combination with intravenous vinblastine in metastatic renal cell cancer.** *Oncology* 1998, **55**(1):10–15.

28. Sidana A, Goyal J, Aggarwal P, Verma P, Rodriguez R: **Determinants of outcomes after resection of renal cell carcinoma with venous involvement.** *Int Urol Nephrol* 2012, **44**(6):1671–1679.

29. Horn T, Thalgott MK, Maurer T, Hauner K, Schulz S, Fingerle A, Retz M, Gschwend JE, Kubler HR: **Presurgical treatment with sunitinib for renal cell carcinoma with a level III/IV vena cava tumour thrombus.** *Anticancer Res* 2012, **32**(5):1729–1735.

30. Garcia JR, Simo M, Huguet M, Ysamat M, Lomena F: **Usefulness of 18-fluorodeoxyglucose positron emission tomography in the evaluation of tumor cardiac thrombus from renal cell carcinoma.** *Clin Transl Oncol* 2006, **8**(2):124–128.

31. Ward TJ, Kadoch MA, Jacobi AH, Lopez PP, Salvo JS, Cham MD: **Magnetic resonance imaging of benign cardiac masses: a pictorial essay.** *J Clin Imaging Sci* 2013, **3**:34.

32. Buck AK, Nekolla S, Ziegler S, Beer A, Krause BJ, Herrmann K, Scheidhauer K, Wester HJ, Rummeny EJ, Schwaiger M, Drzezga A: **Spect/Ct.** *J Nucl Med* 2008, **49**(8):1305–1319.

33. Escudier B, Albiges L, Sonpavde G: **Optimal management of metastatic renal cell carcinoma: current status.** *Drugs* 2013, **73**(5):427–438.

34. Paule B, Brion N: **Sunitinib re-challenge in metastatic renal cell carcinoma treated sequentially with tyrosine kinase inhibitors and everolimus.** *Anticancer Res* 2011, **31**(10):3507–3510.

35. Porta C, Paglino C, Grunwald V: **Sunitinib re-challenge in advanced renal-cell carcinoma.** *Br J Cancer* 2014, http://www.nature.com/bjc/journal/vaop/ncurrent/full/bjc2014214a.html.

36. Paglino C, Procopio G, Sabbatini R, Bellmunt J, Schmidinger M, Bearz A, Bamias A, Melichar B, Imarisio I, Tinelli C, Porta C: **A retrospective analysis of two different sequences of therapy lines for advanced kidney cancer.** *Anticancer Res* 2013, **33**(11):4999–5004.

37. Maute L, Grunwald V, Weikert S, Kube U, Gauler T, Kahl C, Burkholder I, Bergmann L: **Therapy of mRCC beyond mTOR-inhibition in clinical practice: results of a retrospective analysis.** *J Cancer Res Clin Oncol* 2014, **140**(5):823–827.

38. Zama IN, Hutson TE, Elson P, Cleary JM, Choueiri TK, Heng DY, Ramaiya N, Michaelson MD, Garcia JA, Knox JJ, Escudier B, Rini BI: **Sunitinib rechallenge in metastatic renal cell carcinoma patients.** *Cancer* 2010, **116**(23):5400–5406.

39. Nozawa M, Yamamoto Y, Minami T, Shimizu N, Hatanaka Y, Tsuji H, Uemura H: **Sorafenib rechallenge in patients with metastatic renal cell carcinoma.** *BJU Int* 2012, **110**(6 Pt B):E228–234.

40. Buczek M, Escudier B, Bartnik E, Szczylik C, Czarnecka A: **Resistance to tyrosine kinase inhibitors in clear cell renal cell carcinoma: from the patient's bed to molecular mechanisms.** *Biochim Biophys Acta* 2014, **1845**(1):31–41.

41. Bielecka ZF, Czarnecka AM, Solarek W, Kornakiewicz A, Szczylik C: **Mechanisms of acquired resistance to tyrosine kinase inhibitors in clear -cell renal cell carcinoma (ccRCC).** *Curr Signal Transduct Ther* 2013, **8**:219–228.

42. Grunwald V, Weikert S, Seidel C, Busch J, Johannsen A, Fenner M, Reuter C, Ganser A, Johannsen M: **Efficacy of sunitinib re-exposure after failure of an mTOR inhibitor in patients with metastatic RCC.** *Onkologie* 2011, **34**(6):310–314.

43. Porta C, Szczylik C, Escudier B: **Combination or sequencing strategies to improve the outcome of metastatic renal cell carcinoma patients: a critical review.** *Crit Rev Oncol Hematol* 2012, **82**(3):323–337.

14

Primary renal squamous cell carcinoma mimicking the renal cyst

Peng Jiang[1], Chaojun Wang[1], Shanwen Chen[1], Jun Li[2], Jianjian Xiang[3*] and Liping Xie[1*]

Abstract

Background: Renal squamous cell carcinoma is a rare neoplasm with poor prognosis. Chronic irritation from nephrolithiasis and/or pyelonephritis is the leading cause.

Case presentation: We described a 51-year-old male patient who was admitted because of left flank pain. Ultrasonography showed a renal cyst containing calculus. However, contrast-enhanced ultrasonography and CT scan revealed an irregular-shaped mass derived from a calculi-containing cyst. Ultrasound guided biopsy confirmed the diagnosis of renal squamous cell carcinoma. The patient refused any further therapeutic management and died six months later.

Conclusions: Our present case emphasizes that the careful diagnostic work-up and use of multiple imaging modalities in cases of unusual renal calculi is quite necessary, since they may carry the risk of co-existing hidden malignancy.

Keywords: Kidney, Squamous cell carcinoma

Background

Squamous cell carcinoma (SCC) of the renal pelvis is a rare neoplasm, accounting only 0.5 to 0.8 % of malignant renal tumors [1]. The predisposing factors leading to development of SCC of the renal pelvis include renal calculi, infections, endogenous and exogenous chemicals, vitamin A deficiency, hormonal imbalance and radiotherapy [2–4]. We reported a case of primary SCC of the renal pelvis, which was unsuspected before biopsy, and the most recent related literatures were reviewed as well.

Case presentation

An otherwise healthy 51-year-old male suffering from persist left flank pain for one week and was referred to the urology department. Physical examination revealed mild left costovertebral angle tenderness but was otherwise normal. Routine diagnostic work-up including chest

* Correspondence: ultraxjj@126.com; xielp@zju.edu.cn
[3]Department of Ultrasonography, The First Affiliated Hospital, School of Medicine, Zhejiang University, Hangzhou, Zhejiang Province, China
[1]Department of Urology, The First Affiliated Hospital, School of Medicine, Zhejiang University, Qingchun Road 79, Hangzhou 310003, Zhejiang Province, China
Full list of author information is available at the end of the article

X-ray and laboratory investigations were all within the normal range, but ultrasonography revealed a renal cyst containing calculus. Further computed tomography (CT) of the kidneys revealed an irregular-shaped homogeneous mass derived from the cyst was found. The mass enveloped the renal pedicle, aorta and inferior vena cava (Fig. 1). The mass was biopsied percutaneously under ultrasonographic guidance. The histological examination revealed squamous cell carcinoma (Fig. 2). Considering that the mass was un-resectable, the patient refused any other treatment. He returned to home hospice and unfortunately died six months later.

Discussion

The kidney is an unusual site for SCC. Renal SCC, most of which is known to arise from collecting system, is a rare clinical entity representing only 0.5 to 0.8 % of malignant renal tumors [1]. It usually occurs in late adulthood and is reported of an equal incidence in men and women [5]. However, according to the recent literatures (Table 1), men bear a higher incidence of renal SCC, probably because of higher incidence of nephrolithiasis in men [2, 6–20]. Long-standing nephrolithiasis and/or chronic pyelonephritis are the most common causes for

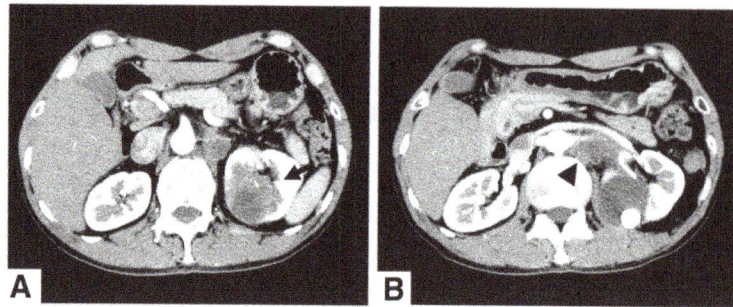

Fig 1 CT showed an irregular-shaped homogeneous mass (arrow) derived from the cyst and enveloped the renal pedicle

renal SCC. Other potential etiology have been described in the literatures, including exogenous and endogenous chemicals (e.g. arsenic), vitamin A deficiency, and prior surgery for renal stones, analgesic abuse, radiotherapy or chronic rejection in a transplant kidney [2–4]. Chronic irritation can cause squamous metaplasia of the renal collecting system, which may subsequently progress to leukoplakia and neoplasia of the urothelium, resulting in SCC of the renal pelvis. In our case, we speculated that the tumor has arisen in a chronically inflamed hydronephrotic calyx or a calyceal diverticulum with long term irritation by calculi.

Patients with renal SCC may present with flank or abdominal pain, microscopic or gross hematuria, fever, weight loss or a palpable abdominal mass (Table 1). It could also be the incidental finding on radiographic imaging for other reasons. Establishing the diagnosis of renal SCC by imaging techniques before biopsy or surgery is a clinical dilemma. Conventional ultrasonography is the choice of imaging modality for renal diseases evaluation, but renal SCC lacks specific echoic pattern in ultrasonography. Real-time CEUS was supposed to provide additional information for improving the diagnosis [21]. CT may play a crucial role in diagnosis and staging of the tumor. The radiologic evidences of renal SCC are diverse and may appear as a solid mass with irregular shape, hydronephrosis, calcifications, or as a renal pelvic infiltrative lesion without evidence of a distinct mass. The most helpful feature in CT of renal SCC is presence of enhancing extra-luminal and exophytic mass in some cases, with an intra-luminal component [16]. Lack of specific clinical and radiologic features in renal SCC would result in diagnostic confusion. Thus, the precise histological diagnosis was usually established after nephrectomy. For the un-resectable cases, both endoscopic and percutaneous biopsy could be applied to obtain the specimen. In our case, we chose ultrasound-guided biopsy because the CT scan presented the feature of extensive peritumoral vascular invasion, which indicated that the tumor was un-resectable.

Surgical resection is regarded as the mainstay of treatment for renal SCC [18]. However, the renal SCC is aggressive in nature and concealed. Most cases usually present at an advanced stage-pT3 or higher [16]. Therefore, for the treatment of advanced disease, a multidisciplinary approach comprising of surgical treatment and adjuvant chemoradiotherapy should be applied. Still, the prognosis of renal SCC is generally poor. According to the literatures, the outcome of renal SCC is dismal with a median survival of only several months postoperatively. Holmäng *et al.* reported that the prognosis of renal SCC is usually poor with a mean survival period of 7 months [5]. The 5-year survival rate is reported less than 10 % [14]. Thus, early diagnosis, monitoring of patients with longstanding nephrolithiasis, and new treatment modalities are urgently needed to improve patients' outcomes.

Conclusions

For patient with unusual renal calculi, the careful diagnostic work-up with multiple imaging modalities should be applied to exclude the co-existing hidden malignancy.

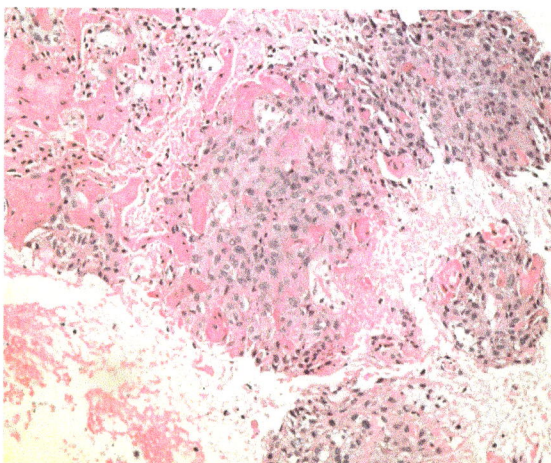

Fig 2 Biopsy pathology showing a high power view of squamous cell carcinoma (H&E x200)

Table 1 Characteristics of the reported cases from recent 5 years

Author	Sex	Age	Presentation	Ultrasonographic/radiological feature	Treatment	Prognosis
Bandyopadhyay et al. [6]	M	58	Heaviness and swelling in the left upper abdomen	Hydronephrosis	Nephrectomy	N/A[a]
Imriaco et al. [7]	M	69	Left flank abdominal pain	A solid mass within the left side of a horseshoe kidney, with associated large renal stones	Partial left nephrectomy	N/A
Mathur et al. [20]	M	52	Heaviness and swelling in the left upper abdomen	Non-functional kidney with dilation of renal calyces	Nephrectomy	N/A
Jain et al. [10]	M	50	Right flank pain	Staghorn calculi with right renal hydronephrosis	Nephrectomy	N/A
	M	87	Left lower abdomen pain	Left nephrolithiasis with staghorn calculi and hydronephrosis	Nephrectomy	Die in hospital because of coronary complication
	F	50	Left flank pain	Left renal and ureteric calculi with absence of corticomedullary distinction	Nephrectomy + cisplatin-based chemotherapy	Alive at 3 months after surgery
	M	53	Bilateral flank pain	Right renal calculi with hydronephrosis	Nephrectomy + cisplatin-based chemotherapy	Alive at 5 months after surgery
Paonessa et al. [11]	F	70	Vague abdominal pain	Multiple calcified areas within superior pole of the left kidney	Nephrectomy	N/A
Baseskioğlu et al. [13]	M	56	Left flank pain and fever	Hydronephrosis, staghorn calculi	Nephrectomy + radiation	Local recurrence, died 3 years later
Verma et al. [12]	M	62	Intermittent colicky pain at the right lumbar region	Right pyonephrosis with nephrolithiasis	Pyelithotomy (Palliative) + chemotherapy	N/A
Ham et al. [15]	M	69	Swelling and pain of right upper abdomen	Severe hydronephrosis with calyceal stones	Nephrectomy + Chemo	Died 7 months later
Bhajiee [14]	F	77	Weight loss and severe anemia	Left upper pole renal mass, staghorn calculus and renal vein thrombus	Nephrectomy	Asymptomatic with no evidence of recurrent or metastatic disease 6 months after surgery
Kalayci et al. [16]	M	63	10 kg weight loss	Big, non-functioning right kidney with staghorn calculi and a hypodense mass within the renal parenchyma extending to the upper pole of the right kidney	Nephrectomy	N/A
Palmer et al. [17]	F	46	Incidental finding	Large Coarse calculi with dilated renal collecting systems	Nephrectomy	Died on postoperative day 8
Wu et al. [19]	M	66	Intermittent melena, nausea, malaise, and abdominal pain	Heterogeneous renal mass containing a staghorn stone	Exploratory operation + biopsy	Died less than 5 months
Lin et al. [18]	M	56	Hematuria	Right renal staghorn calculi	Debulking surgery	Asymptomatic with no evidence of recurrent or metastatic disease 6 months after surgery
Hameed et al. [2]	F	41	Chronic backache in the right gluteal region	Complete staghorn calculus with sacral bone metastasis	Chemotherapy	Died 2 weeks after the 3rd cycle of chemotherapy

[a]N/A = Not Available

Consent

Written informed consent was obtained from the patient for publication of this case report and any accompanying images.

Abbreviations

SCC: Squamous cell carcinoma; CEUS: Contrast-enhanced ultrasonography; CT: Computed tomography.

Competing interests

The authors declare that they have no competing interests.

Authors' contributions

PJ and JJX drafted the manuscript. JJX provided imaging description and figures. CJW, SWC and JL assisted with manuscript preparation and literatures collection. LPX revised the manuscript. All authors have read and approved the final manuscript.

Author details

[1]Department of Urology, The First Affiliated Hospital, School of Medicine, Zhejiang University, Qingchun Road 79, Hangzhou 310003, Zhejiang Province, China. [2]Department of Pathology, The First Affiliated Hospital, School of Medicine, Zhejiang University, Hangzhou, Zhejiang Province, China. [3]Department of Ultrasonography, The First Affiliated Hospital, School of Medicine, Zhejiang University, Hangzhou, Zhejiang Province, China.

References

1. Li MK, Cheung WL. Squamous cell carcinoma of the renal pelvis. J Urol. 1987;138(2):269–71.
2. Hameed ZB, Pillai SB, Hegde P, Talengala BS. Squamous cell carcinoma of the renal pelvis presenting as sacral bone metastasis. BMJ Case Rep. 2014;2014. doi:10.1136/bcr-2013-201719.
3. Schena S, Bogetti D, Setty S, Kadkol S, Bruno A, Testa G, et al. Squamous cell carcinoma in a chronically rejected renal allograft. Am J Transplant. 2004;4(7):1208–11.
4. Papadopoulos I, Wirth B, Weichert-Jacobsen K, Loch T, Wacker HH. Primary squamous cell carcinoma of the ureter and squamous adenocarcinoma of the renal pelvis: 2 case reports. J Urol. 1996;155(1):288–9.
5. Holmang S, Lele SM, Johansson SL. Squamous cell carcinoma of the renal pelvis and ureter: incidence, symptoms, treatment and outcome. J Urol. 2007;178(1):51–6.
6. Bandyopadhyay R, Biswas S, Nag D, Ghosh AK. Squamous cell carcinoma of the renal pelvis presenting as hydronephrosis. J Cancer Res Ther. 2010;6(4):537–9.
7. Imbriaco M, Iodice D, Erra P, Terlizzi A, Di Carlo R, Di Vito C, et al. Squamous cell carcinoma within a horseshoe kidney with associated renal stones detected by computed tomography and magnetic resonance imaging. Urology. 2011;78(1):54–5.
8. Soni HC, Jadav VJ, Sumariya B, Venkateshwaran KN, Patel N, Arya A. Primary malignancy in crossed fused ectopic kidney. Abdom Imaging. 2012;37(4):659–63.
9. Hsieh TC, Wu YC, Sun SS, Chiang IP, Yang CF, Yen KY, et al. Synchronous squamous cell carcinomas of the esophagus and renal pelvis. Clin Nucl Med. 2011;36(11):e171–174.
10. Jain A, Mittal D, Jindal A, Solanki R, Khatri S, Parikh A, et al. Incidentally detected squamous cell carcinoma of renal pelvis in patients with staghorn calculi: case series with review of the literature. ISRN Oncol. 2011;2011:620574.
11. Paonessa J, Beck H, Cook S. Squamous cell carcinoma of the renal pelvis associated with kidney stones: a case report. Med Oncol. 2011;28 Suppl 1:S392–394.
12. Verma N, Yadav G, Dhawan N, Kumar A. Squamous cell carcinoma of kidney co-existing with renal calculi: a rare tumour. BMJ Case Rep. 2011;2011.
13. Baseskioglu B, Yenilmez A, Acikalin M, Can C, Donmez T. Verrucous carcinoma of the renal pelvis with a focus of conventional squamous cell carcinoma. Urol Int. 2012;88(1):115–7.
14. Bhaijee F. Squamous cell carcinoma of the renal pelvis. Ann Diagn Pathol. 2012;16(2):124–7.
15. Ham BK, Kim JW, Yoon JH, Oh M, Bae JH, Park HS, et al. Squamous cell carcinoma must be considered in patients with long standing upper ureteral stone and pyonephrosis. Urol Res. 2012;40(4):425–8.
16. Kalayci OT, Bozdag Z, Sonmezgoz F, Sahin N. Squamous cell carcinoma of the renal pelvis associated with kidney stones: radiologic imaging features with gross and histopathological correlation. J Clin Imaging Sci. 2013;3:14.
17. Palmer CJ, Atty C, Sekosan M, Hollowell CM, Wille MA. Squamous cell carcinoma of the renal pelvis. Urology. 2014;84(1):8–11.
18. Lin Z, Chng JK, Chong TT, Soo KC. Renal pelvis squamous cell carcinoma with inferior vena cava infiltration: Case report and review of the literature. Int J Surg Case Rep. 2014;5(8):444–7.
19. Hui Wu J, Xu Y, Qiang Xu Z, Yang K, Qiang Yang S, Shun Ma H. Severe anemia and melena caused by pyeloduodenal fistula due to renal stone-associated squamous cell carcinoma. Pak J Med Sci. 2014;30(2):443–5.
20. Mathur S, Rana P, Singh S, Goyal V, Sangwan M. Incidentally detected squamous cell carcinoma in non-functioning kidney presenting as multi-cystic mass. J Surg Case Rep. 2011;9:8.
21. Li X, Liang P, Guo M, Yu J, Yu X, Cheng Z, et al. Real-time contrast-enhanced ultrasound in diagnosis of solid renal lesions. Discov Med. 2013;16(86):15–25.

15

Prolonged CT urography in duplex kidney

Honghan Gong*, Lei Gao, Xi-Jian Dai, Fuqing Zhou, Ning Zhang, Xianjun Zeng, Jian Jiang and Laichang He

Abstract

Background: Duplex kidney is a common anomaly that is frequently associated with multiple complications. Typical computed tomography urography (CTU) includes four phases (unenhanced, arterial, parenchymal and excretory) and has been suggested to considerably aid in the duplex kidney diagnosi. Unfortunately, regarding duplex kidney with prolonged dilatation, the affected parenchyma and tortuous ureters demonstrate a lack of or delayed excretory opacification. We used prolonged-delay CTU, which consists of another prolonged-delay phase (1- to 72-h delay; mean delay: 24 h) to opacify the duplicated ureters and affected parenchyma.

Methods: Seventeen patients (9 males and 8 females; age range: 2.5–56 y; mean age: 40.4 y) with duplex kidney were included in this study. Unenhanced scans did not find typical characteristics of duplex kidney, except for irregular perirenal morphology. Duplex kidney could not be confirmed on typical four-phase CTU, whereas it could be easily diagnosed in axial and CT-3D reconstruction using prolonged CTU (prolonged-delay phase).

Results: Between January 2005 and October 2010, in this review board-approved study (with waived informed consent), 17 patients (9 males and 8 females; age range: 2.5 ~ 56 y; mean age: 40.4 y) with suspicious duplex kidney underwent prolonged CTU to opacify the duplicated ureters and confirm the diagnosis.

Conclusion: Our results suggest the validity of prolonged CTU to aid in the evaluation of the function of the affected parenchyma and in the demonstration of urinary tract malformations.

Keywords: Duplex kidney, Duplicated ureters, Prolonged-delay contrast enhancement, Multi-slice spiral CT urography

Background

Duplex kidney is a common anomaly of the urinary system [1]. Most patients are asymptomatic, with this anomaly being detected incidentally on imaging studies performed for other reasons. Symptomatic patients usually have complete ureteric duplication in which the ureters are prone to developing obstruction, reflux, and infection. Despite being easily detected on excretory urography, ultrasonography, computed tomography (CT) and magnetic resonance imaging (MRI), the affected parenchymal function and anatomic variations of duplex kidney are frequently difficult to assess using these imaging modalities [2]. Assessment of the affected parenchymal function and visualization of the entire duplicated ureters/collecting systems are particularly important for surgical planning and long-term follow-up.

Croitoru et al. [3] have previously reported percutaneous injection of iodinated contrast medium into the dilated collecting systems, and intravenous contrast administration was performed. The resultant 3D images clearly showed the entire ectopic ureter in various planes. This method is very useful when evaluating duplicated ureter-related abnormities. However, this method cannot reveal the function of the affected duplex kidney, and the method is also invasive.

In the current study, we first presented prolonged-delay CT urography (CTU), which is a promising protocol to evaluate renal resorption and outline anatomic variations and urinary tract obstruction. We next summarized and discussed the prolonged findings of 17 patients with duplex kidney at our hospital since 2001.

Methods
Subjects

The institutional review board of the First Affiliated Hospital of Nanchang University approved this retrospective

* Correspondence: honghan_gong@sina.com
Department of Radiology, the First Affiliated Hospital of Nanchang University, 17 Yongwai Zheng Street, Donghu District, Nanchang, Jiangxi 330006, China

study and waived the requirement for patient informed consent. Between January 2005 and October 2010, seventeen patients (9 males and 8 females; age range: 2.5 ~ 56 y; mean age: 40.4 y) with duplex kidney were included in this study. These patients demonstrated a renal mass on sonography, MRI or CT. Two blinded abdominal radiologists (Honghan Gong with 40 years of experiences and one of three others, each with up to five years of experiences) independently reviewed the images for the systemic evaluation and diagnosis. Of the seventeen patients with duplex kidney in our study, 15 presented with urinary tract infection and 2 with ectopic ureteral orifice for hospital visits.

CT

Prolonged-delay CTU images were obtained from two CT scanners: Somatom Sensation 16 (Siemens Medical Solutions, Forchheim, Germany) and Aquilion 64 (Toshiba Medical Systems, Tokyo, Japan). The CT scanner calibration was checked weekly and adjusted if needed. CTU images were obtained using varying tube current (150–180 mA from the scanner depending on the patient size) and 120 ~ 140 kVp. The scans were performed with a pitch of 1.0–1.4, a rotation time of 0.5 to 0.8 s, a section thickness of 5–10 mm, a table speed of 7–10 mm/s, and a standard reconstruction algorithm. The target area was from the top of the kidneys to pubic symphysis for each phase. Oral hydration was used for the children prior to scanning.

We first performed unenhanced scanning, and then CTU after a 20-s delay from the beginning of the single-bolus administration of the intravenous contrast agent. Each patient received 90–100 ml of a contrast agent with 300 mg of iodine per milliliter (iopromide 76 %; Iopromide 300; Bayer Schering Pharma AG) at a rate of 3.5–4 ml/s using a power injector (MEORAO-Stellant; MEORAO Company, Germany). CTU included four-phase (unenhanced, arterial, parenchymal and excretory) scanning. After CTU, the radiologist checked each phase immediately to decide whether a prolonged-delayed phase was needed.

Depending on the excretory opacification of duplex kidney, prolonged CTU scanning was performed 1–72 h (mean duration: 24 h) after typical CTU. Each patient received 2–4 (mean: 3 times) prolonged-delay scans using the same scanning parameters as those for typical CTU. Delayed imaging was restricted to the abdomen and was performed about one hour after the initial administration of the bolus using the same imaging parameters. Prescan scout CT images were obtained prior to prolonged-delayed scanning to ensure complete contrast opacification of the duplicated ureters.

Image and data analyses

Multi-planar reconstruction (MPR), volume rendering (VR), maximum intensity projection (MIP), curved-planar reconstruction (CPR) and blood vessel probing were performed using a work station (vitrea@2 version 3.7.0).

Results

The demographic characteristics are summarized in Table 1. Among the 17 confirmed duplex kidneys, 13 were unilateral duplex kidneys, and four were bilateral duplex kidneys; 11 cases were confirmed surgically, and six cases were confirmed at the follow-up.

Unenhanced scanning did not find typical characteristics of duplex kidney, except for irregular perirenal morphology. Duplex kidney could not be confirmed on typical four-phase CTU, whereas duplex kidney was easily diagnosed in axial and 3D reconstruction on prolonged-delay CTU (prolonged delay phase). All 17 cases had irregular perirenal morphology, 7/17 had irregular small kidney-Megaureter malformation or ectopic ureterocele, renal pelvis or ureter malformations, and 5/17 had bladder-ureter malformation (Figs. 1-5). Renal function of duplex kidney could be well assessed in prolonged-delay CTU (Figs. 1-5).

Discussion

Ureteral duplication is often associated with vesicoureteral reflux, ureterocele, or ectopic ureter opening [4]. In most cases, the duplex kidney is divided into two parts—the upper and inferior poles—each with its separate collecting systems. In some cases, however, the kidney is entirely separated into two independent parts, each with its own renal pelvis and ureter. The diagnosis of duplicated ureters was previously based on excretory urography and retrograde ureteropyelography, and now has been replaced by CTU. Ultrasonography, CT and MRI have certain value in the evaluation of duplex kidney [5]. Ultrasonography can display the nonfunctioning upper pole and would be useful to differentiate renal cyst from renal pelvic diverticulum. CTU and MRU can delineate essentially all abnormalities of the collecting systems, ectopic ureter, and ureterocele that benefit the

Table 1 Demographic characteristics of 17 patients with duplex kidney

Patient demographics	
Age	2.5 ~ 56y, mean 40.4y
Sex	9 male/8 female
Category	13 unilateral/4 bilateral
Irregular small kidney/Megaureter malformation Ectopic ureterocele	7
Renal pelvis/Ureter malformations	5
Bladder-ureter malformation	5

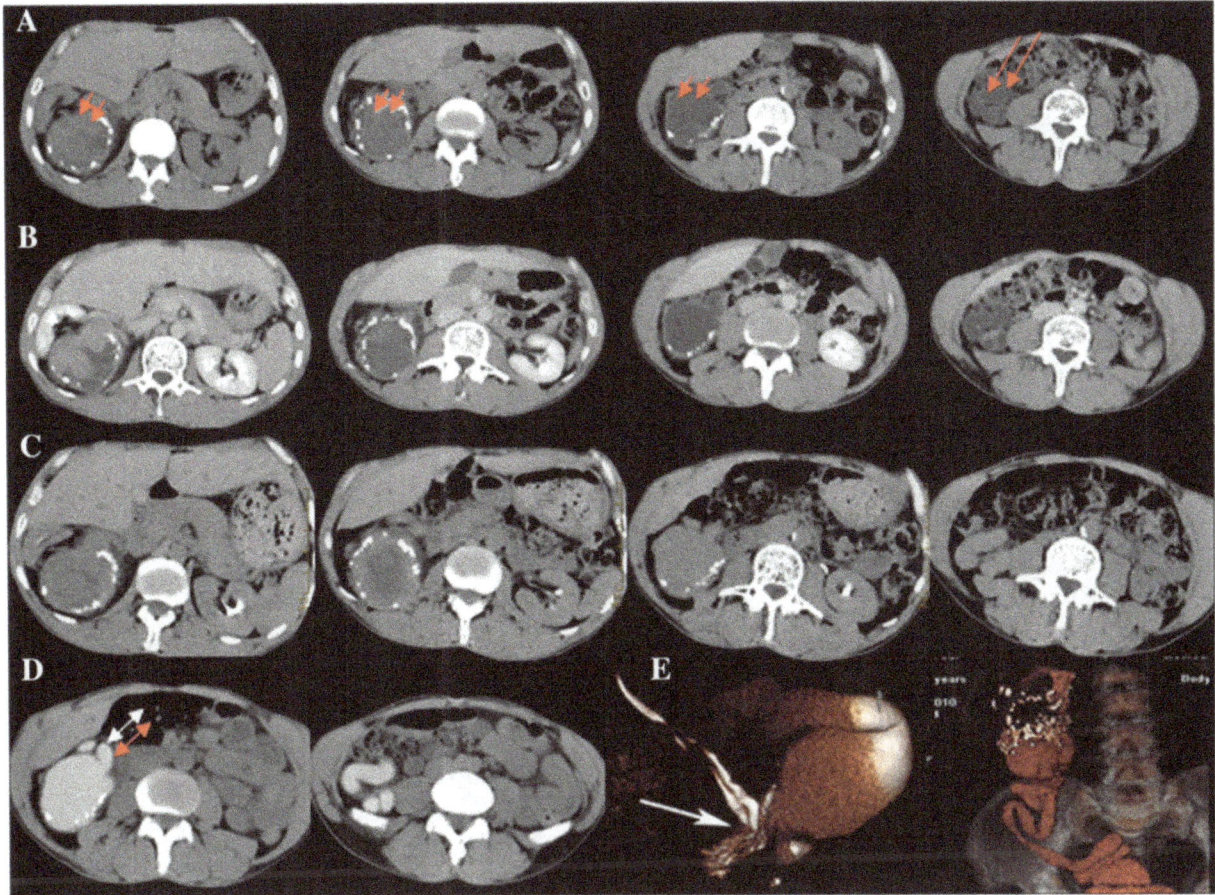

Fig. 1 Case 1. A 56-year-old male patient with right side duplex kidney. Unenhanced supine axial CT (**a**) shows a solitary round, iso-dense, soft-tissue mass with a clear boundary (*short arrow*). The irregularly annular calcified shadow around the mass was equivalent to multiple annular low-density shadows in the ileocecal junction (*long arrow*). The mass was not clearly intensified after contrast enhancement (**b**) and one-hour delayed (**c**) CTU scanning. Interestingly, it was obviously strengthened after 18-h delay (**d**), confirming duplex kidney. Furthermore, we found a band of high-density shadows that was confirmed to be duplicated ureters (*double-headed arrow*). Reformatted 3D CTU after segmentation of bone structures also showed the entire course of the dilated ureters (**e**)

diagnosis of duplicated and ectopic ureter [6–8]. However, these protocols are mainly useful in evaluating duplex kidney with approximately normal function and simple anomaly [5]. However, in some cases, because of poor function and obstruction, a lack of or delayed excretory opacification limits the complete diagnostic features. Duplex kidney can be misdiagnosed as a renal or perirenal neoplasm, a renal cyst, a kidney tumor, or, occasionally, adrenal gland neoplasms. When presented with various complicated complications, duplicated ureters can be misdiagnosed as a cyst, an ectopic ureter, a ureterocele or ureteral obstruction. The opening of duplicated ureters may be outside the bladder or even extracorporal. It is difficult to show an ectopic opening from cystoscopy. Additionally, ultrasonography, CT or MRU can not effectively display the tortuous ureter and ectopic

ureter openings, particularly in duplex kidney with prolonged dilatation.

CTU has basically replaced excretory urography for its advantages in anatomical details, fast imaging, high-quality 3D reconstruction and safety. The CT Urography Working Group of the European Society of Urogenital Radiology (ESUR) has proposed a clear definition of CTU in their Society Meeting in 2006 [9]. An issue was raised concerning the number of phases, including four-phase CTU (unenhanced, arterial, parenchymal and excretory), three-phase CTU (unenhanced, nephrographic and excretory), and two-phase CTU (unenhanced and combined nephroexcretory). In the present study, we reviewed a group of 17 patients who had duplex kidney malformations and various ureteral abnormal complications with enhanced/delay CTU (see Figs. 1-5). Prolonged CTU must include: (a) unenhanced axial scan; (b) arterial enhancement

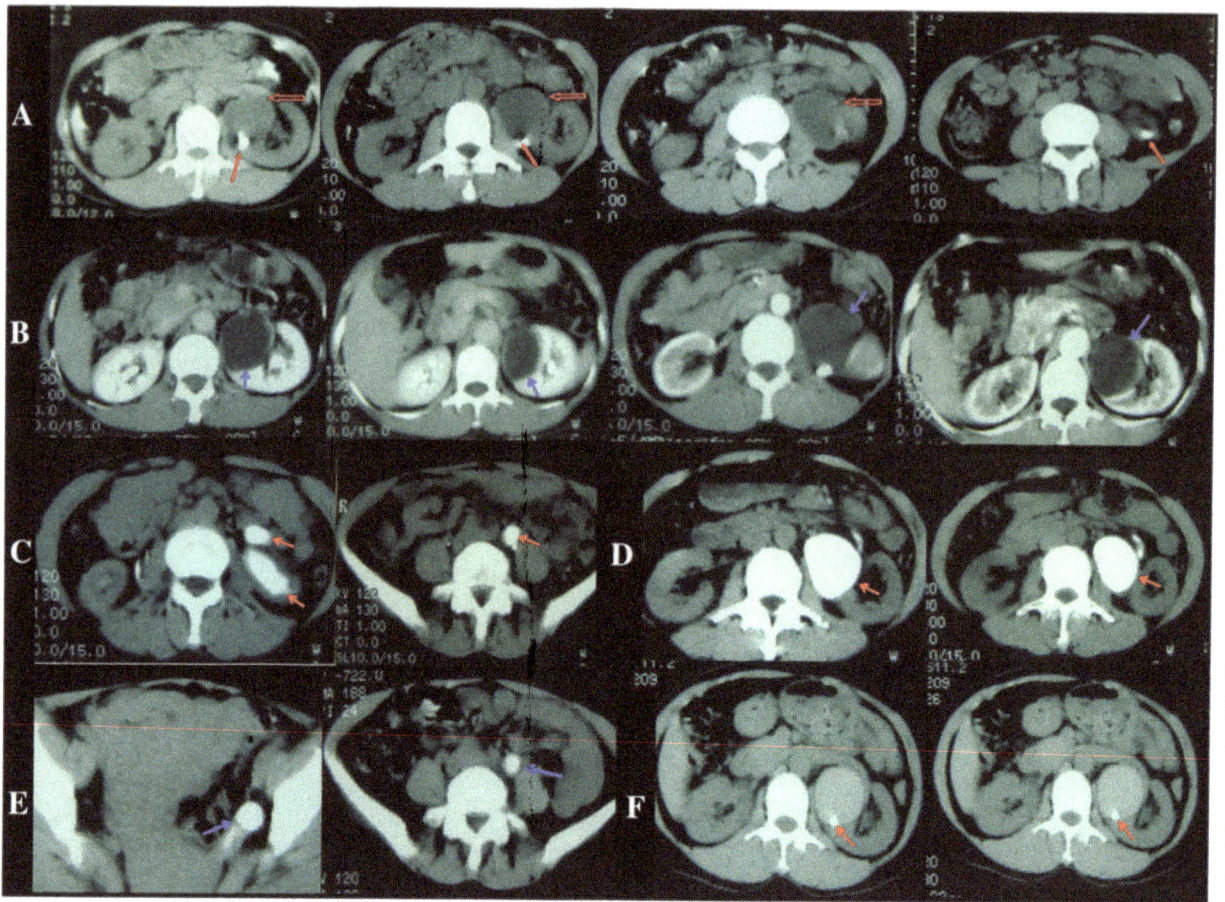

Fig. 2 Case 2. CT scans obtained in a 46-year-old woman with left duplex kidney & ectopic ureter openings. Non- enhanced scan obtained at the level of the upper-middle pole of the left kidney shows areas of abnormal low-density (*red faint arrow*) and stone shadow (*red solid arrow*) (**a**). Contrast-enhanced scans obtained at the same level as in (**a**). The upper-middle pole of the left kidney (blue arrow) shows no enhancement on the 6-min scan (**b**) and abnormal low density enhancement on the 3 h (**c**), 18 h (**d**), 24 h (**e**) and 45 h (**f**) scan, and ectopic ureter openings can be seen in (**e**) (blue arrow)

phase; (c) parenchymal phase; (d) excretory phase and a (e) prolonged-delay enhanced excretory period. Thus, the full course of prolonged-delay CTU includes five phases, differing from the ESUR-recommended or Croitoru et al. protocol reported previously [3]. (1) Our prolonged CTU adopted a single-bolus administration rather than two bolus injections of 300 mg/kg. (2) The delayed duration should be 72 h as the longest and 1 h as the shortest, not just several minutes of delay; in our experience, satisfactory opacification can be achieved 24 h after CTU in most cases. (3) Confine the X-ray beam to the target area to reduce the exposure of X-ray. For the duplex kidney with normal renal function, the ESUR-recommended CTU is sufficient to evaluate the malformations and related complications; in our case, the scanning can be terminated in the excretory phase. The main significance of prolonged-delay enhanced CTU is that there is sufficient delay time for duplex kidney with poor function to secrete contrast

to the duplicated ureters; however, other considerations include the following: (1) confirming the duplex kidney malformation near the normal kidney; (2) exposing the entire course of the duplicated ureters and existing complications; (3) extending the period helps reflect the parenchymal function of duplex kidney.

Ectopic ureter is likely to occur with dysfunction, making it difficult to detect the ureter in complete duplex kidney with duplicated ureters with poor function. 3D reconstruction is a good method in delayed excretory urography, and a large amount of axial plane data has been condensed to the coronal plane to better display the dilated collecting systems.

Our preliminary results indicate that duplex-collecting system abnormalities can be successfully displayed by prolonged CTU. Given that prolonged-delay enhanced CTU is sensitive to duplex kidney with poor function, 3D reconstruction can clearly display

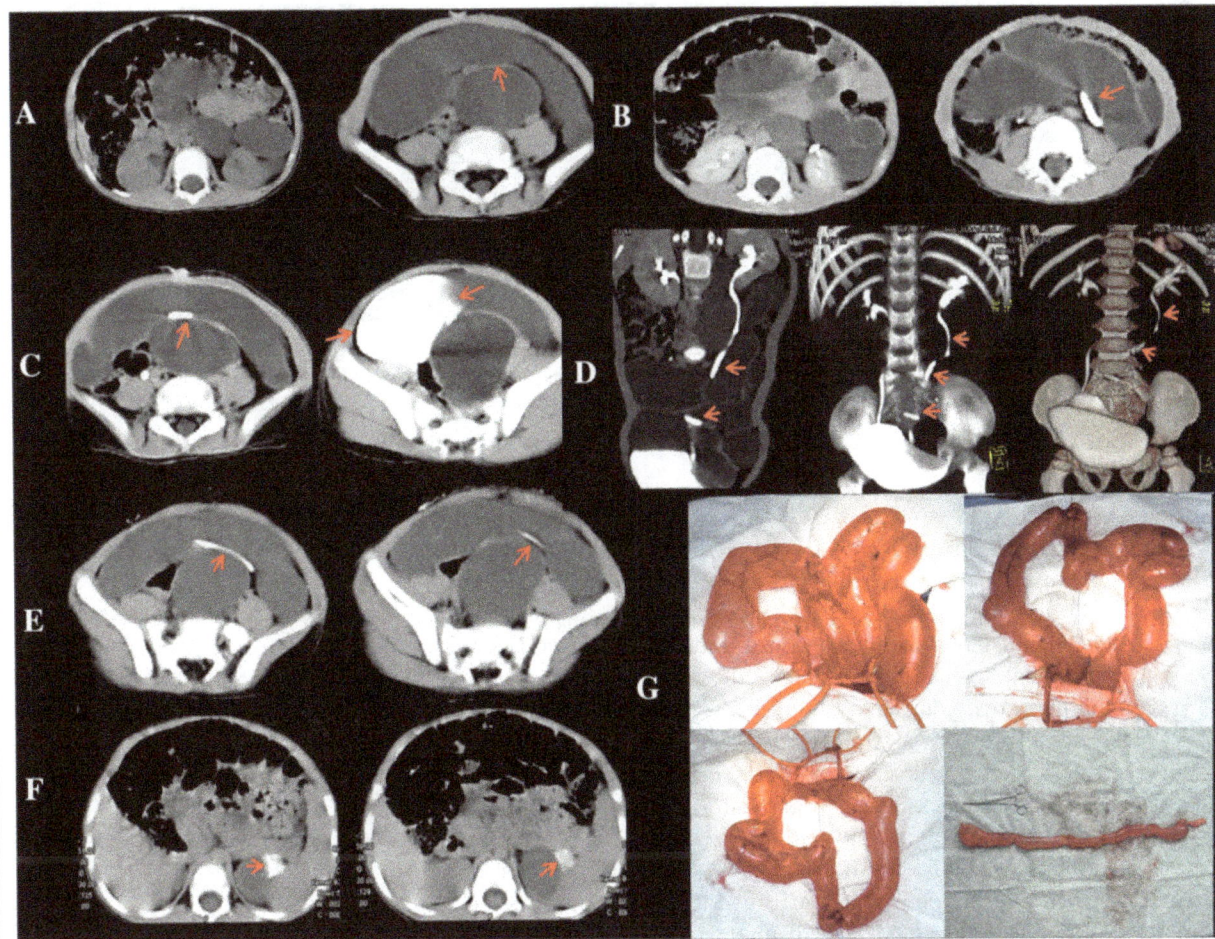

Fig. 3 Case 3. CT obtained in a 3.5-year-old boy with left duplex kidney & ureters, and congenital megaflop-ureter. Non- enhanced scan obtained at the abdomen & pelvis shows fluid-filled loops, the normal bowel loops are compressed to the right side of the abdominal wall, and a tendon-like shadow can be seen in the bowel loop-like areas (red arrow) (**a**). The tendon-like shadow was intensified as the normal ureter (red arrow) (**b**), and the normal bladder was also intensified in the left side pelvis (red arrow) on the 54-min scan (**c**). Meanwhile, MIP reconstruction shows the position and course of left ureter changed (red arrow) (**d**). The left ureter shows delayed enhancement on the 3-h and 13-min scan (**e**). The area of the left side kidney shows a little irregular enhancement on the 23 h and 9-min scan (red arrow) (**f**). Operation findings (**g**)

the entire course of the ureter in multi-planes. Our results suggest that prolonged CTU has more advantages over other imaging modalities. Despite the relatively small sample in the current study, we have successfully examined the 17 cases of duplex kidney and its complications. We believe that prolonged CTU is a better choice in evaluating duplex kidney with poor function.

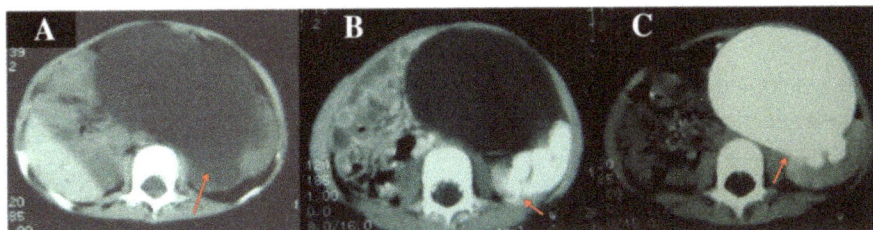

Fig. 4 Case 4. CT scans obtained in a 2.5-year-old girl with left duplex ureters and congenital megalo-ureter. Non-enhanced scan obtained at the level of the inferior-middle pole of the left kidney shows a huge round-like area of low density (red arrow) (**a**). Contrast-enhanced scans were obtained at the same level as in (**a**), this area showed no enhancement on (**b**) the 26-h scan, and the tortuous contrast agent can be seen retroperitoneally (red arrow) (**b**). The huge round-like area of low density was intensified on the 48-h scan (red arrow) (**c**)

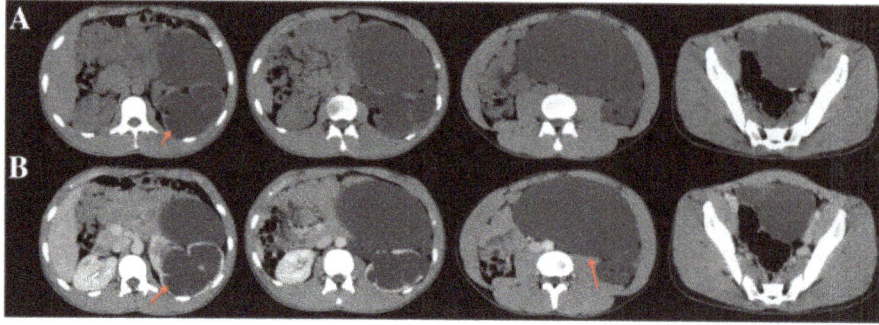

Fig. 5 Case 5. CT scans obtained in a 20-year-old man with left congenital megaloureter. Nonenhanced scan obtained at the abdomen & pelvis shows huge fluid-filled loops (*red arrow*), and the normal bowel loops are compressed to the right side of the abdominal wall (**a**). The left renal pelvis and calyces show marked dilation, with parenchyma thinning (*red arrow*) on parenchymal phase enhancement (**b**), for unknown reason the images of prolonged phase were missing

Beyond the benefits of prolonged CTU, a controversy focuses on radiation exposure. Are the radiation and time worthwhile, particularly in children? This is really an issue that must be addressed. Indeed, this practice results in higher radiation exposure and longer time involvement. However, we believe the benefits from this practice outweigh the risks. First, prolonged scanning provides a straightforward avenue to achieve greater, if not maximal, ureteral opacification, avoids detours and improves efficient diagnosis. Second, delayed CTU may be the only way to outline the entire course of the ureters, and, indirectly, index function in the affected parenchyma in the duplex part of the kidney, a feature that other imaging modalities cannot match. Third, a definitive diagnosis is particularly important for surgical planning and long-term follow-up; this advantage is much greater than the radiation risk.

There are several limitations in this study. First, the delayed phases were obtained in a wide spectrum of time intervals (1–72 h); in our experience, satisfactory opacification in this protocol can be achieved 24 h after CTU in most cases; however, in some cases, satisfactory opacification can be faster (1 h) or slower (72 h). Second, this study is retrospectively summarized over a 5-year period on 2 different scanners and a small sample size; larger samples are needed to refine our conclusion.

Conclusions

Our results suggest the validity that prolonged CT urography could aid in the evaluation of the function of the affected parenchyma and in the demonstration of urinary tract malformations.

Ethics approval and consent to participate

The institutional review board of the First Affiliated Hospital of Nanchang University approved this retrospective study and waived the requirement for patient informed consent.

Competing interests

The authors declare that the research was conducted in the absence of any commercial or financial relationships that could be construed as a potential conflict of interest.

Authors' contributions

HG contributed to the conception, design, and radiological expertise, helped to select and assess cases, conducted the data analysis, and drafted and approved the final manuscript. LG contributed to the drafting and revision of the manuscript. FZ, NZ and XJD offered data collection. FZ, LH, XZ and JJ contributed radiological expertise and offered a critical review of the manuscript for intellectual content. All the authors have read and approved the final manuscript.

Acknowledgments

We especially thank the reviewers and editors for their valuable and selfless assistance on our manuscript.

Funding

This work was supported by the National Natural Science Foundations of China (grants 81260217 and 81460263).

References

1. Fernbach SK, Feinstein KA, Spencer K, Lindstrom CA. Ureteral duplication and its complications. Radiographics. 1997;17(1):109–27.
2. Hack K, Pinto PA, Gollub MJ. Targeted delayed scanning at CT urography: a worthwhile use of radiation? Radiology. 2012;265(1):143–50.
3. Croitoru S, Gross M, Barmeir E. Duplicated ectopic ureter with vaginal insertion: 3D CT urography with i.v. and percutaneous contrast administration. AJR Am J Roentgenol. 2007;189(5):W272–4.
4. Stec AA, Baradaran N, Gearhart JP. Congenital renal anomalies in patients with classic bladder exstrophy. Urology. 2012;79(1):207–9.
5. Caoili EM, Cohan RH, Korobkin M, Platt JF, Francis IR, Faerber GJ, Montie JE, Ellis JH. Urinary tract abnormalities: initial experience with multi-detector row CT urography. Radiology. 2002;222(2):353–60.
6. Limura A, Yi SQ, Terayama H, Naito M, Buhe S, Oguchi T, Takahashi T, Miyaki T, Itoh M. Complete ureteral duplication associated with megaureter and ureteropelvic junction dilatation: report on an adult cadaver case with a brief review of the literature. Ann Anat. 2006;188(4):371–5.

7. Van Der Molen AJ, Cowan NC, Mueller-Lisse UG, Nolte-Ernsting CC, Takahashi S, Cohan RH. CT urography: definition, indications and techniques. A guideline for clinical practice. Eur Radiol. 2008;18(1):4–17.

8. Kwatra N, Shalaby-Rana E, Majd M. Scintigraphic features of duplex kidneys on DMSA renal cortical scans. Pediatr Radiol. 2013;43(9):1204–12.

9. Stacul F, Rossi A, Cova MA. CT urography: the end of IVU? Radiol Med. 2008; 113(5):658–69.

Significant response to nivolumab for metastatic chromophobe renal cell carcinoma with sarcomatoid differentiation

Go Noguchi[1*] (iD), Sohgo Tsutsumi[1], Masato Yasui[1], Shinji Ohtake[2], Susumu Umemoto[1], Noboru Nakaigawa[2], Masahiro Yao[2] and Takeshi Kishida[1]

Abstract

Background: The treatment of advanced or metastatic renal cell carcinoma (RCC) has drastically changed since the approval of immune checkpoint therapy. Nivolumab is a treatment option for patients with metastatic RCC, previously treated with targeted antiangiogenic therapy. The efficacy of nivolumab for patients with RCC was established by the Checkmate 025 clinical trial. Chromophobe RCC (CRCC) represents around 5% of RCC cases, but non-clear cell RCC (non-ccRCC) subtypes were excluded from the Checkmate 025 clinical trial. We report a case in which the use of nivolumab as the seventh-line therapy elicited a significant response in the treatment of metastatic CRCC with sarcomatoid differentiation.

Case presentation: We report a case of a 41-year-old woman with metastatic CRCC with sarcomatoid differentiation. She was treated with sunitinib, pazopanib, everolimus, sorafenib, axtinib, and temsirolimus, but treatment was discontinued because of disease progression or strong adverse events. Seventh-line treatment with nivolumab was initiated and significant clinical improvement was noted after 4 cycles. The treatment was well-tolerated with no significant side effects and the patient continues with nivolumab treatment at present.

Conclusions: Nivolumab may be an attractive treatment option for non-ccRCC patients with sarcomatoid differentiation that exhibited aggressive characteristics and poor prognosis. Further investigation is warranted.

Keywords: Non-clear renal cell carcinoma, Sarcomatoid differentiation, Immune-checkpoint inhibitor, Nivolumab

Background

The treatment of advanced or metastatic renal cell carcinoma (RCC) has been drastically changed by the approval of immune checkpoint therapy. Nivolumab, the fully humanized monoclonal immunoglobulin(Ig)-G4 programmed death 1 (PD-1) checkpoint inhibitor, is a treatment option for patients with metastatic RCC previously treated with targeted antiangiogenic therapy. The efficiency of nivolumab for patients with RCC was established by the Checkmate 025 clinical trial [1]. Chromophobe RCC (CRCC) represents a heterogeneous RCC subtype and comprises about 5% of cases of RCC, but non-clear cell subtypes including CRCC were excluded from the Checkmate 025 trial [1]. To date, only one case of CRCC successfully treated with nivolumab has been reported [2]. We present a case of a patient with CRCC with sarcomatoid differentiation who presented a positive response to nivolumab.

Case presentation

A 41-year-old woman with no medical or family history presented with an incidental right renal tumor. Computed tomography (CT) imaging revealed a 9.5-cm tumor with no evidence of metastatic disease. She underwent right nephrectomy in August 2011. Pathological assessment revealed CRCC with sarcomatoid

* Correspondence: noguchig@kcch.jp
[1]Department of Urology, Kanagawa Cancer Center, 2-3-2, Nakao, Asahi-ku, Yokohama, Kanagawa 2418515, Japan
Full list of author information is available at the end of the article

Significant response to nivolumab for metastatic chromophobe renal cell carcinoma with sarcomatoid...

107

differentiation, 10.5-cm in maximal diameter and nuclear grade 4 (Fuhrman grade). The pathological stage was T2bN0M0.

Recurrence first occurred in September 2012 with multiple lung masses revealed on CT imaging. In February and August 2013, she underwent metastasectomy twice for the bilateral lung tumors, but recurrence reappeared in February 2014 with multiple lung masses and lung hilar lymph nodes. The pathological result of the lung tumors was also CRCC with sarcomatoid differentiation.

In January 2015, she initiated first-line sunitinib on the 2/1 schedule (37.5 mg once daily for 2 consecutive weeks on treatment followed by 1-week-off), but a drug eruption appeared and the treatment with sunitinib was discontinued. In February 2015, she initiated second-line treatment with pazopanib, 800 mg daily, but the first tumor assessment showed progression of disease. In March 2015, third-line treatment with everolimus was administered, but the disease progressed. In July 2015, fourth-line treatment with sorafenib was administered, but a drug eruption appeared. In September 2015, fifth-line treatment with axtinib was administered, but the disease progressed. In May 2016, sixth-line treatment with temsirolimus was administered, but again, the disease progressed. Her performance status was declining and the symptom of hoarseness from a recurrent nerve

paralysis was developing. In July 2016, she decided to receive best supportive care.

In October 2016, nivolumab was approved by pharmaceutical and medical devices agencies in Japan. She initiated seventh-line treatment with nivolumab, 3 mg/kg every 2 weeks, in October 2016. After 4 cycles, a partial response was observed and the symptom of hoarseness was not observed. Significant clinical improvement was noted after 12 cycles (Fig. 1). The treatment has been well-tolerated with no significant side effects thus far, and the patient continues with the treatment of nivolumab at present.

Discussion

RCC includes multiple histological subtypes. The most common subtype is clear cell RCC (ccRCC) (80.5%), followed by papillary RCC (PRCC) (14.3%), and CRCC (5.2%) [3]. Several reports have suggested that localized non-ccRCC is more likely to have a favorable prognosis than that of ccRCC. Paradoxically, some series have shown that metastatic, non-ccRCC exhibits significantly lower response rates for systemic treatment and poorer median progression-free and overall survival than those with ccRCC [4, 5].

Nivolumab is a fully human IgG4 PD-1 immune checkpoint inhibitor antibody that selectively blocks the

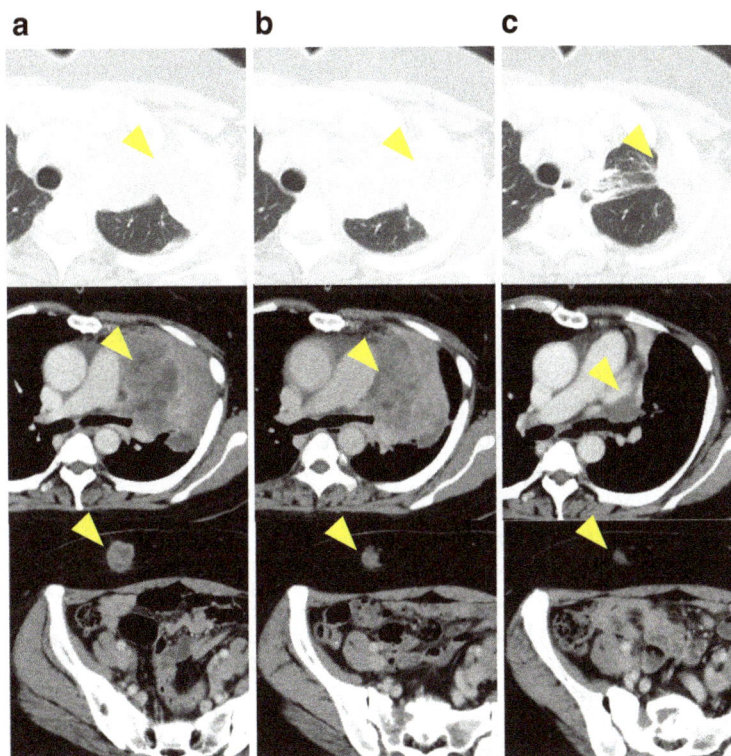

Fig. 1 Computed tomography images demonstrate a decrease in the size of lung nodules, lung hilar lymph node metastases, and skin metastases after four and twelve cycles of nivolumab. **a** Before initiating nivolumab therapy. **b** After four cycles of nivolumab. **c** After twelve cycles of nivolumab

interaction between PD-1 and PD-1 ligands 1 (PD-L1) and 2 [1]. In the CheckMate 025 clinical trial, Motzer et al. suggested a superior response rate with nivolumab versus everolimus (25% vs. 5%, respectively) and longer median overall survival (25.0 months vs. 19.6 months, respectively) [1]. However, non-ccRCC patients were excluded in this study, and no prospective trials on the efficacy of immunotherapy in non-ccRCC have been published previously. Little is known about the efficacy of nivolumab in non-ccRCC. Here, we reported, to the best of our knowledge, the second case of a partial response to nivolumab achieved in a CRCC patient.

Only a few case reports have discussed non-ccRCC treated with immune-checkpoint inhibitors. Rouvinov et al. published the first case report on a CRCC patient with sarcomatoid transformation who exhibited a dramatic response to nivolumab as second-line therapy [2]. Geynisman reported the case of a patient with PRCC with sarcomatoid and rhabdoid features who exhibited an excellent response to nivolumab as third-line therapy [6]. Adra et al. reported the case of a patient with unclassified RCC with sarcomatoid features who demonstrated a significant response to nivolumab as second-line therapy [7].

Sarcomatoid differentiation is expressed in 5.1% of ccRCC and 8.2% of CRCC [3]. It has been reported that the presence of sarcomatoid histologic features in RCC is associated with significantly poor prognosis and outcomes for targeted therapies [8, 9]. On the other hand, Joseph et al. reported that PD-L1 positivity in RCC with sarcomatoid differentiation is detected in 89% of patients with these tumors and they may be good candidates for treatment with anti-PD-1/PD-L1 therapy [9]. It has been reported that PD-L1 expression is detected in 23.9% of ccRCC patients [10] and in 10.9% of non-ccRCC patients (5.6% in CRCC, 10% in PRCC, 30% in Xp11.2 translocation RCC, and 20% in collecting duct carcinoma) [4]; PD-L1 expression in RCC with sarcomatoid differentiation is extremely high.

Although PD-L1 expression is predictive of the response to PD-L1/PD-1 inhibitors in patients with lung cancer and melanoma, this association was not established in patients with ccRCC in the CheckMate 025 trial [1, 11, 12]. However, it is unclear whether PD-L1 expression may be a predictive marker for response to immune checkpoint therapy in patients with non-ccRCC. It has been reported that rapidly growing tumors are very likely to respond to anti-PD-1/PD-L1 therapy; although this is opposite to what has been observed previously in the era of molecular targeted therapy [13], there is a possibility that the prognostic factors established thus far may change greatly. The existence of sarcomatoid differentiation may be a predictive marker for the efficiency of nivolumab in non-ccRCC in the era of immuno-oncology. For patients with non-ccRCC with sarcomatoid differentiation that exhibit aggressive characteristics and poor prognosis, nivolumab may be an effective treatment.

Conclusions

We have reported a case of metastatic CRCC with sarcomatoid differentiation treated with nivolumab as 7th-line therapy with a significant response. Sarcomatoid differentiation may be a predictive marker of the efficiency of nivolumab in patients with non-ccRCC and further investigation is warranted.

Abbreviations

RCC: Renal cell carcinoma; Ig: Immunoglobulin; CRCC: Chromophobe RCC; Non-ccRCC: Non-clear cell RCC; PD-1: Programmed death 1; CT: Computed tomography; ccRCC: Clear cell RCC; PRCC: Papillary RCC; PD-L1: PD-1 ligands 1

Acknowledgements

We would like to thank Editage (www.editage.jp) for English language editing.

Availability of data and materials

Due to ethical restrictions, the raw data underlying this paper is available upon request to the corresponding author.

Authors' contributions

GN was responsible for the concept and drafted the manuscript. ST, MY1, SU and NN gave intellectual content and critically reviewed the manuscript. SO helped to provide patient history and helped in the writing of the manuscript. MY2 and TK treated the patient and helped to draft the manuscript. All authors have read and approved the final manuscript.

Competing interests

The authors declare that they have no competing interests.

Author details

[1]Department of Urology, Kanagawa Cancer Center, 2-3-2, Nakao, Asahi-ku, Yokohama, Kanagawa 2418515, Japan. [2]Department of Urology, Yokohama City University Graduate School of Medicine, Yokohama, Japan.

References

1. Motzer RJ, Escudier B, McDermott DF, George S, Hammers HJ, Srinivas S, Tykodi SS, Sosman JA, Procopio G, Plimack ER, et al. Nivolumab versus Everolimus in advanced renal-cell carcinoma. N Engl J Med. 2015;373(19):1803–13.
2. Rouvinov K, Osyntsov L, Shaco-Levy R, Baram N, Ariad S, Mermershtain W. Rapid response to Nivolumab in a patient with sarcomatoid transformation of Chromophobe renal cell carcinoma. Clin Genitourin Cancer. 2017;15(6):e1127–30.
3. Leibovich BC, Lohse CM, Crispen PL, Boorjian SA, Thompson RH, Blute ML, Cheville JC. Histological subtype is an independent predictor of outcome for patients with renal cell carcinoma. J Urol. 2010;183(4):1309–15.
4. Choueiri TK, Fay AP, Gray KP, Callea M, Ho TH, Albiges L, Bellmunt J, Song J, Carvo I, Lampron M, et al. PD-L1 expression in nonclear-cell renal cell carcinoma. Ann Oncol. 2014;25(11):2178–84.
5. Vera-Badillo FE, Templeton AJ, Duran I, Ocana A, de Gouveia P, Aneja P, Knox JJ, Tannock IF, Escudier B, Amir E. Systemic therapy for non-clear cell renal cell carcinomas: a systematic review and meta-analysis. Eur Urol. 2015; 67(4):740–9.

6. Geynisman DM. Anti-programmed cell death protein 1 (PD-1) antibody Nivolumab leads to a dramatic and rapid response in papillary renal cell carcinoma with Sarcomatoid and Rhabdoid features. Eur Urol. 2015;68(5):912–4.

7. Adra N, Cheng L, Pili R. Unclassified renal cell carcinoma with significant response to Nivolumab. Clin Genitourin Cancer. 2017;15(3):e517–9.

8. Golshayan AR, George S, Heng DY, Elson P, Wood LS, Mekhail TM, Garcia JA, Aydin H, Zhou M, Bukowski RM, et al. Metastatic sarcomatoid renal cell carcinoma treated with vascular endothelial growth factor-targeted therapy. J Clin Oncol. 2009;27(2):235–41.

9. Joseph RW, Millis SZ, Carballido EM, Bryant D, Gatalica Z, Reddy S, Bryce AH, Vogelzang NJ, Stanton ML, Castle EP, et al. PD-1 and PD-L1 expression in renal cell carcinoma with Sarcomatoid differentiation. Cancer Immunol Res. 2015;3(12):1303–7.

10. Thompson RH, Kuntz SM, Leibovich BC, Dong H, Lohse CM, Webster WS, Sengupta S, Frank I, Parker AS, Zincke H, et al. Tumor B7-H1 is associated with poor prognosis in renal cell carcinoma patients with long-term follow-up. Cancer Res. 2006;66(7):3381–5.

11. Reck M, Rodriguez-Abreu D, Robinson AG, Hui R, Csoszi T, Fulop A, Gottfried M, Peled N, Tafreshi A, Cuffe S, et al. Pembrolizumab versus chemotherapy for PD-L1-positive non-small-cell lung Cancer. N Engl J Med. 2016;375(19):1823–33.

12. Larkin J, Chiarion-Sileni V, Gonzalez R, Grob JJ, Cowey CL, Lao CD, Schadendorf D, Dummer R, Smylie M, Rutkowski P, et al. Combined Nivolumab and Ipilimumab or monotherapy in untreated melanoma. N Engl J Med. 2015;373(1):23–34.

13. Champiat S, Dercle L, Ammari S, Massard C, Hollebecque A, Postel-Vinay S, Chaput N, Eggermont A, Marabelle A, Soria JC, et al. Hyperprogressive disease is a new pattern of progression in Cancer patients treated by anti-PD-1/PD-L1. Clin Cancer Res. 2017;23(8):1920–8.

17

Multicystic nephroma masquerading as hydatid cyst: a diagnostic challenge

Abdelmoneim E. M. Kheir[1*], Aziza M. Elnaeema[2], Sara M. A. Gafer[3], Sawsan A. Mohammed[4] and Mustafa E. Bahar[5]

Abstract

Background: Multicystic nephroma is an uncommon, non-familial renal neoplasm that is usually benign. About 200 cases of this lesion have been described in the literature.

Case presentation: We report on a Sudanese child who presented at the age of two and a half years with an abdominal mass, clinical and radiological features favored the diagnosis of hydatid cyst which is endemic in this African tropical country, and the diagnosis of multicystic nephroma was only possible after histopathological examination.

Conclusion: Multicystic nephroma is a rare benign tumour with an excellent prognosis. Clinical and radiological differentiation of multicystic nephroma from hydatid cyst is difficult. Thus, histopathological examination of the surgical specimens seems to be the only feasible method of making the correct diagnosis.

Keywords: Multicystic nephroma, Hydatid cyst, Benign, Sudan, Case report

Background

Multicystic nephroma (MCN) is a rare, non-familial renal tumour, that has a benign nature. About 200 cases of this lesion have been reported so far [1]. Different names have been used to describe this renal mass, including solitary multilocular cyst, multilocular renal cyst, renal cystadenoma, cystic renal hamartoma and partial polycystic kidney. Due to similarities in age, sex and histochemical profile, adult cystic nephroma is now classified within this group of mixed epithelial and stromal tumours, and the world health organization (WHO) renal tumour subcommittee recommended using the term mixed epithelial and stromal tumour family for both entities [2]. As opposed to adult cystic nephroma, paediatric cystic nephroma is now regarded a separate entity with specific DICER1 mutations [3]. MCN can be seen in both infants and adults. Seventy-three percent of the patients are males and aged between 2 and 4 years [4].

The pathogenesis of MCN remains unclear, [5] thus its origin is designated as being dysplastic/hamartomatous/neoplastic. Histologic features include: cysts lined by flat,

cuboidal, or hobnail epithelium and septa variably lined by fibrous and/or ovarian-like stroma. These histological features are quite unique, however confusion does occur with other cystic renal tumours, especially cystic renal cell carcinoma which can lead to conflict in the treatment of this lesion [6].

We describe a Sudanese child who presented at the age of two and a half years with an abdominal mass, clinical and radiological features favored the diagnosis of hydatid cyst and the diagnosis of multicystic nephroma was only possible after histopathological examination. To our knowledge this is the first case report of multicystic nephroma masquerading as hydatid cyst from a tropical country in Africa.

Case presentation

A two and a half year old male child from Darfur province, west of Sudan was brought by his parents because of abdominal distension for 8 months prior to admission. The distension was associated with mild pain and no symptoms related to the urinary or gastrointestinal systems. His past medical history was unremarkable apart from poor socioeconomic status and contact with livestock and sheepdogs. Physical examination revealed a slightly pale child with no jaundice and no lymphadenopathy. Abdomen was grossly distended with bulging of

* Correspondence: moneimkheir62@hotmail.com
[1]Department of Paediatrics and Child Health, Faculty of Medicine, University of Khartoum and Soba University Hospital, P.O. Box 102, Khartoum, Sudan
Full list of author information is available at the end of the article

the right flank, there was umbilical hernia. There were cautery marks, striae, and superficial veins (Fig. 1). Superficially abdomen was tense with palpable right sided abdominal mass extending from the right renal angel to the umbilicus about (15 × 25 cm), no hepatosplenomegaly and negative shifting dullness. His vital signs including blood pressure were normal.

Investigations performed included a full blood count which showed nutritional anaemia, ESR 57 mm/h. His renal and liver function tests were entirely normal. Urine analysis was also normal. CXR was normal.

The first abdominal ultrasound revealed a huge right cystic renal mass, containing small daughter cysts arranged eccentrically as well as few septations with normal left kidney. Findings were compatible with right renal embryonic multi cystic tumor. A repeat ultrasound in a different setup showed the same findings with a strong possibility of hydatid renal disease. Computed tomography (CT) of the chest was normal and CT abdomen showed a large cystic mass arising from the right kidney consistent with hydatid cyst (Fig. 2). The paediatric surgeon was consulted who requested a dynamic renal scan that showed a nonfunctioning right kidney with features of parenchymal effacement. The suspicion for hydatid disease was high based on the radiological findings of a large cystic mass, the geographical prevalence and patient risk factors for hydatid cyst. The child was commenced on Albendazole (antihelminthic drug) and a radical right sided nephrectomy was performed 4 weeks later and the cyst ruptured during the operation (Fig. 3), the dimensions of the mass was 7×13 cm. Histopathological examination showed multiple cysts separated from renal tissue by fibrous tissue, the cysts were

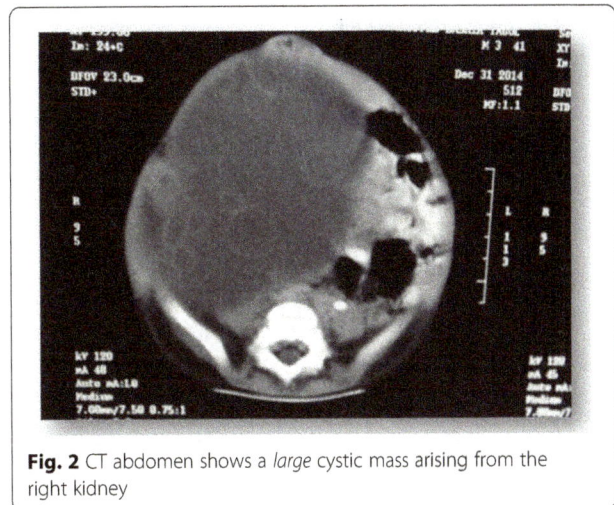

Fig. 2 CT abdomen shows a *large* cystic mass arising from the right kidney

lined by flattened to columnar epithelium, some showing hobnail pattern (Fig. 4). The renal tissue was composed of hyalinized glomeruli, atrophied tubules and mixed inflammatory cellular infiltration. All was consistent with multicystic nephroma. The child had a benign postoperative course and was discharged home in good condition with a view for follow up in outpatient clinic.

Discussion

The first case of MCN in the literature was reported by Edmund et al. as cystic nephroma of the kidney in 1892 [7]. In 1956, Boggs and Kimmelstiel first proposed the true neoplastic nature of the lesions in a case report, suggesting the term benign multilocular cystic nephroma for this condition [8].

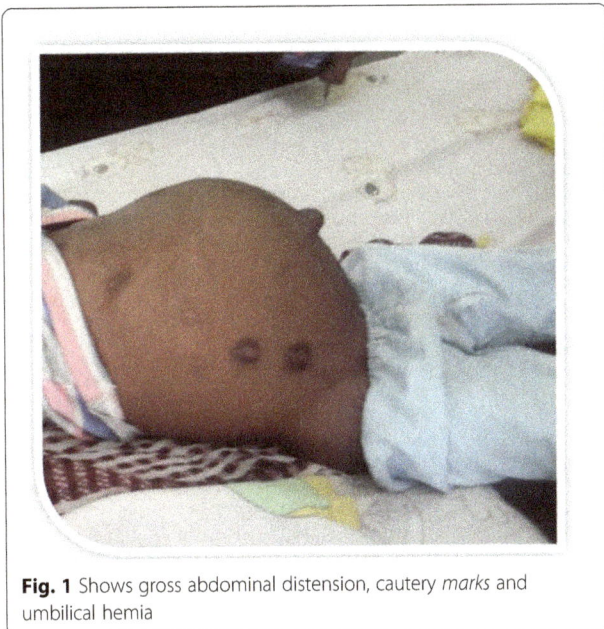

Fig. 1 Shows gross abdominal distension, cautery *marks* and umbilical hemia

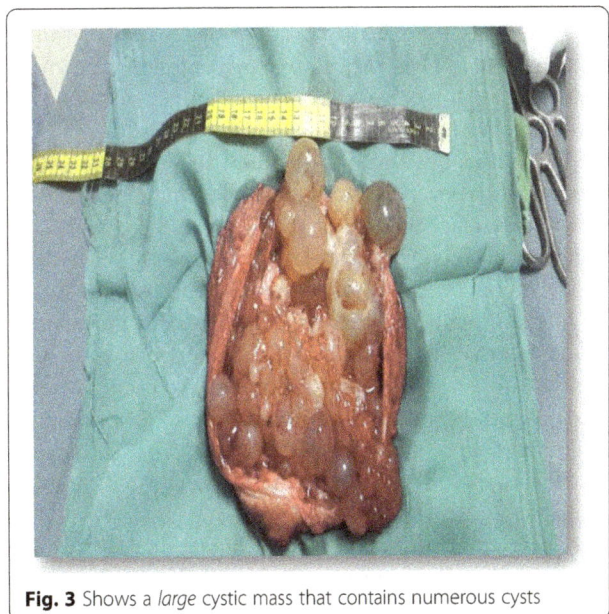

Fig. 3 Shows a *large* cystic mass that contains numerous cysts

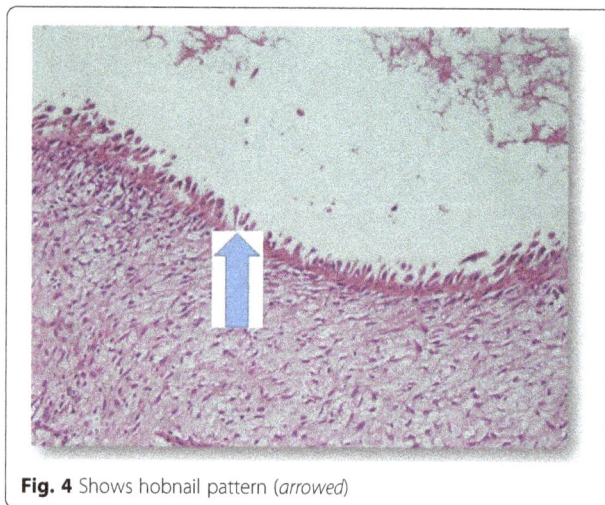

Fig. 4 Shows hobnail pattern (*arrowed*)

MCN is diagnosed by set of criteria as suggested by Powell et al. in 1951 [9] and later modified in 1956 [8]. The diagnostic criteria of cystic nephroma established by Joshi and Beckwith et al. [10] are used widely and include the following: multilocular, solitary, unilateral, noncommunication between the renal pelvis and the cystic lesion, a definite lining of epithelium on the loculi, no nephron in the interlobular septa, and normal residual renal tissue. Our case meets these criteria.

Our case was a two and a half year old male child with unilateral MCN, and this is similar to what is reported in the literature [4], however bilateral cases also have been reported [2]. The usual presentation of MCN is a benign clinical course, asymptomatic abdominal mass, with non-specific symptoms as abdominal pain, hematuria, and urinary tract infection [11]. The main complaint in our case was abdominal mass and pain without haematuria. Haematuria can be seen in all age groups and is thought to be due to extension of tumor into the renal pelvis [12]. Rarely presentation can sometimes be with severe colicky abdominal pain due to spontaneous rupture of the cyst [13].

The background history of our case was poor socio-economic status, poor sanitation and contact with livestock and sheepdogs, all these, together with the radiological findings, favored the diagnosis of hydatid cyst (Echinococcosis) . Cystic echinococcosis is caused by infection with the larvae of Echinococcus granulosus. Areas of the world with noted prevalence are rural regions of Africa, southern Europe, Asia, the Middle East, Central and South America and is principally maintained in a dog–sheep–dog cycle, [14]. Serological tests were not done for our case because they aren't available.

At present there is no reliable clinical or radiographic means to differentiate cystic nephroma from other cystic renal disease in children [15]. The non-specific clinical

findings and the poor contribution of imaging studies make the exact preoperative distinction from other cystic renal neoplasia difficult and as a result

histopathological examination from a resected specimen seems to be the only feasible method of making the correct diagnosis [5].

Because preoperative diagnosis is difficult to achieve and multicystic renal cell carcinoma is suspected, radical nephrectomy is the standard treatment of choice. Our case had a radical right nephrectomy as the diagnosis was uncertain and the dynamic renal scan showed a nonfunctioning right kidney. In cases of solitary, localized, unilateral lesions less than 4 cm with frozen section proven diagnosis, nephron-sparing surgery is advocated [16]. The prognosis is usually good for MCN and surgical excision is curative, however, these cases should be followed up because three cases of local recurrence have been reported [17].

Conclusion

MCN is a rare benign tumour which has a good prognosis. Clinical and radiological differential diagnosis of MCN from hydatid cyst is difficult. Thus, histopathological examination of the surgical specimens seems to be the only feasible method of making the correct diagnosis.

Abbreviations
CT: Computed tomography; MCN: Multicystic nephroma; WHO: World Health Organization

Acknowledgements
We would like to thank the family of the child mentioned in this report for permitting to use of the case details and photographs. Thanks are also extended to the staff of the paediatric ward at Soba University Hospital.

Funding
There was no research grant for this study.

Authors' contributions
AK, AE and SG made substantial contributions to conception and acquisition of data and analysis and interpretation of data. SM and MB helped to draft the manuscript as well as extensive literature search. All authors read and approved the final manuscript.

Competing interests
The authors declare that they have no competing interests.

Author details
[1]Department of Paediatrics and Child Health, Faculty of Medicine, University of Khartoum and Soba University Hospital, P.O. Box 102, Khartoum, Sudan. [2]Paediatric Surgeon and Paediatric Urologist, Soba University Hospital, Ahfad University for Women, Omdurman, Sudan. [3]Department of Paediatrics, Soba University Hospital, Khartoum, Sudan. [4]Department of Histopathology, Soba University Hospital, Khartoum, Sudan. [5]Department of Radiology, Soba University Hospital, Khartoum, Sudan.

References

1. Singh S, Gupta R, Khurana N, Aggarwal SK, Mandal AK. Multicystic nephroma–report of two cases. Indian J Pathol Microbiol. 2004;47:520–3.

2. Moch H, Cubilla AL, Humphrey PA, Reuter VE, Ulbright TM. The 2016 WHO classification of tumours of the urinary system and male genital organs-part a: renal, penile, and testicular tumours. Eur Urol. 2016;70(1):93–105.

3. Doros LA, Rossi CT, Yang J, et al. DICER1 mutations in childhood cystic nephroma and its relationship to DICER1-renal sarcoma. Mod Pathol. 2014; 27:1267–80.

4. Castillo OA, Boyle Jr ET, Kramer SA. Multilocular cysts of kidney. A study of 29 patients and review of literature. Urology. 1991;37:156–62.

5. Sacher P, Willi UV, Niggli F, et al. Cystic nephroma: a rare benign renal tumor. Pediatr Surg Int. 1998;13:197–9.

6. Bonsib SM. Cystic nephroma. Mixed epithelial and stromal tumor. In: Eble JN, Sauter G, Epstein JL, Sesterhenn IA, editors. Pathology and genetics of tumors of the urinary system and male genital organs; WHO classification of tumours. Lyon: IARC Press; 2004. p. 76.

7. Edmunds W. Cystic adenoma of the kidney. Trans Pathol Soc Lond. 1892;43: 89–90.

8. Boggs LK, Kimmelstiel P. Benign multilocular cystic nephroma: report of two cases of so-called multilocular cyst of the kidney. J Urol. 1956;76:530–41.

9. Powell T, Shackman R, Johnson HD. Multilocular cysts of the kidney. Br J Urol. 1951;23:142.

10. Joshi VV, Beckwith JB. Multilocular cyst of the kidney (cystic nephroma) and cystic, partially differentiated nephroblastoma. Terminology and criteria for diagnosis. Cancer. 1989;64:466–79.

11. Agrons GA, Wagner BJ, Davidson AJ, et al. Multilocular cystic renal tumor in children: radiologic pathologic correlation. Radiographics. 1995;15:653–69.

12. Bouhafs A, Cherradi N, Lamaalmi N, Belkacem R, Barahioui M. An unusual case of multilocular cystic nephroma with prominent renal pelvis involvement. Int J Urol. 2006;13(4):436–8.

13. Fujimoto K, Samma S, Fukui Y, Yamaguchi A, Hirayama A, Kikkawa A. Spontaneously ruptured multilocular cystic nephroma. Int J Urol. 2002;9(3): 183–6.

14. Tappe D, Zidowitz S, Demmer P, Kern P, Barth TF, Frosch M. Three-dimensional reconstruction of Echinococcus multilocularis larval growth in human hepatic tissue reveals complex growth patterns. Am J Trop Med Hyg. 2010;82(1):126–7.

15. Boybeyi O, Karnak I, Orhan D, et al. Cystic nephroma and localized renal cystic disease in children: diagnostic clues and management. J Pediatr Surg. 2008;43:1985–9.

16. Kuzgunbay B, Turunc T, Bolat F, Kilinc F. Adult cystic nephroma: a case report and a review of the literature. Urol Oncol. 2009;27(4):407–9.

17. Bastian PJ, Kuhlmann R, Vogel J, Bastian HP, Bastian H. Local recurrence of a unilateral cystic nephroma. Int J Urol. 2004;11:329–31.

18

Intraoperative and postoperative feasibility and safety of total tubeless, tubeless, small-bore tube, and standard percutaneous nephrolithotomy

Joo Yong Lee[1], Seong Uk Jeh[2], Man Deuk Kim[3], Dong Hyuk Kang[4], Jong Kyou Kwon[5], Won Sik Ham[1], Young Deuk Choi[1] and Kang Su Cho[6*]

Abstract

Background: Percutaneous nephrolithotomy (PCNL) is performed to treat relatively large renal stones. Recent publications indicate that tubeless and total tubeless (stentless) PCNL is safe in selected patients. We performed a systematic review and network meta-analysis to evaluate the feasibility and safety of different PCNL procedures, including total tubeless, tubeless with stent, small-bore tube, and large-bore tube PCNLs.

Methods: PubMed, Cochrane Central Register of Controlled Trials, and EMBASE™ databases were searched to identify randomized controlled trials published before December 30, 2013. One researcher examined all titles and abstracts found by the searches. Two investigators independently evaluated the full-text articles to determine whether those met the inclusion criteria. Qualities of included studies were rated with Cochrane's risk-of-bias assessment tool.

Results: Sixteen studies were included in the final syntheses including pairwise and network meta-analyses. Operation time, pain scores, and transfusion rates were not significantly different between PCNL procedures. Network meta-analyses demonstrated that for hemoglobin changes, total tubeless PCNL may be superior to standard PCNL (mean difference [MD] 0.65, 95% CI 0.14–1.13) and tubeless PCNLs with stent (MD -1.14, 95% CI -1.65–-0.62), and small-bore PCNL may be superior to tubeless PCNL with stent (MD 1.30, 95% CI 0.27–2.26). Network meta-analyses also showed that for length of hospital stay, total tubeless (MD 1.33, 95% CI 0.23–2.43) and tubeless PCNLs with stent (MD 0.99, 95% CI 0.19–1.79) may be superior to standard PCNL. In rank probability tests, small-bore tube and total tubeless PCNLs were superior for operation time, pain scores, and hemoglobin changes.

Conclusions: For hemoglobin changes, total tubeless and small-bore PCNLs may be superior to other methods. For hospital stay, total tubeless and tubeless PCNLs with stent may be superior to other procedures.

Keywords: Calculi, Lithotripsy, Nephrostomy, Percutaneous, Meta-analysis, Bayes theorem

* Correspondence: kscho99@yuhs.ac
[6]Department of Urology, Gangnam Severance Hospital, Urological Science Institute, Yonsei University College of Medicine, 211 Eonju-ro, Gangnam-gu, Seoul 06273, South Korea
Full list of author information is available at the end of the article

Background

Urinary stone is one of the most prevalent urological disorders. Reports suggest that up to 12% of people will suffer from urinary tract calculi during their lifetime, and the rates of recurrence is close to 50% [1]. There are several treatment modalities for renal stones, including observation expecting spontaneous passage, extracorporeal shock wave lithotripsy (ESWL), percutaneous nephrolithotomy (PCNL), and retrograde intrarenal surgery (RIRS) using flexible ureterorenoscope [2]. PCNL is currently the standard treatment for large renal stones considered too large for or refractory to shock wave lithotripsy [3, 4]. Conventionally, a 20-24 French nephrostomy catheter is placed routinely after PCNL to provide urine drainage, prevent extravasation of urine, and make tamponade against bleeding [5, 6]. In addition, it can be used as a tract for a second-look PCNL [7]. The need for placing a conventional large-bore nephrostomy catheter has been questioned because of its accompanying increase in postoperative discomfort and other morbidity, and the low incidence of second-look operations [8, 9]. In recent years, tubeless or small-bore PCNL has been widely used, and previously reported systematic reviews have demonstrated the safety and efficacy in these techniques.

The recently introduced network meta-analysis is a meta-analysis in which multiple treatments are compared using both direct comparisons of interventions within randomized controlled trials (RCTs), and indirect comparisons across trials based on a common comparator [10–14]. Thus, we performed a systematic review and network meta-analysis based on published relevant studies to evaluate the feasibility and safety of each PCNL procedure, including total tubeless, tubeless with stent, small-bore tube, and large-bore tube PCNLs, for the treatment of renal stones.

Methods

Inclusion and exclusion criteria

Reported RCTs that fitted the following criteria were selected: (i) a design of each study that involved comparing the feasibility and safety for least two PCNL procedures, including total tubeless, tubeless with stent, small-bore tube, and large-bore tube PCNLs; (ii) the study groups were matched for baseline characteristics, including the total number of subjects and the values of each variable; (iii) at least one of the following outcomes was assessed: operation time, hospital stay length, hemoglobin decrease, return to normal activity, and complication rate; and (iv) the full text of each study was accessible and written in English.

The exclusion criteria were as follows: (i) noncomparative studies; (ii) the trial included children; and (iii) the trial did not exclude patients who underwent bilateral simultaneous PCNL or had complete or partial staghorn stones, more than two nephrostomy tracts, anatomical anomalies, or urinary infection. This report was prepared in compliance with the Preferred Reporting Items for Systematic Reviews and Meta-Analyses (PRISMA) statement (accessible at http://www.prisma-statement.org/) [15].

Search strategy

A literature search was performed to identify RCTS published prior to December 30, 2013 in PubMed, the Cochrane Central Register of Controlled Trials, and EMBASE™ online databases. A cross-reference search of eligible articles was performed to identify additional studies not found by the computerized search. Combinations of the following MeSH and key words were used: percutaneous nephrolithotomy or nephrostomy or percutaneous nephrostomy or nephrolithiasis or PCNL or PCN or PNL, and total tubeless or tubeless or nephrostomy free.

Data extraction

One researcher (J.Y.L.) screened the title and abstract of all articles retrieved using the search strategy. The other two investigators (D.H.K. and H.L.) independently assessed the full text of the articles to determine whether they met the inclusion criteria. For each included study, the following data were extracted independently as follows; authors, date, demographics of included patients, PCNL methods, feasibility, efficacy outcomes, complications, and inclusion of a reference standard. Disagreements arising in the study selection and data extraction processes were resolved by discussion until a consensus was reached or by arbitration employing another researcher (K.S.C.).

Study quality assessment

Once the final group of articles was agreed upon, two researchers (J.Y.L. and D.H.K.) independently examined the quality of each article using the Cochrane's risk-of-bias as a quality assessment tool for RCTs. The assessment involves the assignment of a "yes," "no," or "unclear" rating for each domain, designating a low, high, or unclear risk of bias, respectively. If ≤1 domain was rated "unclear" or "no," the study was classified as having a low risk of bias. If ≥4 domains were rated "unclear" or "no," the study was classified as having a high risk of bias. If 2 or 3 domains were rated "unclear" or "no," the study was classified as having a moderate risk of bias. [16]. Quality assessment was performed using Review Manager 5.2 (RevMan 5.2.11, Cochrane Collaboration, Oxford, UK).

Statistical analyses

Each outcome variable at specific time-points was compared by network meta-analysis using the odds ratio (OR) or mean difference (MD) with 95% confidence interval (CI). A random-effect model was used. Each analysis was based on non-informative priors for effect size and precision. Convergence and lack of auto-correlation were checked and confirmed after four chains and a 50,000-simulation burn-in phase, and direct probability statements were based on an additional 100,000-simulation phase. Calculation of the probability that each group had the lowest rate of clinical events was performed using Bayesian Markov Chain Monte Carlo modeling. Sensitivity analyses were performed by repeating the main computations using a fixed-effect method. Model fit was appraised by computing and comparing estimates for deviance and deviance information criterion. Pairwise inconsistency and inconsistency between direct and indirect effect estimates were assessed with the I^2-statistic, with values <25%, 25% to 50%, and >50% representing mild, moderate, and severe inconsistency, respectively. The extent of small study effects/publication bias was assessed by visual inspection of funnel plots for the pairwise meta-analyses. All statistical analyses were performed using Review Manager 5 and R (R version 3.0.3, R Foundation for Statistical Computing, Vienna, Austria; http://www.r-project.org) [17], and its meta, forestplot, gemtc, and R2WinBUGS packages for pairwise and network meta-analyses using Bayesian Markov Chain Monte Carlo modeling.

Results

Eligible studies

Our database search identified 43 studies that could be potentially included in the meta-analysis. Based on the inclusion and exclusion criteria, 18 articles were excluded during screening of the titles and abstracts because they were retrospective studies (11 articles) or case series (7 articles). This left 25 RCTS that evaluated various types of PCNL procedures for renal stones. After reviewing the full-text articles for these studies, 9 were excluded because they reported irrelevant results. Therefore, 16 RCTs were ultimately included in the qualitative analysis, as well as the quantitative synthesis using pairwise and network meta-analyses (Fig. 1).

There were differences in procedures among the included studies. Five studies included comparisons between standard and total tubeless PCNLs, and five RCTs also compared standard and tubeless PCNLs. Four trials reported on various factors in small-bore and tubeless PCNLs. In two studies, the results of three arms—standard, small-bore, and tubeless PCNLs—were published (Table 1). Finally, the included studies covered four different PCNL procedures: total tubeless, tubeless, standard and small-bore PCNLs (Fig. 2).

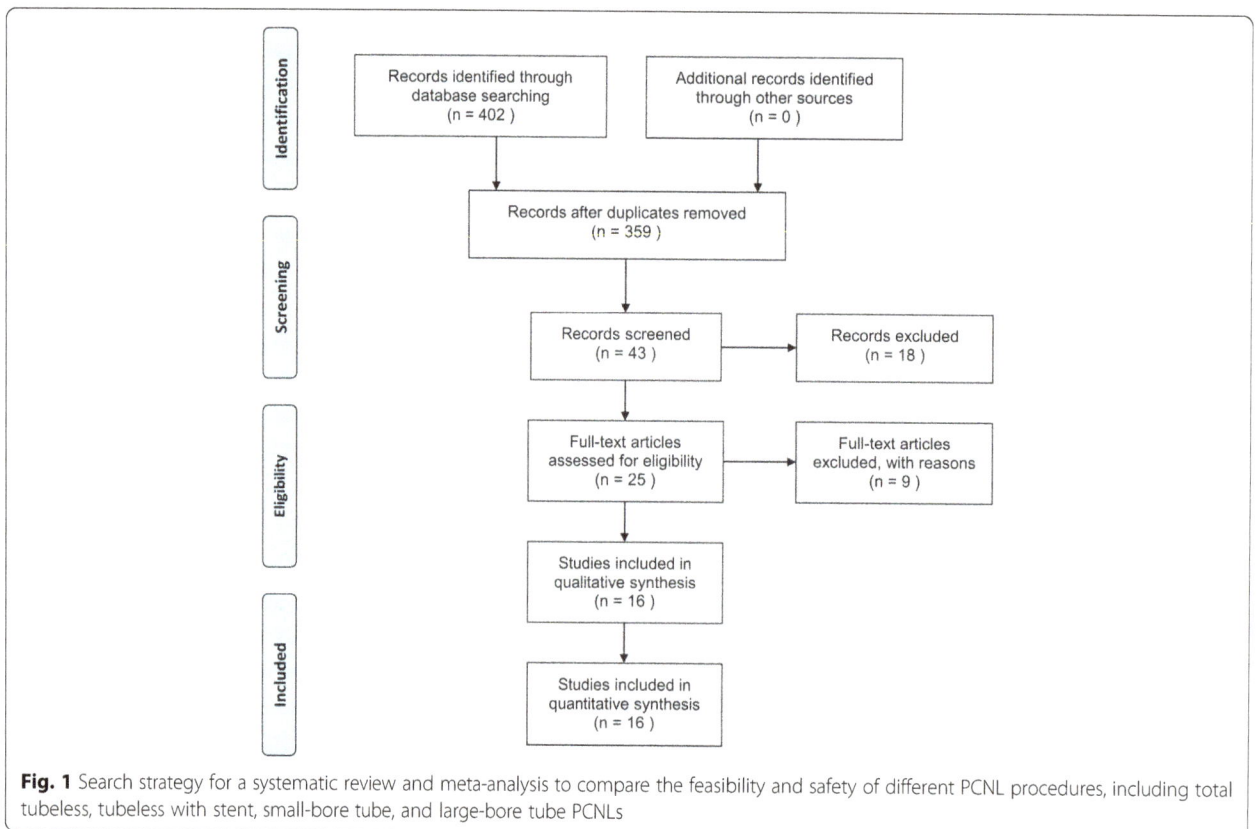

Fig. 1 Search strategy for a systematic review and meta-analysis to compare the feasibility and safety of different PCNL procedures, including total tubeless, tubeless with stent, small-bore tube, and large-bore tube PCNLs

Table 1 Characteristics of included trials

Study	Year	Design	Procedures	Sample size	Age (year)	Stone burden Size	P-value	Tube	Stone-free rate (%)	P-value	Quality assessment
Chang et al. [41].	2011	RCT	Standard	63	58.7	24.86 ± 2.78 mm	0.722	20 Fr (7 Fr)	75%	0.51	Low
			Total tubeless	68	59.2	24.74 ± 2.69 mm		None	74%		
Aghamir et al. [42].	2011	RCT	Standard	35	40	2.87 ± 0.62 cm²	0.66	NA	83%	NA	Low
			Total tubeless	35	38.4	2.81 ± 0.59 cm²		None	86%		
Kara et al. [43].	2010	RCT	Standard	30	66.5	25.6 mm	NA	18 Fr	90%	>0.05	Low
			Total tubeless	30	67.7	22.3 mm		None	96%		
Mishra et al. [44].	2010	RCT	Standard	11	42.5	2737 µL	0.18	20 Fr	81.8%	0.14	Low
			Tubeless	11	42.3	2934.2 µL		None (6 Fr)	72.7%		
Istanbulluoglu et al. [45].	2009	RCT	Standard	45	43.9	432.35 ± 195.97 mm²	0.46	14 Fr	NA	NA	Low
			Total tubeless	45	47.5	448.93 ± 249.13 mm²		None	NA		
Crook et al. [46].	2008	RCT	Standard	25	53	17.5 mm	NA	26 Fr	84%	NA	Low
			Total tubeless	25	52	21.6 mm		None	96%		
Agrawal et al. [47].	2008	RCT	Standard	101	31	NA	NA	16 Fr	100%	–	Low
			Tubeless	101	33	NA		None (6 Fr)	100%		
Singh et al. [48].	2008	RCT	Standard	30	34	800 mm²	>0.05	22 Fr	93.3%	0.64	Moderate
			Tubeless	30	31	750 mm²		None (NA)	90%		
Shah et al. [18].	2008	RCT	Small-bore tube	32	46.7	495.92 mm²	0.88	8Fr	87.5%	0.96	Low
			Tubeless	33	44.1	535.36 mm²		None (6 Fr)	87.9%		
Sofikerim et al. [35].	2007	RCT	Standard	24	54.1	425 mm²	NA	24 Fr or 18 Fr	85% (24 Fr),	0.71	Moderate
			Tubeless	24	47.8	428 mm²		None (6 Fr)	83% (18 Fr), 79%		
Tefekli et al. [49].	2007	RCT	Standard	18	41.32	3.1 cm	NA	14 Fr	89%	>0.05	Moderate
			Tubeless	17	38.4	2.8 cm		None (NA)	94%		
Weiland et al. [50].	2007	RCT	Small-bore tube	9	65	6.7 cm²	0.15	8.3 Fr			Moderate
			Tubeless	9	54	3.2 cm²		None (8.2 Fr)			
Choi et al. [32].	2006	RCT	Small-bore tube	12	47	32.41 mm	0.77	8.2 Fr	91.7%	0.64	High
			Tubeless	12	52.9	28.5 mm		None (6 Fr)	100%		
Desai et al. [51].	2004	RCT	Standard	10	43.4	263.7 mm²	>0.05	20 Fr	100%	–	Moderate
			Small-bore tube	10	44.8	243 mm²		9 Fr	100%		
			Tubeless	10	41.1	249.1 mm²		None (6 Fr)	100%		

Table 1 Characteristics of included trials (Continued)

Study	Year	Type		N								
Marcovich et al. [52].	2004	RCT	Standard	20	58	3.6 cm	0.64	24 Fr		0.63	Moderate
			Small-bore tube	20	61	3 cm		8 Fr			
			Tubeless	20	57	3.4 cm		None (NA)			
Feng et al. [53].	2001	RCT	Standard	10	53	8.4 cm^3	0.75	22 Fr	31.5%	NA	Moderate
			Tubeless	8	62	4.4 cm^3		None (NA)	71.4%		

NA not applicable, *RCT* randomized controlled trial

Fig. 2 Comparison network of included randomized controlled trials. Five studies included comparisons between standard and total tubeless PCNLs, and five RCTs also compared standard and tubeless PCNLs. Four trials reported on various factors in small-bore and tubeless PCNLs. In two studies, the results of three arms—standard, small-bore, and tubeless PCNLs—were published

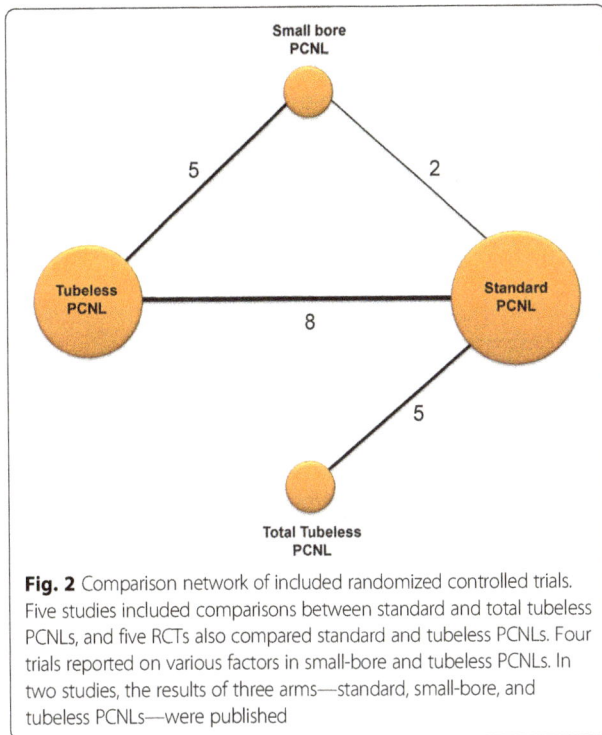

Quality assessment and publication bias

Figures 3 and 4 present the details of quality assessment, as measured by the Cochrane Collaboration risk-of-bias tool. Seven trials exhibited a moderate risk of bias for all quality criteria and only one study was classified as having a high risk of bias (Table 1). For operation time, hemoglobin change, and transfusion rate, little evidence of publication bias was demonstrated on funnel plots; however, for the visual analogue scale (VAS) pain score and hospital stay, moderate evidence of publication bias was demonstrated on these plots (Fig. 5).

Operation time

During the pairwise meta-analysis of operation time between standard and total tubeless PCNLs, there was a significant degree of heterogeneity among these studies, and data were pooled with a random effects model (P = 0.04, I^2 = 69%). There was no statistically significant difference in operation time between standard and total tubeless PCNLs, although the MD was 6.19 (95% CI -0.14 to 12.52) (Fig. 6a). Between standard and tubeless PCNLs with stent, the MD also demonstrated no statistical difference (MD 7.43, 95% CI -1.70 to 16.57) (Fig. 6b). Likewise, the MDs did not exhibit statistically significant differences for standard versus small-bore PCNLs (MD -1.0, 95% CI -11.93 to 9.93) or tubeless versus small-bore PCNLs (MD 0.86, 95% CI -7.95 to 9.68) (Fig. 6c). Using network meta-analysis, there were no significant differences among all procedures (Fig. 7a) (Table 2), although total tubeless and small-bore PCNLs had higher rank probabilities than the other procedures (Fig. 8a).

	Random sequence generation (selection bias)	Allocation concealment (selection bias)	Incomplete outcome data (attrition bias)	Selective reporting (reporting bias)	Other bias
Aghamir 2011	+	+	+	+	+
Agrawal 2008	+	+	+	+	+
Chang 2011	+	?	+	+	+
Choi 2006	−	−	?	−	+
Crook 2008	+	+	+	+	+
Desai 2004	−	+	?	+	+
Feng 2001	−	−	?	+	+
Istanbulluoglu 2009	+	+	+	+	+
Kara 2010	?	+	+	+	+
Marcovich 2004	+	−	?	+	+
Mishra 2010	+	+	?	+	+
Shah 2008	+	+	?	+	+
Singh 2008	−	−	−	+	+
Sofikerim 2007	+	−	?	+	+
Tefekli 2007	−	−	?	+	+
Weiland 2007	−	−	?	+	+

Fig. 3 Risk-of-bias summary: review of the authors' judgments on each risk-of-bias item for each included study

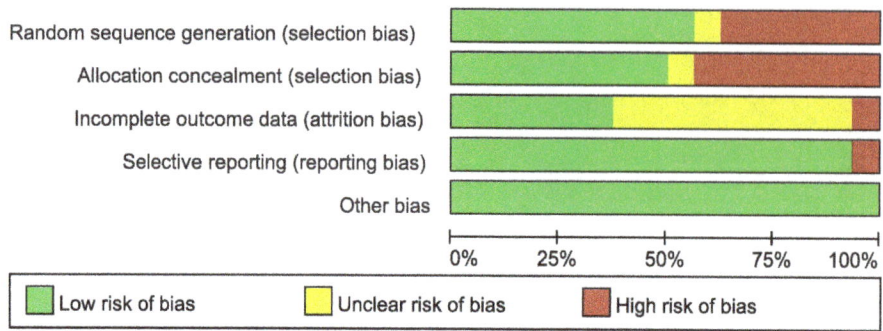

Fig. 4 Risk-of-bias graph: review of the authors' judgments on each risk-of-bias item presented as percentages across all included studies

Visual analogue scale pain score

In the pairwise meta-analysis of VAS pain scores, there was a significant degree of heterogeneity among studies and the data were pooled with a random effects model. There were no statistically significant differences comparing standard versus total tubeless PCNLs with stent (MD 0.06, 95% CI -0.56 to 0.69, $P = 0.84$) (Fig. 9a) or tubeless versus small-bore PCNLs (MD 1.21, 95% CI -0.02 to 2.44, $P = 0.05$) (Fig. 9b). In the network meta-analysis, there were no statistically significant differences among all

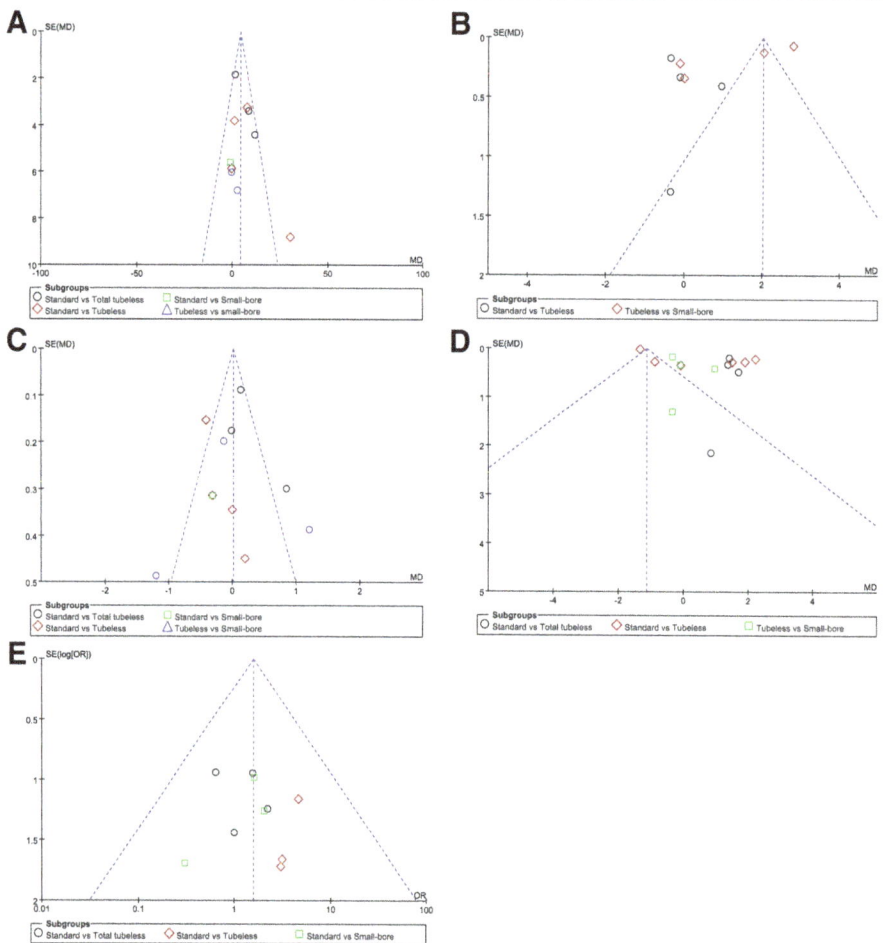

Fig. 5 Funnel plots of each variable. **a** Operation time, **b** visual analogue scale (VAS) pain score, **c** hemoglobin change, **d** length of stay, and **e** transfusion rate. For operation time, hemoglobin change, and transfusion rate, little evidence of publication bias was demonstrated on visual or statistical examination of the funnel plots; however, for VAS scores and hospital stay, moderate evidence of publication bias was demonstrated on visual or statistical examination of the plots

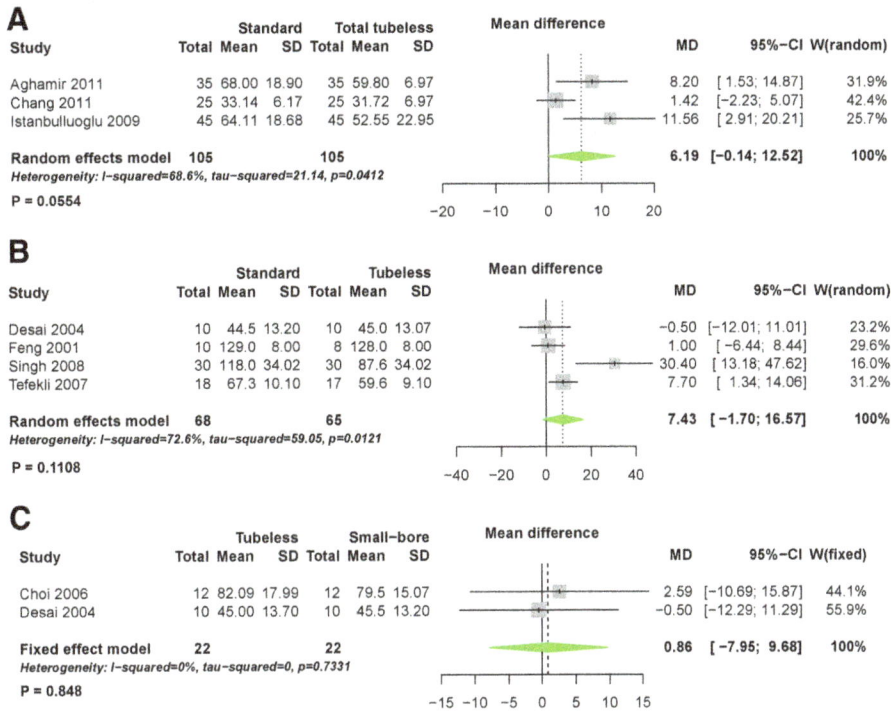

Fig. 6 Forest plots for operation time using pairwise meta-analysis. **a** Standard versus total tubeless PCNLs, **b** standard versus tubeless PCNLs, and **c** tubeless versus small-bore PCNLs. SD, standard deviation; MD, Mean difference; CI, confidence interval; W, Weight

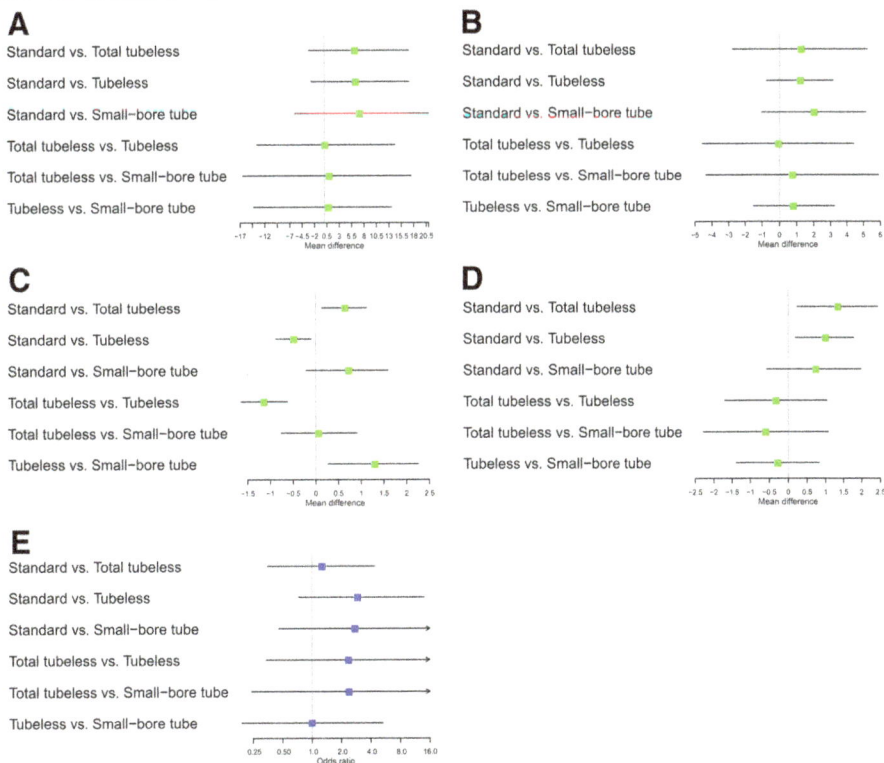

Fig. 7 Forest plots for (**a**) operation time, **b** visual analogue scale, **c** hemoglobin change, **d** hospital stay, and **e** transfusion rate using network meta-analysis

Table 2 Results of network and pairwise meta-analyses comparing procedures for operation time, visual analogue scale pain score, hemoglobin change, and hospital stay

Procedures	Network meta-analysis		Pairwise meta-analysis	
	Mean difference	95% CI	Mean difference	95% CI
Operation time				
Standard				
Total tubeless	6.11	−3.14 – 17.02	6.19[a]	−0.14 – 12.52
Tubeless	6.28	−2.71 – 17.06	7.43[a]	−1.70 – 16.57
Small-bore tube	7.09	−6.03 – 20.95	NA	
Total tubeless				
Tubeless	0.08	−13.60 – 14.27	NA	
Small-bore tube	0.95	−16.46 – 17.52	NA	
Tubeless				
Small-bore tube	0.80	−14.27 – 13.60	0.86[b]	−7.95 – 9.68
Visual analogue scale pain score				
Standard				
Total tubeless	1.25	−2.80 – 5.22	NA	
Tubeless	1.20	−0.75 – 3.14	0.06[a]	−0.56 – 0.69
Small-bore tube	2.00	−1.03 – 5.14	NA	
Total tubeless				
Tubeless	−0.07	−4.58 – 4.41	NA	
Small-bore tube	0.75	−4.37 – 5.89	NA	
Tubeless				
Small-bore tube	0.80	−1.51 – 3.24	1.21[a]	−0.02 – 2.44
Hemoglobin change				
Standard				
Total tubeless	0.65	0.14 – 1.13	0.23[a]	−0.12 – 0.58
Tubeless	−0.48	−0.87 – −0.09	-0.29[a]	−0.53 – −0.05
Small-bore tube	0.73	−0.21 – 1.60	NA	
Total tubeless				
Tubeless	−1.14	−1.65 – −0.62	NA	
Small-bore tube	0.06	−0.76 – 0.92	NA	
Tubeless				
Small-bore tube	1.30	0.27 – 2.26	−0.02[a]	−1.13 – 1.10
Hospital stay				
Standard				
Total tubeless	1.33	0.23 – 2.43	1.42[b]	1.10 – 1.75
Tubeless	0.99	0.19 – 1.79	0.54[a]	−1.03 – 2.11
Small-bore tube	0.73	−0.57 – 1.98	NA	
Total tubeless				
Tubeless	−0.33	−1.71 – 1.04	NA	
Small-bore tube	−0.60	−2.29 – 1.08	NA	
Tubeless				
Small-bore tube	−0.28	−1.39 – 0.83	0.06[a]	−0.56 – 0.69

CI confidence interval, *NA* not applicable
[a]Random-effect model with inverse variance method
[b]Fixed-effect model with inverse variance method

Intraoperative and postoperative feasibility and safety of total tubeless, tubeless, small-bore tube...

123

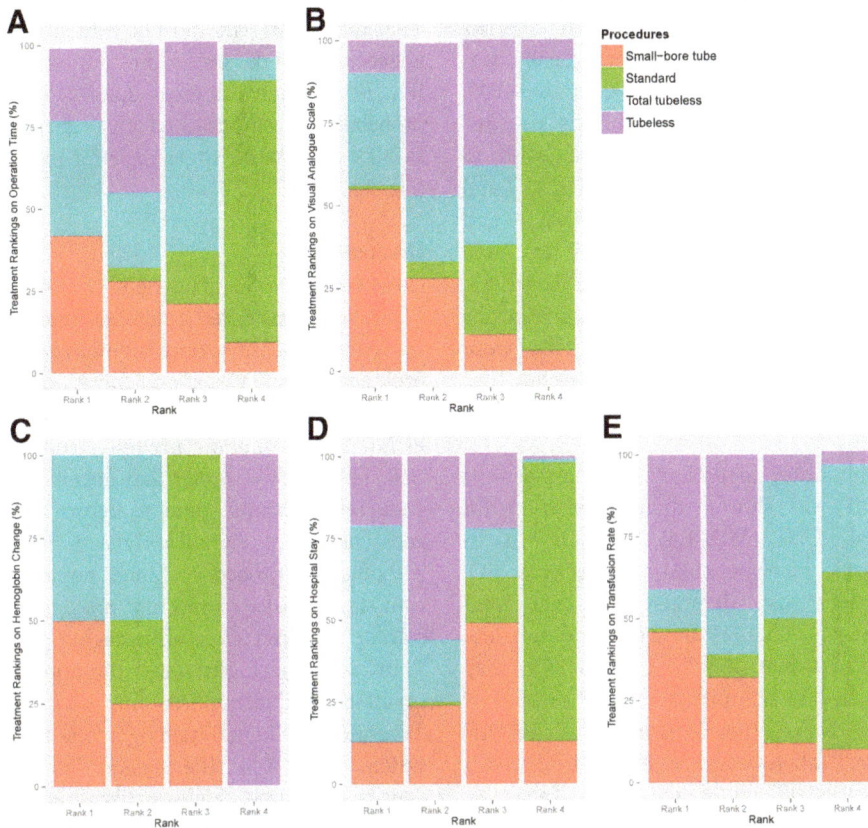

Fig. 8 Rank probability test. **a** Operation time, **b** visual analogue scale, **c** hemoglobin change, **d** hospital stay, and **e** transfusion rate

procedures for VAS pain scores (Fig. 7b) (Table 2), although the rank probabilities demonstrated that small-bore and total tubeless PCNLs may be superior to the other procedures (Fig. 8b).

Hemoglobin change

Using pairwise meta-analysis for hemoglobin change, three comparisons, including standard versus total tubeless PCNLs, standard versus tubeless PCNLs with stent,

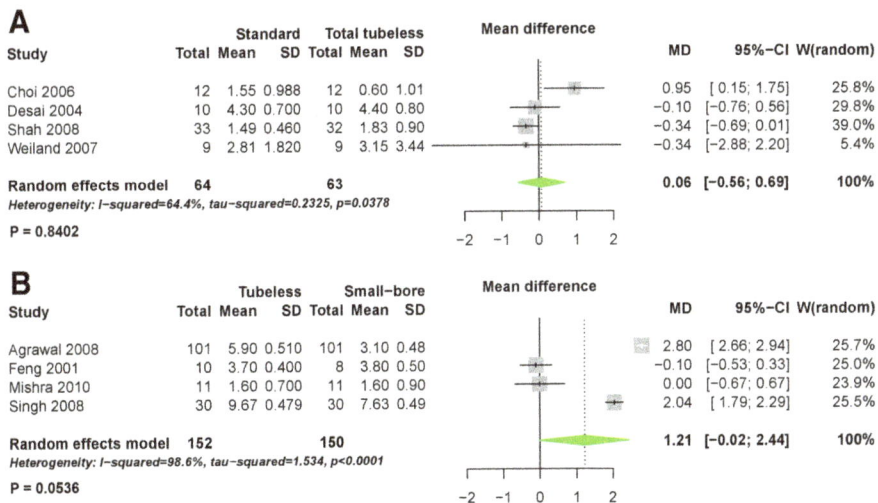

Fig. 9 Forest plots for visual analogue scale pain score using pairwise meta-analysis. **a** Standard versus total tubeless PCNLs, and **b** standard versus tubeless PCNLs, SD, standard deviation; MD, Mean difference; CI, confidence interval; W, Weight

and tubeless versus small-bore PCNLs, were examined (Fig. 10). Only one comparison for standard versus tubeless PCNLs with stent showed a statistically significant difference (MD -0.29, 95% CI -0.53 to −0.05, *P* = 0.02) (Fig. 10b). Network meta-analysis demonstrated that total tubeless PCNL may be superior to standard PCNL (MD 0.65, 95% CI 0.14 to 1.13). Total tubeless (MD -1.14, 95% CI -1.65 to −0.62), and small-bore PCNLs (MD 1.30, 95% CI 0.27 to 2.26) were also superior to tubeless PCNL with stent for hemoglobin change (Fig. 7c) (Table 2). In rank probabilities, total tubeless and small-bore PCNLs were ranked higher than the other procedures (Fig. 8c).

Hospital stay

The length of hospital stay in patients who underwent total tubeless PCNL was shorter than for those who underwent standard PCNL (MD 1.42, 95% CI 1.10 to 1.75, *P* < 0.01) during pairwise meta-analysis (Fig. 11). Network meta-analysis also demonstrated that total tubeless (MD 1.33, 95% CI 0.23 to 2.43) and tubeless PCNLs with stent (MD 0.99, 95% CI 0.19 to 1.79) may be superior to standard PCNL, producing a shorter hospital stay (Fig. 7d). However, there was no significant difference between total tubeless and tubeless PCNLs with stent (MD -0.33, 95% CI -1.71 to 1.04) (Table 2), although total tubeless PCNL showed the highest rank probability of all procedures (Fig. 8d).

Transfusion rate

The transfusion rate did not exhibit significant differences between any of the procedures during both pairwise analysis (Fig. 12) and network meta-analysis (Fig. 7e) (Table 3). Rank probabilities demonstrated that small-bore and tubeless PCNLs with stent may be superior to the other procedures (Fig. 8e).

Discussion

Conventionally, the placement of a nephrostomy tube after PCNL was considered a necessary safety option. However, the use of a nephrostomy tube has been associated with a prolonged hospital stay and more postoperative pain [18]. In 1997, Bellman et al. first reported the use of tubeless PCNL using a double-J ureteral stent and Council catheter [19]. They demonstrated that hospital length of stay, analgesia requirements, time to return to normal activities, and cost were significantly less with this procedure. Although the procedure gained popularity, tubeless PCNL with stent had two important problems: ureteral stent discomfort and loss of the advantages of a nephrostomy tube. Thus, some urologists used the approach of placing the smallest possible nephrostomy tube to minimize patient discomfort while maintaining access to the renal collecting system [20]. With the recent development of a high-density telescope, high-quality lithotripters, and radiological interventional techniques to embolize blood vessels, several investigators reported that tubeless and total

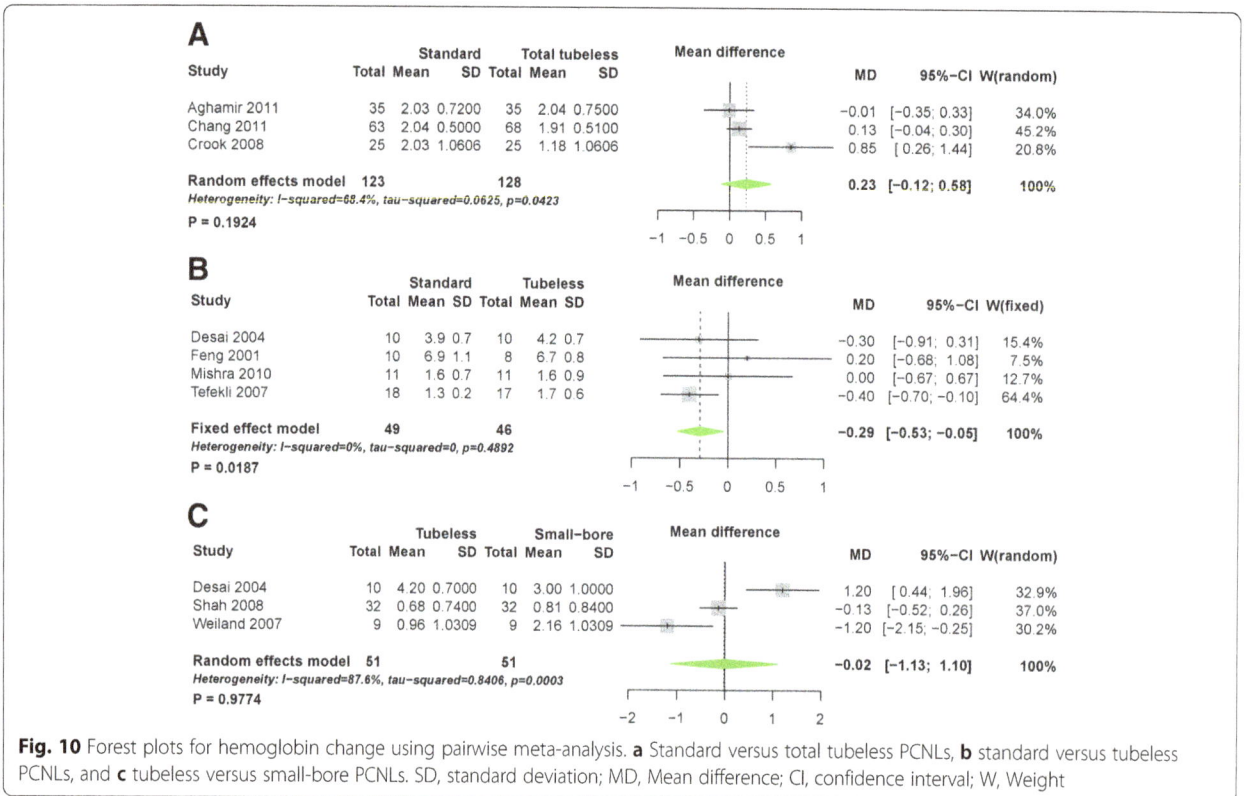

Fig. 10 Forest plots for hemoglobin change using pairwise meta-analysis. **a** Standard versus total tubeless PCNLs, **b** standard versus tubeless PCNLs, and **c** tubeless versus small-bore PCNLs. SD, standard deviation; MD, Mean difference; CI, confidence interval; W, Weight

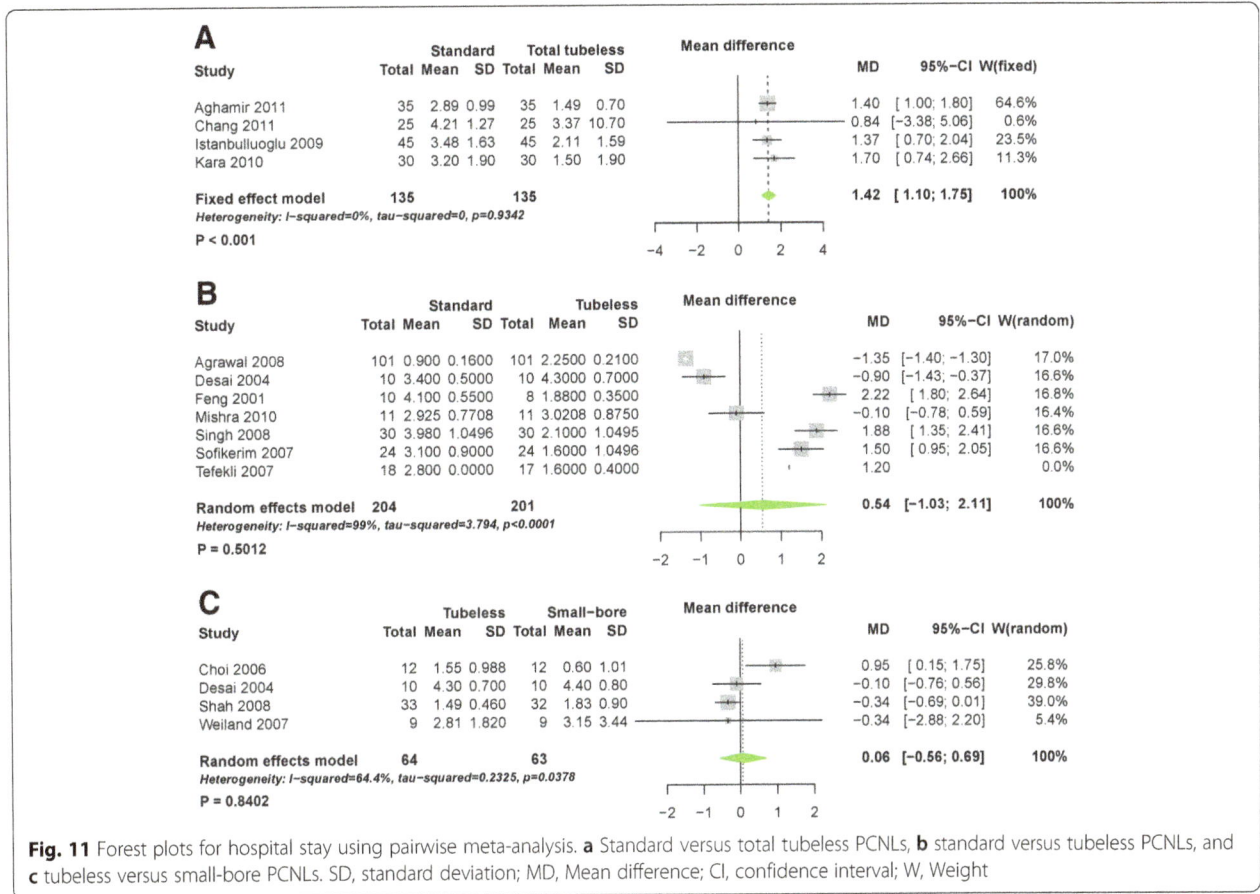

Fig. 11 Forest plots for hospital stay using pairwise meta-analysis. **a** Standard versus total tubeless PCNLs, **b** standard versus tubeless PCNLs, and **c** tubeless versus small-bore PCNLs. SD, standard deviation; MD, Mean difference; CI, confidence interval; W, Weight

tubeless (stentless) PCNL in selected patients was safe and associated with a reduced hospital length of stay and analgesic requirements.

The results of RCTs for each PCNL procedure have been reported, and previous systematic reviews and meta-analyses have been published. However, most of the studies reported in the previous meta-analyses compared standard PCNL versus tubeless PCNL with stent or standard PCNL versus total tubeless PCNL [21–25]. Therefore, an integrated analysis of standard, small-bore tube, tubeless with stent, and total tubeless PCNLs has not yet been published.

In our study, using network meta-analysis, there were no significant differences in operation time for the four procedures. It is known that large stones increase operation time and complication rates [26, 27], and operation times vary depending on the size and characteristics of the stone.

We also detected no statistically significant differences between methods for the VAS pain scores. No significant differences were observed between standard versus total tubeless PCNLs and tubeless versus small-bore tube PCNLs not only during the network meta-analysis, but even during pairwise meta-analyses. Operation-related factors that may prolong pain after PCNL include the

nephrostomy tube size [28] and stent discomfort caused by a double-J stent [29], but statistically significant differences between procedures were not observed. This finding is presumably due to the relatively small sample size (only eight studies reported the VAS pain scores), and the possibility of publication bias, as suggested by the asymmetric funnel plot (Fig. 5b). However, in the rank probability test of pain scores using Bayesian Markov Chain Monte Carlo modeling, small-bore tube PCNL was ranked highest, followed by the total tubeless PCNL and then tubeless PCNL with stent (Fig. 8b). Additional RCTs are necessary in the future to more definitively address this issue.

With regard to the hemoglobin changes, network meta-analysis showed that total tubeless and small-bore tube PCNLs were superior, and tubeless with stent PCNL was the worst. In addition, total tubeless and small-bore PCNLs showed similar superiority in the network meta-analysis and rank probability test (Fig. 8c). Considering that all enrolled studies were RCTs, the possibility of selection bias between patients who had total tubeless or small-bore tube PCNLs and other procedures should be relatively low. For tubeless PCNLs, the possibility of bleeding caused by ureteral stenting should be considered. In previous studies, hematuria

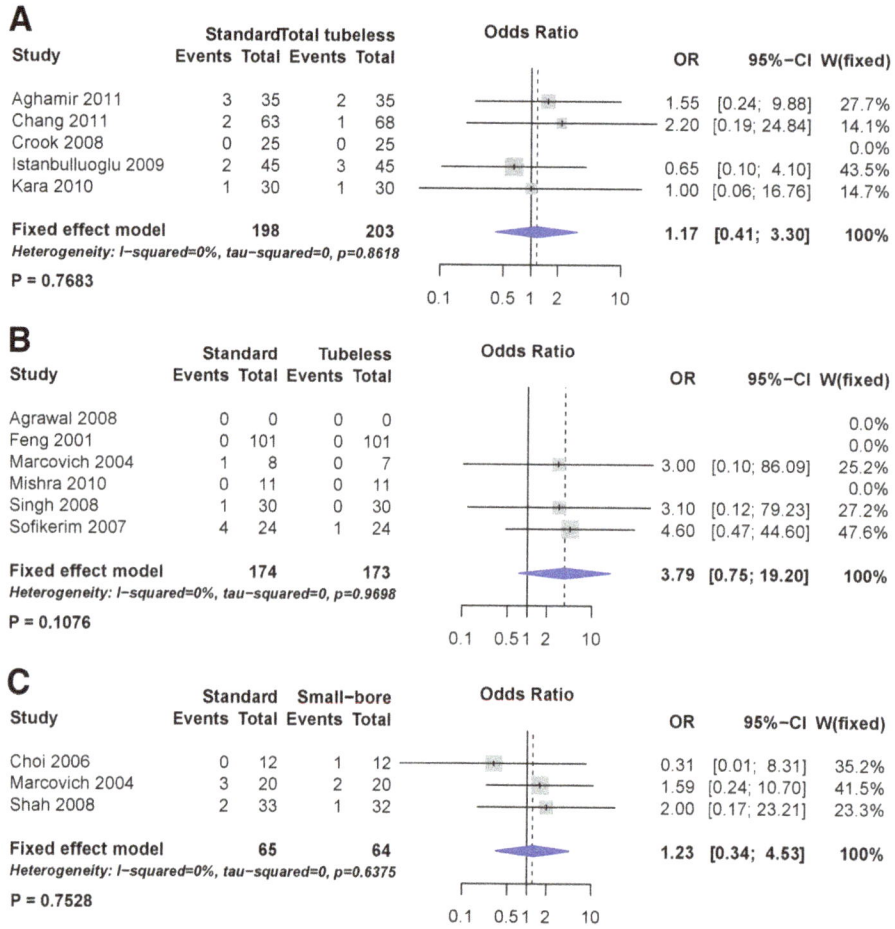

Fig. 12 Forest plots for transfusion rate using pairwise meta-analysis. **a** Standard versus total tubeless PCNLs, **b** standard versus tubeless PCNLs, and **c** tubeless versus small-bore PCNLs. OR, Odds ratio; CI, confidence interval; W, Weight

accounted for 13.6% of early complications and 18.1% of late complications after tubeless PCNL with stent [29]. In contrast to the hemoglobin changes, transfusion rates were not different between the four procedures. This

Table 3 Results of network and pairwise meta-analyses comparing procedures for transfusion rate

Procedures	Network meta-analysis		Pairwise meta-analysis[a]	
	OR	95% CI	OR	95% CI
Standard				
Total tubeless	1.27	0.35–4.40	1.17	0.41–3.30
Tubeless	2.94	0.73–14.06	3.79	0.75–19.20
Small-bore tube	2.76	0.46–24.52	NA	
Total tubeless				
Tubeless	2.37	0.34–18.19	NA	
Small-bore tube	2.39	0.24–22.21	NA	
Tubeless				
Small-bore tube	1.00	0.19–5.30	1.23	0.34–4.53

CI confidence interval, OR odds ratio
[a]Fixed-effect model with Mantel-Haenszel method

lack of difference is likely due to the development of high-quality surgical skills and patient monitoring approaches because of the popularity of PCNL procedures.

For the length of hospital stay, the total tubeless and tubeless PCNLs showed superiority. We assumed that this is because these methods do not require additional procedures, such as nephrostomy tube removal or tract revision.

During the rank probability for each variable, small-bore and tubeless PCNLs were ranked higher for operation time, VAS pain scores, and hemoglobin change. In addition, total tubeless PCNL was ranked highest for hospital stay and transfusion rate. Notably, total tubeless PCNL was ranked highest for each item. However, total tubeless PCNL has not been in widespread use, even considering the potential benefits of this approach, because of concerns that potentially fatal complications, such as massive bleeding without a nephrostomy tube in place, may occur [30]. Because omitting a nephrostomy catheter may potentially increase the risk of bleeding and serious complications, various methods have been used in an attempt to seal the tract. Milkahi and colleagues were the first to describe the instillation of the hemostatic agent Tiseel° into the nephrostomy tract [31]. However, they were unable to determine whether this diminished postoperative bleeding or urinary extravasation following tubeless PCNL. Choi et al. instilled gel matrix thrombin (Floseal°) into the tract whenever persistent bleeding was observed after omitting the nephrostomy catheter [32]. Okeke et al. explored cryoablation of the nephrostomy tract after tubeless PCNL, where they inserted a cryoprobe into the access tract and performed a 10-min freeze-thaw cycle at a temperature -20 °C. This method did not significantly affect the rate of delayed bleeding or urinary extravasation [33]. Recently, a randomized study by Cormio et al. showed that TachoSil° provided better tract control and a shorter hospital stay than nephrostomy tube placement, although it did not reduce pain or analgesic requirements [34].

Total tubeless PCNL is advocated by leading surgeons in the field of endourology. The future role of tubed PCNL will likely reside primarily in cases of severe intraoperative bleeding or major damage to the collecting system, and when there is the possibility of a second-look operation. However, some controversies remain about the feasibility and efficacy of tubeless PCNLs in certain clinical settings. In their prospective randomized study, Shoma et al. suggested that the tubeless approach might not be suitable for patients with chronic kidney disease or those who require a supracostal approach [30]. However, Shah et al. reported the successful use of a tubeless technique in a patient with chronic kidney disease. Likewise, Sofikerim et al. reported that tubeless PCNL is a safe and effective technique, even for supracostal access, and is associated with less postoperative pain and shorter hospital stay [35]. Resorlu et al. maintained that single or no nephrostomy drainage following multitract PCNL offered the potential advantages of decreased postoperative analgesic requirements and shorter hospital stay, without increasing the rate of complications [36].

A limitation of our study was that we did not perform subgroup analyses based on the size of the stone. We also did not compare success rates because the success rates were high in each study. In addition, there was some degree of publication bias. However, in the review of 48 articles from the Cochrane Database of Systematic Reviews performed by Sutton et al., publication or related biases were noted to be common within the sample of assessed meta-analyses, but did not affect the conclusions in most cases [37]. Additionally, the position of the patient during PCNL (prone or supine position) can influence the outcomes of a tubeless or not tubeless procedure. Anesthesiologists prefer the supine position because of better airway control during procedures. Another advan-

tage of the supine position is that there is no need for position changes when performing additional endoscopic procedures, such as cystoscopic or ureteroscopic operations [38]. Endoscopic combined intrarenal surgery is also a novel way of performing PCNL in the supine position [39]. Better visualization with the procedure allows for correct puncture of the kidney, and thus, can improve the safety and feasibility of a tubeless or total tubeless procedure.

Despite these limitations and shortcomings, our study has the substantial advantage of including larger samples from each study than the previously conducted pairwise meta-analyses [40]. Moreover, this is the first study to use network meta-analysis to compare PCNL methods, which enhances the statistical confidence and overcomes the limitations of pairwise meta-analyses.

Conclusions
In comparing each procedure through network meta-analysis, total tubeless and small-bore PCNLs were superior in terms of hemoglobin change, and total tubeless and tubeless PCNLs were superior with regard to the length of hospital stay. These findings indicate that conventional PCNL can be replaced with other techniques, especially total tubeless PCNL, in selected patients.

Abbreviations
PCNL: Percutaneous nephrolithotomy; RCT: Randomized controlled trial; VAS: Visual analogue scale

Funding
This study was supported by a faculty research grant from the Yonsei University College of Medicine for 2014 (6-2014-0156).

Authors' contributions
Systematic review and meta-analysis JYL, SUJ, MDK, DHK, JKK, WSH, YDC, KSC. Identification of studies, critical evaluation and discussion. JYL, KSC, DHK, WSH, YDC. All authors read and approved the final manuscript.

Competing interests
All the authors declare that they have no competing interests.

Author details
[1]Department of Urology, Severance Hospital, Urological Science Institute, Yonsei University College of Medicine, Seoul, South Korea. [2]Department of Urology, Gyeongsang National University Hospital, Gyeongsang National University School of Medicine, Jinju, South Korea. [3]Department of Radiology, Severance Hospital, Research Institute of Radiological Science, Yonsei University College of Medicine, Seoul, South Korea. [4]Department of Urology, Inha University School of Medicine, Incheon, South Korea. [5]Department of

Urology, Severance Check-Up, Yonsei University Health System, Seoul, South Korea. [6]Department of Urology, Gangnam Severance Hospital, Urological Science Institute, Yonsei University College of Medicine, 211 Eonju-ro, Gangnam-gu, Seoul 06273, South Korea.

References

1. Teichman JM. Clinical practice. Acute renal colic from ureteral calculus. N Engl J Med. 2004;350:684–93.

2. Lee JW, Park J, Lee SB, Son H, Cho SY, Jeong H. Mini-percutaneous Nephrolithotomy vs Retrograde Intrarenal Surgery for Renal Stones Larger Than 10 mm: A Prospective Randomized Controlled Trial. Urology. 2015;86:873–7.

3. Sivalingam S, Al-Essawi T, Hosking D. Percutaneous nephrolithotomy with retrograde nephrostomy access: a forgotten technique revisited. J Urol. 2013;189:1753–6.

4. Jung GH, Jung JH, Ahn TS, Lee JS, Cho SY, Jeong CW, et al. Comparison of retrograde intrarenal surgery versus a single-session percutaneous nephrolithotomy for lower-pole stones with a diameter of 15 to 30 mm: A propensity score-matching study. Korean J Urol. 2015;56:525–32.

5. Istanbulluoglu MO, Cicek T, Ozturk B, Gonen M, Ozkardes H. Percutaneous nephrolithotomy: nephrostomy or tubeless or totally tubeless? Urology. 2010;75:1043–6.

6. Paul EM, Marcovich R, Lee BR, Smith AD. Choosing the ideal nephrostomy tube. BJU Int. 2003;92:672–7.

7. Shah HN, Kausik VB, Hegde SS, Shah JN, Bansal MB. Tubeless percutaneous nephrolithotomy: a prospective feasibility study and review of previous reports. BJU Int. 2005;96:879–83.

8. Akman T, Binbay M, Yuruk E, Sari E, Seyrek M, Kaba M, et al. Tubeless Procedure is Most Important Factor in Reducing Length of Hospitalization After Percutaneous Nephrolithotomy: Results of Univariable and Multivariable Models. Urology. 2011;77:299–304.

9. Li H, Zhang Z, Li H, Xing Y, Zhang G, Kong X. Ultrasonography-guided percutaneous nephrolithotomy for the treatment of urolithiasis in patients with scoliosis. Int Surg. 2012;97:182–8.

10. Caldwell DM, Ades AE, Higgins JP. Simultaneous comparison of multiple treatments: combining direct and indirect evidence. BMJ. 2005;331:897–900.

11. Mills EJ, Thorlund K, Ioannidis JP. Demystifying trial networks and network meta-analysis. BMJ. 2013;346:f2914.

12. Yuan J, Zhang R, Yang Z, Lee J, Liu Y, Tian J, et al. Comparative effectiveness and safety of oral phosphodiesterase type 5 inhibitors for erectile dysfunction: a systematic review and network meta-analysis. Eur Urol. 2013;63:902–12.

13. Kwon JK, Cho KS, Oh CK, Kang DH, Lee H, Ham WS, et al. The beneficial effect of alpha-blockers for ureteral stent-related discomfort: systematic review and network meta-analysis for alfuzosin versus tamsulosin versus placebo. BMC Urol. 2015;15:55.

14. Lee JY, Cho KS, Kang DH, Jung HD, Kwon JK, Oh CK, et al. A network meta-analysis of therapeutic outcomes after new image technology-assisted transurethral resection for non-muscle invasive bladder cancer: 5-aminolaevulinic acid fluorescence vs hexylaminolevulinate fluorescence vs narrow band imaging. BMC Cancer. 2015;15:566.

15. Moher D, Liberati A, Tetzlaff J, Altman DG. Preferred reporting items for systematic reviews and meta-analyses: the PRISMA statement. PLoS Med. 2009;6:e1000097.

16. Chung JH, Lee SW. Assessing the quality of randomized controlled urological trials conducted by korean medical institutions. Korean J Urol. 2013;54:289–96.

17. R Development Core Team. R: A language and environment for statistical computing. Vienna: R Foundation for Statistical Computing; 2011. Accessed at www.R-project.org on 18 Mar 2013

18. Shah HN, Sodha HS, Khandkar AA, Kharodawala S, Hegde SS, Bansal MB. A randomized trial evaluating type of nephrostomy drainage after percutaneous nephrolithotomy: small bore v tubeless. J Endourol. 2008;22:1433–9.

19. Bellman GC, Davidoff R, Candela J, Gerspach J, Kurtz S, Stout L. Tubeless percutaneous renal surgery. J Urol. 1997;157:1578–82.

20. Kim SC, Tinmouth WW, Kuo RL, Paterson RF, Lingeman JE. Using and choosing a nephrostomy tube after percutaneous nephrolithotomy for large or complex stone disease: a treatment strategy. J Endourol. 2005;19:348–52.

21. Zhong Q, Zheng C, Mo J, Piao Y, Zhou Y, Jiang Q. Total tubeless versus standard percutaneous nephrolithotomy: a meta-analysis. J Endourol. 2013;27:420–6.

22. Yuan H, Zheng S, Liu L, Han P, Wang J, Wei Q. The efficacy and safety of tubeless percutaneous nephrolithotomy: a systematic review and meta-analysis. Urol Res. 2011;39:401–10.

23. Wang J, Zhao C, Zhang C, Fan X, Lin Y, Jiang Q. Tubeless vs standard percutaneous nephrolithotomy: a meta-analysis. BJU Int. 2012;109:918–24.

24. Shen P, Liu Y, Wang J. Nephrostomy tube-free versus nephrostomy tube for renal drainage after percutaneous nephrolithotomy: a systematic review and meta-analysis. Urol Int. 2012;88:298–306.

25. Borges CF, Fregonesi A, Silva DC, Sasse AD. Systematic Review and Meta-Analysis of Nephrostomy Placement Versus Tubeless Percutaneous Nephrolithotomy. J Endourol. 2010;24:1739–46.

26. Michel MS, Trojan L, Rassweiler JJ. Complications in percutaneous nephrolithotomy. Eur Urol. 2007;51:899–906. discussion

27. Lee JK, Kim BS, Park YK. Predictive factors for bleeding during percutaneous nephrolithotomy. Korean J Urol. 2013;54:448–53.

28. Pietrow PK, Auge BK, Lallas CD, Santa-Cruz RW, Newman GE, Albala DM, et al. Pain after percutaneous nephrolithotomy: impact of nephrostomy tube size. J Endourol. 2003;17:411–4.

29. Damiano R, Oliva A, Esposito C, De Sio M, Autorino R, D'Armiento M. Early and late complications of double pigtail ureteral stent. Urol Int. 2002;69:136–40.

30. Shoma AM, Elshal AM. Nephrostomy tube placement after percutaneous nephrolithotomy: critical evaluation through a prospective randomized study. Urology. 2012;79:771–6.

31. Mikhail AA, Kaptein JS, Bellman GC. Use of fibrin glue in percutaneous nephrolithotomy. Urology. 2003;61:910–4. discussion 4

32. Choi M, Brusky J, Weaver J, Amantia M, Bellman GC. Randomized trial comparing modified tubeless percutaneous nephrolithotomy with tailed stent with percutaneous nephrostomy with small-bore tube. J Endourol. 2006;20:766–70.

33. Okeke Z, Lee BR. Small renal masses: the case for cryoablation. J Endourol. 2008;22:1921–3.

34. Cormio L, Perrone A, Di Fino G, Ruocco N, De Siati M, de la Rosette J, et al. TachoSil((R)) sealed tubeless percutaneous nephrolithotomy to reduce urine leakage and bleeding: outcome of a randomized controlled study. J Urol. 2012;188:145–50.

35. Sofikerim M, Demirci D, Huri E, Ersekerci E, Karacagil M. Tubeless percutaneous nephrolithotomy: safe even in supracostal access. J Endourol. 2007;21:967–72.

36. Resorlu B, Kara C, Sahin E, Unsal A. Comparison of nephrostomy drainage types following percutaneous nephrolithotomy requiring multiple tracts: single tube versus multiple tubes versus tubeless. Urol Int. 2011;87:23–7.

37. Sutton AJ, Duval SJ, Tweedie RL, Abrams KR, Jones DR. Empirical assessment of effect of publication bias on meta-analyses. BMJ. 2000;320:1574–7.

38. Chung DY, Lee JY, Kim KH, Choi JH, Cho KS. Feasibility and efficacy of intermediate-supine percutaneous nephrolithotomy: initial experience. Chonnam Med J. 2014;50:52–7.

39. Cracco CM, Scoffone CM. ECIRS (Endoscopic Combined Intrarenal Surgery) in the Galdakao-modified supine Valdivia position: a new life for percutaneous surgery? World J Urol. 2011;29:821–7.

40. Li K, Lin T, Zhang C, Fan X, Xu K, Bi L, et al. Optimal frequency of shock wave lithotripsy in urolithiasis treatment: a systematic review and meta-analysis of randomized controlled trials. J Urol. 2013;190:1260–7.

41. Chang CH, Wang CJ, Huang SW. Totally tubeless percutaneous nephrolithotomy: a prospective randomized controlled study. Urol Res. 2011;39:459–65.

42. Aghamir SM, Modaresi SS, Aloosh M, Tajik A. Totally tubeless percutaneous nephrolithotomy for upper pole renal stone using subcostal access. J Endourol. 2011;25:583–6.

43. Kara C, Resorlu B, Bayindir M, Unsal A. A randomized comparison of totally tubeless and standard percutaneous nephrolithotomy in elderly patients. Urology. 2010;76:289–93.

44. Mishra S, Sabnis RB, Kurien A, Ganpule A, Muthu V, Desai M. Questioning the wisdom of tubeless percutaneous nephrolithotomy (PCNL): a prospective randomized controlled study of early tube removal vs tubeless PCNL. BJU Int. 2010;106:1045–8. discussion 8–9

45. Istanbulluoglu MO, Ozturk B, Gonen M, Cicek T, Ozkardes H. Effectiveness of totally tubeless percutaneous nephrolithotomy in selected patients: a prospective randomized study. Int Urol Nephrol. 2009;41:541–5.

46. Crook TJ, Lockyer CR, Keoghane SR, Walmsley BH. A randomized controlled trial of nephrostomy placement versus tubeless percutaneous nephrolithotomy. J Urol. 2008;180:612–4.

47. Agrawal MS, Agrawal M, Gupta A, Bansal S, Yadav A, Goyal J. A randomized comparison of tubeless and standard percutaneous nephrolithotomy. J Endourol. 2008;22:439–42.

48. Singh I, Singh A, Mittal G. Tubeless percutaneous nephrolithotomy: is it really less morbid? J Endourol. 2008;22:427–34.

49. Tefekli A, Altunrende F, Tepeler K, Tas A, Aydin S, Muslumanoglu AY. Tubeless percutaneous nephrolithotomy in selected patients: a prospective randomized comparison. Int Urol Nephrol. 2007;39:57–63.

50. Weiland D, Pedro RN, Anderson JK, Best SL, Lee C, Hendlin K, et al. Randomized prospective evaluation of nephrostomy tube configuration: impact on postoperative pain. Int Braz J Urol. 2007;33:313–8. discussion 9–22

51. Desai MR, Kukreja RA, Desai MM, Mhaskar SS, Wani KA, Patel SH, et al. A prospective randomized comparison of type of nephrostomy drainage following percutaneous nephrostolithotomy: large bore versus small bore versus tubeless. J Urol. 2004;172:565–7.

52. Marcovich R, Jacobson AI, Singh J, Shah D, El-Hakim A, Lee BR, et al. No panacea for drainage after percutaneous nephrolithotomy. J Endourol. 2004;18:743–7.

53. Feng MI, Tamaddon K, Mikhail A, Kaptein JS, Bellman GC. Prospective randomized study of various techniques of percutaneous nephrolithotomy. Urology. 2001;58:345–50.

19

Metastatic renal cell carcinoma initially presenting with hematochezia and subsequently with vaginal bleeding

Simon Ouellet[1*], Audrey Binette[2], Alexander Nguyen[1], Perrine Garde-Granger[3] and Robert Sabbagh[1]

Abstract

Background: We report an unusual case of a synchronous rectal and metachronous vaginal metastatic renal cell carcinoma.

Case presentation: A 78-year-old woman presented with hematochezia and a colonoscopy revealed a metastatic clear-cell renal cell carcinoma rectal polyp biopsy-proven. Abdominal computed tomography identified a 9.0-cm left renal mass with renal vein thrombosis, for which she underwent a laparoscopic radical nephrectomy. Histopathological examination confirmed a pT_{3a} clear-cell renal cell carcinoma. Seven months later, the patient presented with vaginal bleeding. Physical examination revealed a vaginal polypoid mass and biopsy confirmed a clear-cell renal cell carcinoma metastasis.

Conclusions: This case represents unusual manifestations of metastatic renal cell carcinoma and is a reminder of the wide spectrum of clinical course of this disease.

Keywords: Renal cell carcinoma, Rectal metastasis, Vaginal metastasis

Background

Renal cell carcinoma (RCC) frequently metastasizes to the lungs, lymph nodes, bones and liver. Although RCCs have been shown to metastasize to virtually all organs, both rectal and vaginal metastases are exceptional. To our best knowledge, this is the fifth reported case of RCC metastasis to the rectum and the first one in a patient without a prior diagnosis of RCC [1–4]. Herein, we report a rare case of two unusual sites of metastatic clear-cell RCC (ccRCC) in a 78-year-old woman who initially presented with hematochezia and subsequently with vaginal bleeding due to synchronous rectal and metachronous vaginal metastases.

Case presentation

A 78-year-old woman consulted the gastroenterology outpatient clinic for painless hematochezia. She had no gross hematuria or abdominal pain. Her familial and past medical histories were unremarkable. Except for the presence of red stained stool on the digital rectal examination, the physical examination and laboratory investigations were within normal limits. A colonoscopy showed a 1-cm rectal polyp that was completely removed with a snare. Macroscopic examination of the specimen revealed an ulcerated rectal polypoid lesion with granulation tissue on its surface. Histologic examination exhibited proliferation of tumor cells disposed in layers and pseudo-glandular structures. The lesion was highly vascularized. The

* Correspondence: simon.ouellet3@usherbrooke.ca
[1]Department of Surgery, Division of Urology, Université de Sherbrooke, Centre Hospitalier Universitaire de Sherbrooke (CHUS), 3001 12e avenue Nord, Sherbrooke, QC J1H 5N4, Canada
Full list of author information is available at the end of the article

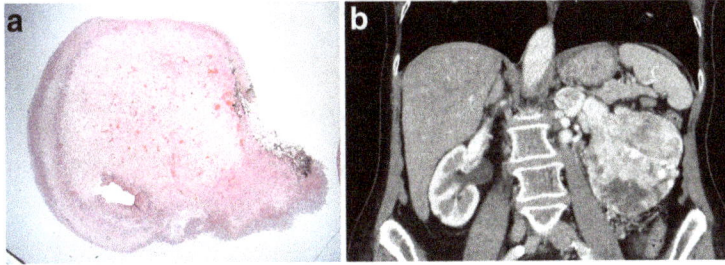

Fig. 1 a Microscopic imaging (hematoxylin and eosin stain; 4×) of the tumoral proliferation with clear cytoplasm, infiltrating the rectal submucosal. b An abdominal computed tomography (CT) revealed a 9-cm heterogeneous and enhancing left renal mass with a 3-cm renal vein thrombosis

tumor cells had central nuclei, distinct borders and a clear cytoplasm suggesting clear cell carcinoma (Fig. 1a). Immunohistochemical studies of the tumor were positive for pankeratin, CD10, EMA and RCC-ma, confirming metastatic ccRCC. An abdominal computed tomography (CT) revealed a 9-cm heterogeneous and enhancing left renal mass with a 3-cm renal vein thrombosis (Fig. 1b). A chest CT was within normal limits.

The patient then underwent a left radical laparoscopic nephrectomy, leading to the diagnosis of a clear-cell RCC (Fig. 2). The tumor measured 8 cm and was characterized as Fuhrman Grade III/IV and associated with a renal vein thrombus of 1.5 cm. The renal vein margin, the peri-renal fat and the left adrenal gland were not invaded and therefore the final pathological stage was pT3aR0. A pulmonary embolism complicated the postoperative period and the patient was started on anticoagulotherapy. The patient was considered cancer-free and no systemic adjuvant

treatment was given. Chest and abdominal CT showed no signs of recurrence at 3 and 6 months.

Seven months after the surgery, she presented with weakness, loss of appetite and sporadic vaginal spotting. Vaginal examination revealed a 3 and a 6-mm fragile polypoid lesion, both originating from anterior vaginal wall. There was no evidence of adenopathy or involvement of the vulva or cervix. Vaginal cytology was negative. A cystoscopy was performed to rule out a urethral diverticulum and was negative. A biopsy of both polyps was performed. Pathological analysis exhibited mucosal fragments containing foci of clear cell tumor, showing identical immunohistochemical staining features with primary tumor, such as diffuse staining with pankeratin, CD10 and RCC-ma (Fig. 3a and b). No systemic treatments were considered for the patient given her poor performance status.

Five months following the initial episode of vaginal bleeding, the patient was admitted to the hospital for persistent heavy bleeding. Physical examination revealed an important increase in size of the vaginal metastases. Laboratory tests were unremarkable, except for a hemoglobin level of 105 g/l. The patient received external beam radiotherapy with 20 Gray in 5 fractions directed to the vaginal lesions. Bleeding then diminished substantially. However, the patient expired 6 months later because of a rapid progression of her metastatic ccRCC (Table 1).

Discussion and conclusions

Renal cell carcinoma (RCC) accounts for 3% of all adult malignancies and 85% of all primary renal tumors. RCC can present with a variety of symptoms due to local invasion, paraneoplasic syndrome and metastasis. Approximately 30% of patients with RCC present with metastatic disease at the time of diagnosis and 20 to 40% of those with initially localized disease will eventually develop metastasis [5]. RCC

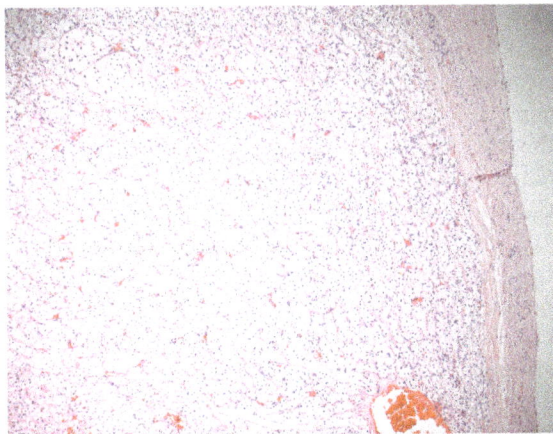

Fig. 2 Microscopic imaging (hematoxylin and eosin stain; 100×) of the primary renal tumor

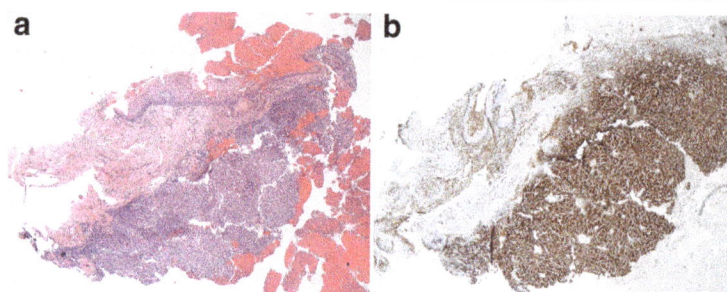

Fig. 3 a Microscopic imaging (hematoxylin and eosin stain; 4×) showing islands of epithelial cells with clear cytoplasm nested in hemorrhagic fields under vaginal mucosa. **b** Immunohistochemical study demonstrating CD10 immunoreactivity. Tumour cells were negative for keratin 7

distant metastasis spread is lymphatic, haematogenous, transcoelomic or by direct invasion [6]. Frequent sites of metastasis from RCC include lungs, lymph nodes, bones and liver. Unusual sites of metastasis from RCC include thyroid, orbit, nasal structures, vagina, gallbladder, pancreas, sublingual tissues and soft tissues of distal extremities [6].

Gastrointestinal tract is rarely the site of metastatic lesions, although melanoma, ovarian and bladder cancer are most commonly involved [7]. Digestive RCC metastases are rare and tend to be present in patients with known RCC. The duodenum is the most commonly intestinal segment involved given its close location to the right kidney [8]. Upper gastrointestinal bleeding secondary to stomach and pancreatico-duodenal metastases have been described [5]. Only 13 cases of colon metastasis are reported and most of these patients presented with hematochezia [8, 9]. Rectal bleeding as the patient's initial symptom of mRCC was seen in only one case [8]. Symptoms from bowel metastasis tend to occur more frequently in patients with know metastatic disease or in patients with a remote history of nephrectomy for RCC. Treatments for bowel metastasis include segmental resections, trans-catheter embolization, palliative derivation and endoscopic resection [5]. Endoscopic

resection can be both diagnostic and therapeutic when the lesion is small as in this case.

Rectal metastasis from RCC is a very unusual event with only four cases in the literature (Table 2) [1–4].

All patients had prior nephrectomy for RCC. Reported survival after initial symptoms is poor. Herein we present the first case of metastatic RCC initially presenting with hematochezia secondary to rectal metastasis.

Later in the course of the disease the patient presented with vaginal bleeding secondary to anterior vaginal wall metastases. Since primary adenocarcinoma of the vagina comprises less than 10% of all vaginal neoplasms, they should be considered metastatic until proven otherwise [10]. Metastatic adenocarcinoma of the vagina may develop from the cervix, endometrium, colon or ovary in 65% of cases [11]. Rarely, the primary tumor originates from the pancreas, the stomach, or exceptionally the kidney [10]. To date less than 100 cases of vaginal RCC metastasis have been reported in the literature [12]. In most of these cases, the vaginal lesion is typically solitary and located in the lower third of the anterior wall of the vagina [12]. Interestingly, the primary renal lesion is typically on the left side [11]. Retrograde venous dissemination seems the most plausible cause at the origin of vaginal metastasis, especially in our case with the presence of a renal vein thrombus. Immunohistochemically, metastatic clear cell carcinomas (CCC) to the gynecologic tract show constant positivity of CD10, which is in sharp contrast with the constant negativity of all primary gynecologic CCC, regardless of the site of origin. No conclusive data exist in the literature regarding the value of cervicovaginal cytology both in the diagnosis and the follow-up of these patients. Local excision and/or radiotherapy have been advocated as therapeutic interventions, although literature is limited [12].

In conclusion, we describe a rare case of synchronous metastatic RCC in a patient initially presenting

Table 1 Timeline

Time	Events
2007 – March	Painless rectal bleeding
2007- April	Colonoscopy and biopsy of a rectal polyp revealing metastatic ccRCC
2007 – May	Left radical laparoscopic nephrectomy – final pathology: ccRCC pT3a
2007 – December	Vaginal bleeding from a vaginal ccRCC metastasis
2008 – May	Significant vaginal bleeding from metastasis treated with external beam radiotherapy (20 Gray in 5 fractions)
2008 – October	Patient expired from disease progression

Table 2 Clinical characteristics of previous cases of rectal metastasis of RCC

Author/Year	Sex/Age	Presenting symptom of rectal lesion	Prior nephrectomy	Timing after initial nephrectomy	Survival after initial GI bleeding
Current case	80/F	Hematochezia	No	–	18 months
Rosito et al., 2002 [2]	55/M	Anal bleeding	Yes	9 months	18 months
Dellon and Gangarosa, 2006 [1]	70/M	Hematochezia	Yes	28 years	11 months
Maehata et al., 2016 [3]	61/M	Hematochezia	Yes	NR	NR
Zheng et al., 2017 [4]	65/M	During follow-up for a benign rectal polyp	Yes	10 years	Alive with lungs, lymph nodes and bone metastasis

NR Not Reported

with hematochezia secondary to metastatic involvement of the rectum. Subsequently the patient presented with vaginal bleeding secondary to metachronous vaginal metastases. This case illustrates the wide variability in RCC presentation and contributes to a better understanding of metastases to the rectum and the vagina.

Abbreviations
CCC: Clear cell carcinoma; ccRCC: Clear-cell renal cell carcinoma; RCC: Renal cell carcinoma

Acknowledgements
None

Funding
NA

Availability of data and materials
NA

Authors' contributions
SO: drafted the manuscript. AB: drafted part of the manuscript and reviewed the manuscript. AN: provided the clinical information and reviewed the manuscript. PGG: drafted the pathologic section and reviewed the manuscript. RS: surgeon how performed the nephrectomy and reviewed the manuscript. All authors read and approved the final manuscript.

Competing interests
The authors declare that they have no competing interests.

Author details
¹Department of Surgery, Division of Urology, Université de Sherbrooke, Centre Hospitalier Universitaire de Sherbrooke (CHUS), 3001 12e avenue Nord, Sherbrooke, QC J1H 5N4, Canada. ²Department of Obstetrics and Gynaecology, Université de Sherbrooke, Centre Hospitalier Universitaire de Sherbrooke (CHUS), 3001 12e avenue Nord, Sherbrooke, Canada. ³Department of Pathology, Université de Sherbrooke, Centre Hospitalier Universitaire de Sherbrooke (CHUS), 3001 12e avenue Nord, Sherbrooke, Canada.

References
1. Dellon ES, Gangarosa LM. Hematochezia due to a renal cell carcinoma metastasis to the rectum: a case report and review of the literature. Rev Gastroenterol Mex. 2006;71:316–8.
2. Rosito MA, Damin DC, Lazzaron AR, André C, Schwartsmann G. Metastatic renal cell carcinoma involving the rectum. Int J Color Dis. 2002;17:359–61.
3. Maehata Y, Esaki M, Fujita K, Hirahashi M. Solitary rectal metastasis from renal cell carcinoma treated by endoscopic resection. Dig Liver Dis. 2016;48:566.
4. Zheng G, Li H, Li J, Zhang X, Zhang Y, Wu X. Metastatic renal cell clear cell carcinoma to the rectum, lungs, ilium and lymph nodes: a case report. Medicine (Baltimore). 2017;96:5720.
5. Bukowski RM. Natural history and therapy of metastatic renal cell carcinoma: the role of interleukin-2. Cancer. 1997;80:1198–220.
6. Sadler GJ, Anderson MR, Moss MS, Wilson PG. Metastases from renal cell carcinoma presenting as gastrointestinal bleeding: two case reports and a review of the literature. BMC Gastroenterol. 2007;7:4.
7. Washington K, McDonagh D. Secondary tumors of the gastrointestinal tract: surgical pathologic findings and comparison with autopsy survey. Mod Pathol. 1995;8:427–33.
8. Short TP, Thomas E, Joshi PN, Martin A, Mullins R. Occult gastrointestinal bleeding in renal cell carcinoma: value of endoscopic evaluation. Am J Gastroenterol. 1993;88:300–2.
9. Zhao WP, Yu YL, Chen ZQ, Huang XF, Zhang ZG. Colon metastasis of chromophobe renal cell carcinoma with sarcomatoid change. Chin Med J. 2012;125:3352–4.
10. Perez CA, Gersell DJ, McGuire WP, et al. Vaginal cancer. In: Hoskins WJ, Perez CA, Young RC, editors. Principles and practice of gynecologic oncology. Philadelphia, PA: Lippincott, Williams and Wilkins; 2000. p. 811–40.
11. Allard JE, McBroom JW, Zahn CM, McLeod D, Maxwell GL. Vaginal metastasis and thrombocytopenia from renal cell carcinoma. Gynecol Oncol. 2004;92:970–3.
12. Mendese GW, Ayvazian PJ, Li C. Renal cell carcinoma presenting as a perineal mass: case report and review of the literature. Urology. 2006;67:847.

20

Pazopanib as a second-line treatment for non-cytokine-treated metastatic renal cell carcinoma

Victor C. Kok[1,2]* and Jung-Tsung Kuo[3]

Abstract

Background: The currently recommended treatment algorithm for patients with advanced renal cell carcinoma who fail the first-line targeted therapy does not normally include pazopanib as a second-line treatment option. It would therefore be of interest to determine the efficiency of pazopanib in this setting in terms of the partial response rate (PRR), disease control rate (DCR), and progression-free survival (PFS).

Methods: Peer-reviewed clinical reports without language restriction, both full papers and conference abstracts, which assessed the second-line use of pazopanib following failure of first-line non-cytokine-targeted therapy, were included. After the literature retrieval, we conducted a Preferred Reporting Items for Systematic reviews and Meta-Analyses (PRISMA)-compliant systematic review of the literature and meta-analysis of the size of the effect of each outcome measure (PRR, DCR, and PFS). The effect size and 95 % confidence interval (CI) were calculated using fixed-effect or random-effects models based on the heterogeneity represented by I^2 of selected studies. Meta-analysis forest plots with a fixed-effect model showing the PRR and DCR were created.

Results: Our results show that there are no available comparative studies on pazopanib second-line treatment. Only phase II trials or retrospective analysis reports were retrievable. Six studies (comprising 217 patients) were included in the qualitative and quantitative analysis. Pazopanib as a second-line treatment resulted in a PRR of 23 % (95 % CI, 17–31 %; $I^2 = 52.6$ %) and a DCR of 73 % (95 % CI, 65–80 %; $I^2 = 0.00$ %). The meta-analysis with fixed-effect model revealed that PFS was 6.5 months (95 % CI, 5.6–7.5 months; $I^2 = 86.2$ %).

Conclusions: In conclusion, the effectiveness and indication of pazopanib for use in the second-line setting has not yet been examined in-depth; however, this meta-analysis has shown that the treatment effects in terms of PRR, DCR, and PFS may be similar to other well-studied second-line targeted therapies. Rigorous comparative phase III trials testing this hypothesis are required.

Keywords: Pazopanib, Second-line therapy, Meta-analysis, Renal cell carcinoma, Targeted therapy

* Correspondence: victorkok@asia.edu.tw
[1]Division of Medical Oncology, Cancer Center of Kuang Tien General Hospital, 117 Shatien Rd, Taichung 43303, Taiwan
[2]Department of Biomedical Informatics, Asia University, Taichung 41354, Taiwan
Full list of author information is available at the end of the article

Background

Before the advent of targeted therapies, patients with advanced renal cell carcinoma (RCC) were treated with cytokine immunotherapy using interferon or interleukin-2. Although some long-term remission was achieved, most patients did not benefit from this treatment, but instead suffered from significant adverse effects from the immunotherapy. Health-related quality of life has been shown to be significantly poorer in patients receiving immunotherapy [1].

Up until early September 2015, at least seven targeted agents (sunitinib, sorafenib, pazopanib, axitinib, everolimus, temsirolimus, and bevacizumab) have been approved for treatment of metastatic RCC (mRCC) by the US Food and Drug Administration (FDA) [2]. In late August 2015, the FDA granted the use of lenvatinib, a multiple tyrosine kinase inhibitor, for investigational use only in patients with advanced or mRCC who had failed or did not tolerate the first-line targeted therapy [3]. Non-cytokine targeted therapy has become the first-line choice because of its favorable toxicity profiles and ease of administration in ambulatory settings. Based on limited evidence from clinical trials, expert opinions, and consensus meetings, practice guidelines on how to select these agents in sequential order and in defined risk groups have been established [4]. The rationale behind the sequential monotherapy for mRCC is mainly driven by research results from well-designed clinical trials. Treatment with combination therapeutics has been deemed to be unfeasible due to toxicity profiles, or has not been shown to be more effective than sequential monotherapy. Several population-based studies have demonstrated that sequential targeted monotherapy improves overall survival [5–7]. Nevertheless, the optimal sequencing of targeted agents to treat mRCC and maximize the patients' survival is still under rigorous investigations [8, 9].

Pazopanib was approved by the FDA in 2009 for treatment-naïve or cytokine-failed patients with advanced RCC. Pazopanib is an oral agent that inhibits vascular endothelial growth factor (VEGF), PDGF, and C-Kit tyrosine kinase receptors. However, pazopanib as a second-line treatment for advanced RCC that is non-responsive to previous treatment with VEGF-targeted drugs has not received adequate investigation, and has never proceeded to phase III trials.

The present study involved a systematic review of the current literature with the aim of providing a more precise estimate of the treatment effects, such as the partial response rate (PRR), disease control rate (DCR), and progression-free survival (PFS) of pazopanib used in the second-line setting after a non-cytokine VEGF-targeted therapy.

Methods

This systematic review and meta-analysis of treatment effect is reported according to the preferred reporting items for systematic reviews and meta-analyses (PRISMA) guidelines [10]. The research was performed in accordance with the Declaration of Helsinki after approval by the Kuang Tien General Hospital accredited in-house institutional review board (certificate no. KTGH-10431).

Eligibility criteria

Peer-reviewed clinical reports without language restriction- either full papers or conference abstracts- assessing the second-line use of pazopanib after failed first-line non-cytokine-targeted therapy were included. An explicit statement of questions being addressed with reference to participants, interventions, comparisons, outcomes, and study design (PICOS) was established as follows: P- patients with metastatic or advanced RCC failing first-line non-cytokine targeted therapy; I- pazopanib as the second-line drug; C- placebo or other antineoplastic agent when regarding comparative trials; O- response rate, DCR, PFS, and overall survival (OS); S- phase III or phase II comparative or non-comparative trials and retrospective analyses would all qualify for review. Inclusion criteria were studies reporting the treatment effect in terms of response rate, DCR, PFS and/or OS, with a starting dose of pazopanib of 800 mg per day. Studies involving pure cytokine treatment prior to pazopanib treatment were excluded from the analysis.

Search methods

Full electronic searches were performed in the PubMed biomedical literature database using medical subject headings (MeSH), a controlled vocabulary thesaurus and Boolean logic operators. The search phrase was (((("Carcinoma, Renal Cell"[Mesh]) AND pazopanib)) AND ((second-line) OR sequential OR (second line)E). Additional searches were carried out in the EMBASE database using the search terms: "pazopanib AND second AND line AND renal AND cell AND carcinoma AND ([article]/lim OR [article in press]/lim OR [conference abstract]/lim OR [conference paper]/lim OR [conference review]/lim OR [editorial]/lim OR [letter]/lim) AND [humans]/lim AND [embase]/lim." Conference abstracts published in the annual meeting of the American Society of Clinical Oncology (ASCO) and that of the European Society for Medical Oncology (ESMO) are included in the EMBASE database. The date of the last search was 20 May 2015.

Study selection

Duplicate records from searches of both databases were excluded. The remaining records were screened by title and abstract content for suitability of inclusion for further analysis. Although potentially confirming the existence of unpublished studies, abstracts were excluded if they did not contain enough information for this systematic review.

Data extraction

The name of the first author, year of publication, study setting (phase II or retrospective), number of individuals in the study, proportion of male patients, median age with range, histology type of RCC, status of previous nephrectomy, 3-tier risk category such as Memorial Sloan-Kettering Cancer Center (MSKCC) risk group, Motzer, Heng, or International Metastatic RCC Database Consortium (IMDC) risk category; the first-line agent used, complete response rate, partial response rate (PRR), DCR, and PFS time were recorded. Mean age and standard deviation data were calculated when missing [11].

PFS was defined as the time from the initiation of pazopanib treatment to the date of documented progressive disease (PD) based on the Response Evaluation Criteria in Solid Tumors (RECIST) 1.0 or 1.1 criteria or death from any cause. DCR was defined as the proportion of patients who obtained an objective tumor response [complete response (CR) or partial response (PR)] or those who had achieved stable disease (SD) based on RECIST version 1.0 or version 1.1 criteria. Both older and newer versions of RECIST criteria have been widely accepted for objectively assessing responses to therapy in patients with RCC treated with targeted therapy. In a recent study investigating the concordance between RECIST 1.1 and RECIST 1.0 in patients with advanced RCC receiving VEGR-targeted therapy, Krajewski, K. M. et al. reported that response assessments were, overall, highly concordant between the two criteria and there was no evidence of a difference in time–to-progression (TTP) between the two criteria [12].

Data synthesis and statistical analysis
Measuring the treatment effect

To improve the precision and the generalizability of the estimated treatment effect, data synthesis from selected studies using meta-analysis was planned. Studies were weighted before pooling. The meta-analysis forest plot using the fixed-effect model was used at the outset to calculate the rate of partial remission and DCR with 95 % confidence intervals (CI). The fixed-effect model was adopted based upon the assumption that all of the studies to be examined as a whole were considered to have been conducted under similar conditions (second-line treatment following failure of non-cytokine first-line treatment) with similar subjects (advanced/metastatic RCC); in other words, the only difference between the selected studies was their effectiveness in detecting the outcome of interest.

Heterogeneity analysis

Heterogeneity analysis refers to the analysis of the variation in study outcomes between studies selected for the

meta-analysis. Non-combinability testing for measuring heterogeneity in meta-analysis was presented using I^2 (=100 % x (Q-df)/Q) [13]. I^2 is an intuitive and simple expression of the inconsistency across studies and its confidence interval is constructed using the test-based method of Higgins and Thompson. An I^2 value ≤ 24 % was considered as having minimal heterogeneity. An I^2 value between 25 and 49 % was regarded as having low heterogeneity; an I^2 value between 50 and 74 % had moderate heterogeneity, and an I^2 value ≥ 75 % was regarded as having high heterogeneity. If the I^2-value was ≥ 50 %, the random-effects model was used. The statistical software StatsDirect (StatsDirect Ltd, England) and Comprehensive Meta-Analysis software were used to generate the summary figures and pooled effect sizes and CI used in the meta-analysis.

Results

A total of 60 studies were identified from the PubMed ($N = 45$) and EMBASE ($N = 15$) databases. After removing duplicates, 51 retrieved records were screened according to the title and abstract for further eligibility, which subsequently excluded 41 records that did not qualify. The remaining 10 records were then assessed in detail according to the full-text with regard to eligibility for further qualitative and quantitative synthesis, which subsequently excluded four reports; thus, six studies were eventually considered to be eligible for the meta-analysis (Fig. 1). Motives for exclusion included pazopanib being used beyond second-line treatment, cytokine pretreatment, systematic review article reporting secondary results, and missing data. Figure 1 displays the PRISMA flow diagram for study selection and consists of four consecutive steps from identification in databases, screening the records, checking eligibility against the criteria for inclusion, and the final inclusion step.

There were no phase IIb or III comparative clinical trials testing pazopanib in the second-line treatment for mRCC. Six records, of which five were journal articles and one was a conference abstract, were retrieved for analysis [14–19]. All the non-comparative studies were published between 2013 and 2015. Only phase II trial data ($N = 140$), case-series, and registry data were retrievable. The total number of patients in these six studies was 217; 156 of patients, from four studies, were included for meta-analysis of the PRR, 154 from three studies for meta-analysis of the disease control rate, and 203 from five studies were included for the meta-analysis of PFS (Table 1).

Information on patient age was retrievable in five out of the six studies (Table 1). Meta-analysis for mean age with the random-effects model [11] revealed that the mean age was 62 years (95 % CI, 60–64; range, 40–85 years). Overall, there were more male patients (range, 61–76 %). Sunitinib was used as a first-line treatment in

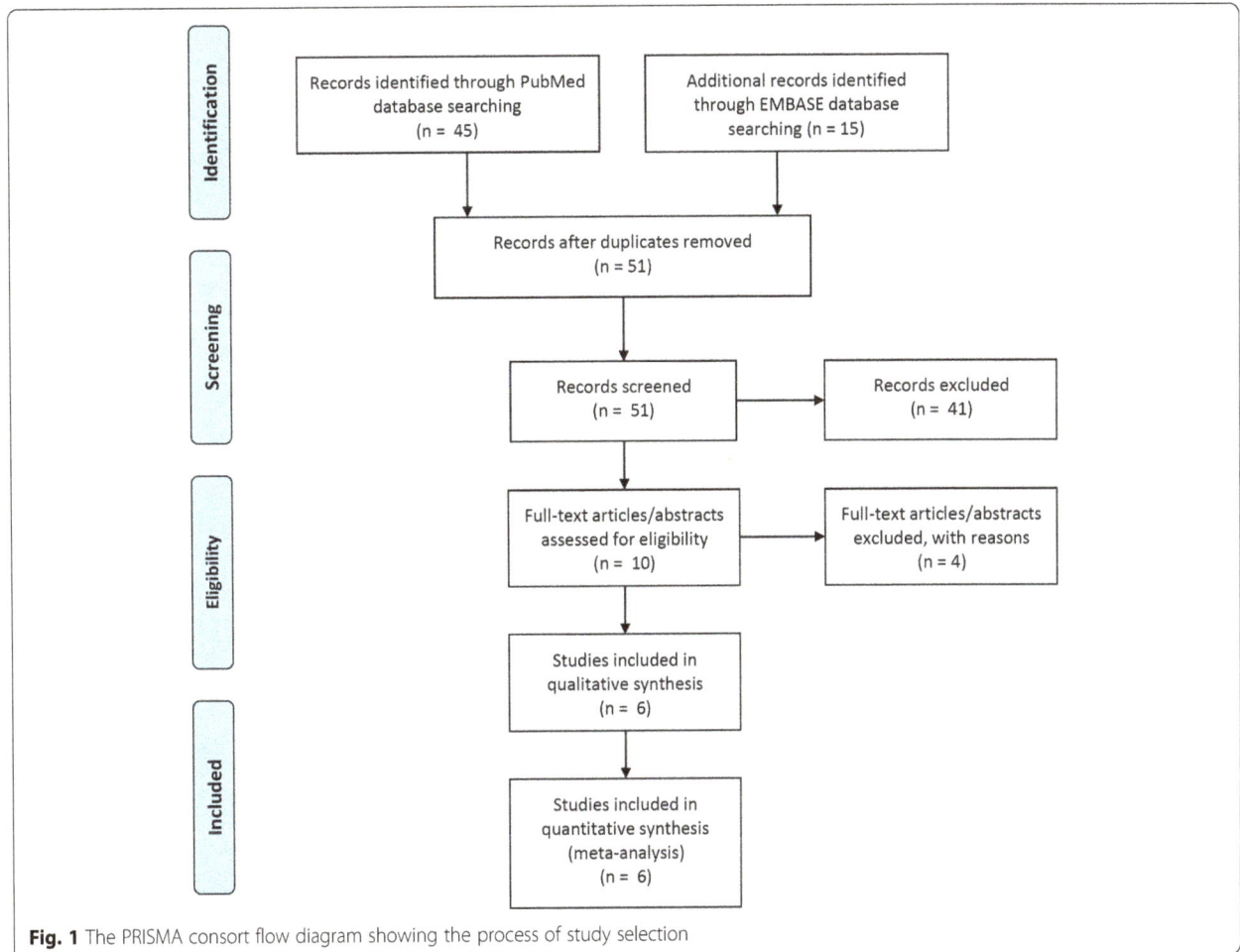

Fig. 1 The PRISMA consort flow diagram showing the process of study selection

187 patients and bevacizumab in 16 patients. Overall response rates (CR + PR) to the first-line targeted therapy have been reported in four studies showing a rate from 16 to 33 %, with an average of 23 % [14, 15, 17, 19].

None of the patients achieved a complete response from second-line pazopanib treatment. Figure 2 displays a meta-analysis forest plot with a fixed-effect model of the PRR as the best response obtained after pazopanib used as the second-line agent. A total of four studies (comprising 156 patients) explicitly presented this rate [14, 15, 17, 19]. The reported PRR in these four studies ranged from 15.3 to 42.9 %. The fixed-effect model derived an estimated PRR of 23 % (95 % CI, 17–31 %). A heterogeneity test with I^2 was 52.6 %, indicating the existence of a moderate degree of inconsistency across the studies. With the random-effects model, an estimated PRR would be 24.5 % (95 % CI, 14.5–38.4 %).

Pazopanib as a second-line treatment showed a DCR of 73 % (95 % CI, 65–80 %; $I^2 = 0.00$ %). Three studies reported the DCR with point estimates ranging from 70.6 to 77 % in a pool of 154 patients (Fig. 3) [15, 17, 19].

In the meta-analysis with a fixed-effect model for studies on PFS that pooled five studies- containing 203 patients-

revealed a PFS of 6.3 months (95 % CI, 5.4–7.2 months; $I^2 = 83.7$ %). With a relatively high degree of heterogeneity, a random-effects model was adopted, which showed a PFS of 7.6 months (95 % CI, 5.0–10.1 months) (Table 2).

Discussion

Pazopanib as a second-line therapy after a non-cytokine targeted therapy in patients with mRCC has not been thoroughly evaluated. Oncologists who wish to prescribe pazopanib in the second-line setting after previous use of a targeted agent would therefore be unable to find adequate information regarding the treatment effects of pazopanib. This meta-analysis of a total of 217 patients worldwide found a PRR of 23 % (95 % CI, 17–31 %), a DCR of 73 % (95 % CI, 65–80 %), and a PFS time of 6.3 months (5.4–7.2 months).

In two recent phase III trials, axitinib therapy (5 mg twice daily), when compared with sorafenib (400 mg twice daily) as the second-line treatment in patients with metastatic clear-cell RCC, resulted in a PFS of 8.3 months (95 % CI, 6.7–9.2) in a population of globally-recruited patients (with 35 % of the patients

Table 1 Selected studies pooling 205 patients for systematic review and meta-analysis and display of main patient characteristics

First author	Year publ.	Setting	N	Gender, % men	Age, median (range)	Clear cell type, %	Previous nephrectomy	Poor risk percent	First-line targeted therapy	PRR	DCR	PFS (months)
Xie	2015	Phase II	85	72 %	63 (41–85)	100 %	81 %	24.4 %[a]	sunitinib	15.3 % (11.2–23.9 %)	70.6 %	5.6 (4.1–6.7)
Hainsworth	2013	Phase II	55	76 %	60 (41–82)	100 %	89 %	29 %[b]	sunitinib (N = 39) or bevacizumab (N = 16)	27 % (?-?)	76 %	7.5 (5.4–9.4)
Sanchez	2013	Retrospective	32	65 %	NA	81 %	74 %	28.3 %[c]	sunitinib	NA	NA	13 (9.0–17.0)
Matrana	2013	Retrospective	17	69 %	65 (45–83)	100 %	89 %	34 % (MSKCC)	sunitinib	NA	NA	3.5 (1.0–15.5)
Rautiola	2013	Retrospective	14	61 %	65 (40–82)	90 %	90 %	19 %[c]	sunitinib	43 %	77 %	11 (4.6–15.6)
Al-Marrawi	2013	Retrospective	14	NA	50 (44–78)	92 %	90 %	17 %[c]	VEGF inhibitor[d]	0 % (0/2)[e]	NA	NA

DCR disease control rate, *mo* months, *MSKCC* Memorial Sloan Kettering Cancer Center risk category, *NA* data not available, *N* number of patients, *PFS* progression-free survival, *PRR* partial response rate

[a]International Metastatic Renal Cell Carcinoma Database Consortium (IMDC) prognostic model

[b]Motzer risk category

[c]Heng risk category

[d]Either one of sunitinib, sorafenib, or bevacizumab

[e]Denominator based on the availability of tumor response information

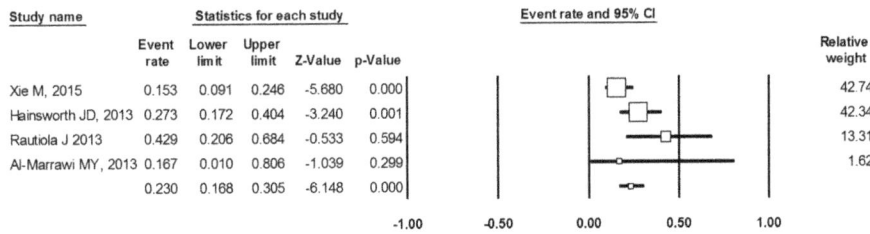

Fig. 2 Meta-analysis forest plot with a fixed-effect model showing the partial response rate (PRR), which is 23 % with a 95 % CI of 17–31 %. The total number of individuals included in the analysis was 156. $I^2 = 52.6$ %. The random-effects model estimated a PRR of 24.5 % (95 % CI, 14.5–38.4 %)

failing to respond to first-line cytokine therapy); [20] and 6.5 months (95 % CI, 4.7–9.1) in all Asian patients (with up to 51 % of the patients failing to respond to first-line cytokine therapy) [21]. Sorafenib in these two trials gave a PFS of 5.7 months (95 % CI, 4.7–6.5) for globally-recruited patients and 4.8 months (95 % CI, 3.0–6.5) in the Asian-only population. In the Asian trial, the overall response rate was reported as 23.7 % (17–32 %), which is very similar to the current meta-analysis result [21].

PRR and PFS data for second-line non-pazopanib targeted agents following non-cytokine first-line therapy are available from the recently reported SWITCH study (only 3 % of all patients previously received cytokine treatment) [8]. The SWITCH study is a European multicenter, randomized phase III trial assessing sorafenib (first-line)-sunitinib (second-line) *vs.* sunitinib-sorafenib (i.e. in the reverse sequence) in patients with mRCC of MSKCC favorable and intermediate risk. The overall response rate in the second-line setting was 17 % in the sorafenib-sunitinib arm and 6.6 % in the sunitinib-sorafenib arm. The magnitude of the ORR is nearly halved compared to the ORR attained in the first-line targeted therapy, which was, on average 23 %, as previously mentioned. The DCR in the second-line setting regarding the sorafenib-sunitinib arm was 49 %, whereas the DCR in the sunitinib-sorafenib arm was 32 %. The

PFS in the second-line setting was 5.4 months (95 % CI, 3.0–5.5 months) in the sorafenib-sunitinib sequence arm, and 2.8 months (95 % CI, 2.7–2.9 months) in the sunitinib-sorafenib sequence arm [8].

Although direct comparison of the above-mentioned studies with the current work is not recommended or correct, the study's intention was to show the possible non-inferiority of pazopanib as a second-line therapy despite previous targeted therapy failure. Evidence-based clinical practice guidelines such as the latest 2014 European Society for Medical Oncology guidelines for diagnosis, treatment and follow-up of RCC suggest pazopanib as a second-line agent only in the setting of first-line cytokine failure [4]. Recommended second-line agents after prior targeted therapy intolerance or failure do not include pazopanib, not because of its ineffectiveness, but solely because there is not yet enough evidence available from randomized controlled trials.

What are the potential advantages when pazopanib is chosen as a second-line drug in terms of anti-neoplastic mechanisms and tolerability to prolonged use of pazopanib? Generally, pazopanib is relatively well tolerated. The most commonly reported treatment-related adverse events include diarrhea (52 %, any grade), hypertension (40 %, any grade), hair color changes (38 %, any grade), nausea (26 %, any grade), and anorexia (24 %, any grade), which tend to be fairly manageable [22]. An interesting

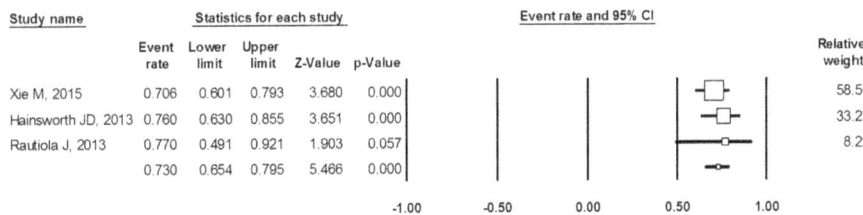

Meta-Analysis of the Disease Control Rate for the Second Line Pazopanib

Fig. 3 Meta-analysis forest plot with a fixed-effect model showing the disease control rate (DCR), which is 73 % with a 95 % CI of 65–80 %. The total number of individuals included in the analysis was 154. $I^2 = 0.000$

Table 2 Meta-analysis with a fixed-effect model for pooling studies on 203 patients on progression-free survival (PFS)

Study name	Statistics for each study							
	Mean[a]	Standard error	Variance	Lower limit	Upper limit	Z value	P value	Total[b]
Rautiola, 2013	11.0	2.222	4.937	6.65	15.36	4.951	0.000	14
Matrana, 2013	3.50	1.203	1.447	1.14	5.86	2.910	0.004	17
Sanchez, 2013	13.00	1.961	3.847	9.16	16.84	6.628	0.000	32
Hainsworth, 2013	7.50	0.973	0.946	5.59	9.41	7.711	0.000	55
Xie, 2015	5.60	0.578	0.334	4.47	6.73	9.684	0.000	85
pooled synthesis	**6.29**	**0.438**	**0.192**	**5.43**	**7.15**	**14.339**	0.000	203
	$I^2 = 83.7 \%$							

Random-effects model estimates a median PFS of 7.6 months (95 % CI, 5.0–10.1)
[a]PFS in months; [b]number of patients in each study; Data in bold-type are the result of data synthesis

cross-over trial demonstrated that pazopanib was superior to sunitinib in health-related quality of life (HRQoL) measures, and significantly more patients reported a preference for pazopanib over sunitinib with HRQoL and safety as the main concerns [23].

The results of the present study could be generalized to a subset of patients with mRCC whose mean age is between 60 and 64 and of the clear cell type, for whom the first-line agent was sunitinib or sorafenib. Ethnicity and prognostic risk category are irrelevant when considering generalizability. Nevertheless, in the meta-analysis, the proportion of patients with poor risk was only around 17 to 34 % representing a minority subgroup of the patients. At the time of writing, we are still lacking adequate evidence-based information on the effectiveness of each second-line targeted agent for this particular poor-risk group.

There are several notable limitations to this study. The number of studies available for the purposes of the meta-analysis was limited and mostly includes small-size studies which may lead to underpowering of the analysis. With the exception of the meta-analysis of the DCR, which had a negligible degree of heterogeneity ($I^2 = 0.000$), the degree of heterogeneity of the studies was moderate when synthesizing the PRR results, and high in the meta-analysis of PFS. The two main reasons for this are that three of the selected studies had fewer than 20 patients, and four of the selected studies were retrospective analyses, while two were phase II clinical trials. The percentage of poor-risk patients in this cohort of mRCC patients was 25 %, which is similar to most of the clinical trial data with unselected patients by risk category. It was not possible to perform subgroup meta-analysis or stratify patients by risk group.

Poor-risk patients have very poor survival, with a median OS of approximately 4 months following diagnosis prior to the era of targeted therapy. With the advent of targeted therapy, a study was performed by Heng et al., in which a model of three risk categories incorporating the MSKCC model with the addition of neutrophil and platelet counts was developed and validated. In the study, the poor-risk group ($N = 152$) having 3–6 prognostic factors, had a median OS of 8.8 months and a 2-year OS of 7 % [24]. The role of pazopanib in this critical clinical scenario requires further investigations.

Currently, having no solid data such as that derived from a randomized controlled trial, pazopanib is not routinely recommended for patients with advanced or mRCC as a second-line targeted therapy after failing a prior targeted agent out of the clinical trial setting.

Conclusion

Pazopanib as a second-line therapy for metastatic renal cell carcinoma following therapy with a targeted agent may be a viable option when other recommended drugs are less suitable for a variety of reasons, such as the patient's inability to tolerate treatment. This meta-analysis of non-comparative studies pooling a total of 217 patients gives a more precise estimate of the treatment effects of pazopanib, such as partial response rate, disease control rate, and progression-free survival in the second-line setting.

Acknowledgements

The authors would like to thank BioMed Proofreading LLC for the language editing of this manuscript by native English-speaking experts.

Authors' contributions

VCK conceived the study, participated in its design and coordination and wrote the manuscript. JTK participated in acquiring the data, performed the statistical analyses and interpreted the data. All authors read and approved the final manuscript. VCK gave final approval of the version to be published.

Authors' information

VCK is the head of the Cancer Center and the Division of Medical Oncology, Kuang Tien General Hospital, Taichung, Taiwan. In 2014, he joined Asia University Taiwan as an Assistant Professor. VCK is a Fellow of the American College of Physicians and a certified member of the European Society for Medical Oncology, as well as a member of the American Society of Clinical Oncology. VCK's research interests include cancer epidemiology, medical oncology and therapeutics, internal medicine, palliative care and population-health informatics. VCK is a review editor of Frontiers in Oncology. JTK graduated from the Department of Applied Mathematics of the National Sun Yat-Sen University of Taiwan and his Master's degree was in Statistics at the same department. He then changed study field into Biostatistics at the Institute of Public Health, School of Medicine, National Yang-Ming University in Taipei, Taiwan.

Competing interests
The authors declare that they have no competing interests.

Consent for publication
Not applicable.

Author details
[1]Division of Medical Oncology, Cancer Center of Kuang Tien General Hospital, 117 Shatien Rd, Taichung 43303, Taiwan. [2]Department of Biomedical Informatics, Asia University, Taichung 41354, Taiwan. [3]Division of Biostatistics, Institute of Public Health, School of Medicine, National Yang-Ming University, Taipei 11221, Taiwan.

References
1. Cella D, Li JZ, Cappelleri JC, Bushmakin A, Charbonneau C, Kim ST, Chen I, Motzer RJ. Quality of life in patients with metastatic renal cell carcinoma treated with sunitinib or interferon alfa: results from a phase III randomized trial. J Clin Oncol. 2008;26(22):3763–9.
2. Su D, Stamatakis L, Singer EA, Srinivasan R. Renal cell carcinoma: molecular biology and targeted therapy. Curr Opin Oncol. 2014;26(3):321–7.
3. Molina AM, Hutson TE, Larkin J, Gold AM, Wood K, Carter D, Motzer R, Michaelson MD. A phase 1b clinical trial of the multi-targeted tyrosine kinase inhibitor lenvatinib (E7080) in combination with everolimus for treatment of metastatic renal cell carcinoma (RCC). Cancer Chemother Pharmacol. 2014;73(1):181–9.
4. Escudier B, Porta C, Schmidinger M, Algaba F, Patard JJ, Khoo V, Eisen T, Horwich A, Group EGW. Renal cell carcinoma: ESMO Clinical Practice Guidelines for diagnosis, treatment and follow-up. Ann Oncol. 2014;25 Suppl 3:iii49–56.
5. Iacovelli R, Carteni G, Sternberg CN, Milella M, Santoni M, Di Lorenzo G, Ortega C, Sabbatini R, Ricotta R, Messina C et al. Clinical outcomes in patients receiving three lines of targeted therapy for metastatic renal cell carcinoma: results from a large patient cohort. Eur J Cancer. 2013;49(9):2134–42.
6. Jurgens H, Tiigi R, Ojamaa K, Pokker H, Innos K, Padrik P. A population-based analysis of changes in therapy of metastatic renal cell carcinoma (mRCC). In: Journal of clinical oncology, vol. 2014. 2014.
7. Soerensen AV, Donskov F, Hermann GG, Jensen NV, Petersen A, Spliid H, Sandin R, Fode K, Geertsen PF. Improved overall survival after implementation of targeted therapy for patients with metastatic renal cell carcinoma: results from the Danish Renal Cancer Group (DARENCA) study-2. Eur J Cancer. 2014; 50(3):553–62.
8. Eichelberg C, Vervenne WL, De Santis M, Fischer Von Weikersthal L, Goebell PJ, Lerchenmuller C, Zimmermann U, Bos MM, Freier W, Schirrmacher-Memmel S et al. SWITCH: A Randomised, Sequential, Open-label Study to Evaluate the Efficacy and Safety of Sorafenib-sunitinib Versus Sunitinib-sorafenib in the Treatment of Metastatic Renal Cell Cancer. Eur Urol. 2015;68(5):837–47.
9. Felici A, Bria E, Tortora G, Cognetti F, Milella M. Sequential therapy in metastatic clear cell renal carcinoma: TKI-TKI vs TKI-mTOR. Expert Rev Anticancer Ther. 2012;12(12):1545–57.
10. Moher D, Liberati A, Tetzlaff J, Altman DG, Group P. Preferred reporting items for systematic reviews and meta-analyses: the PRISMA statement. BMJ. 2009;339:b2535.
11. Hozo SP, Djulbegovic B, Hozo I. Estimating the mean and variance from the median, range, and the size of a sample. BMC Med Res Methodol. 2005;5:13.
12. Krajewski KM, Nishino M, Ramaiya NH, Choueiri TK. RECIST 1.1 compared with RECIST 1.0 in patients with advanced renal cell carcinoma receiving vascular endothelial growth factor-targeted therapy. AJR Am J Roentgenol. 2015;204(3):W282–288.
13. Higgins JP, Thompson SG, Deeks JJ, Altman DG. Measuring inconsistency in meta-analyses. BMJ. 2003;327(7414):557–60.
14. Al-Marrawi MY, Rini BI, Harshman LC, Bjarnason G, Wood L, Vaishampayan U, MacKenzie M, Knox JJ, Agarwal N, Al-Harbi H et al. The association of clinical outcome to first-line VEGF-targeted therapy with clinical outcome to second-line VEGF-targeted therapy in metastatic renal cell carcinoma patients. Targ Oncol. 2013;8(3):203–9.
15. Hainsworth JD, Rubin MS, Arrowsmith ER, Khatcheressian J, Crane EJ, Franco LA. Pazopanib as second-line treatment after sunitinib or bevacizumab in patients with advanced renal cell carcinoma: a Sarah Cannon Oncology Research Consortium Phase II Trial. Clin Genitourin Cancer. 2013;11(3):270–5.
16. Matrana MR, Duran C, Shetty A, Xiao L, Atkinson BJ, Corn P, Pagliaro LC, Millikan RE, Charnsangave C, Jonasch E et al. Outcomes of patients with metastatic clear-cell renal cell carcinoma treated with pazopanib after disease progression with other targeted therapies. Eur J Cancer. 2013;49(15):3169–75.
17. Rautiola J, Utriainen T, Peltola K, Joensuu H, Bono P. Pazopanib after sunitinib failure in patients with metastatic renal cell carcinoma. Acta Oncol. 2014;53(1):113–8.
18. Rodriguez Sanchez A, Garcia Dominguez R, De Velasco G, Pinto A, Puente J, Rubio G, Vazquez-Estevez S, Juan M, Constenla M, Lopez Brea M et al. Pazopanib in metastatic renal carcinoma (mRC): Experience of 31 centers in Spain in first, second, third, or subsequent lines in daily clinical practice. ASCO Meeting Abstracts. 2013;31(15_suppl):e15609.
19. Xie M, He CS, Huang JK, Lin QZ. Phase II study of pazopanib as second-line treatment after sunitinib in patients with metastatic renal cell carcinoma: a Southern China Urology Cancer Consortium Trial. Eur J Cancer. 2015;51(5): 595–603.
20. Motzer RJ, Escudier B, Tomczak P, Hutson TE, Michaelson MD, Negrier S, Oudard S, Gore ME, Tarazi J, Hariharan S et al. Axitinib versus sorafenib as second-line treatment for advanced renal cell carcinoma: overall survival analysis and updated results from a randomised phase 3 trial. Lancet Oncol. 2013;14(6):552–62.
21. Qin S, Bi F, Jin J, Cheng Y, Guo J, Ren X, Huang Y, Tarazi J, Tang J, Chen C et al. Axitinib versus sorafenib as a second-line therapy in Asian patients with metastatic renal cell carcinoma: results from a randomized registrational study. Onco Targets Ther. 2015;8:1363–73.
22. Sternberg CN, Hawkins RE, Wagstaff J, Salman P, Mardiak J, Barrios CH, Zarba JJ, Gladkov OA, Lee E, Szczylik C et al. A randomised, double-blind phase III study of pazopanib in patients with advanced and/or metastatic renal cell carcinoma: final overall survival results and safety update. Eur J Cancer. 2013;49(6):1287–96.
23. Escudier B, Porta C, Bono P, Powles T, Eisen T, Sternberg CN, Gschwend JE, De Giorgi U, Parikh O, Hawkins R et al. Randomized, controlled, double-blind, cross-over trial assessing treatment preference for pazopanib versus sunitinib in patients with metastatic renal cell carcinoma: PISCES Study. J Clin Oncol. 2014;32(14):1412–8.
24. Heng DY, Xie W, Regan MM, Warren MA, Golshayan AR, Sahi C, Eigl BJ, Ruether JD, Cheng T, North S et al. Prognostic factors for overall survival in patients with metastatic renal cell carcinoma treated with vascular endothelial growth factor-targeted agents: results from a large, multicenter study. J Clin Oncol. 2009;27(34):5794–9.

21

Nephron-sparing management of Xanthogranulomatous pyelonephritis presenting as spontaneous renal hemorrhage

William Keith Ballentine III[1]*[iD], Fernandino Vilson[2], Raymond B Dyer[3] and Majid Mirzazadeh[1]

Abstract

Background: Xanthogranulomatous pyelonephritis (XGP) is an uncommon infectious disease of the kidney known to mimic other renal maladies. A rare presentation of this uncommon disease is spontaneous renal hemorrhage (SRH).

Case presentation: We report a case of XGP in a 58 year old woman who presented with abdominal pain, hematuria, and radiating left flank pain. CT scan was felt to be consistent with perirenal hemorrhage abutting a fat-containing renal mass. The patient was eventually taken to surgery for left partial nephrectomy. Pathology report returned as XGP, and the patient has no complications from this disease process at 8 month follow up.

Conclusion: Our search of the literature shows XGP presenting as SRH to be a rare clinical entity. Furthermore, this is the first such case managed with a nephron-sparing approach. The "great imitator" XGP should be added to the differential for patients presenting with spontaneous renal hemorrhage.

Keywords: Xanthogranulomatous pyelonephritis, Spontaneous renal hemorrhage, Wunderlich syndrome, Subcapsular renal hematoma, Case report

Background

XGP is an uncommon infectious disease of the kidney first described in 1918 by Schlagenhaufer and characterized by chronic obstruction and inflammation [1]. The chronic inflammatory renal mass invades the renal parenchyma, replacing it with lipid laden macrophages. Pathologically, the lipid laden macrophages give the renal parenchyma a "tan-yellow" appearance [2]. SRH is defined as a non-traumatic, spontaneous renal bleed into the subcapsular and/or perirenal space. It was first observed by Bonet in 1679 and further described by Wunderlich in 1856 [3, 4]. This is only the 5th case report of XGP presenting as SRH.

Herein, we reported a female presenting with abdominal pain and hematuria with radiographic findings consistent with SRH who was found to have XGP as the underlying cause of her illness. We also review the epidemiology, diagnosis, and management of these two conditions.

Case presentation

A 58 year old female presented with hematuria and left flank pain that radiated to the abdomen. Computed tomography (CT) scan demonstrated a heterogeneous 8.3 X 6.5 X 4.9 cm fat-containing mass arising from the lower pole of the left kidney (Fig. 1c). CT also demonstrated an asymmetrically enlarged left psoas muscle (Fig. 1b), soft tissue stranding (Figs. 1a & 2), mild hydronephrosis, and splenomegaly (Fig. 2). Further evaluation of the CT scan goes on to reveal extensive fascial

---

* Correspondence: wballent@wakehealth.edu
[1]Department of Urology, Wake Forest Baptist Health, Medical Center Blvd, Winston-Salem, NC 27157, USA
Full list of author information is available at the end of the article

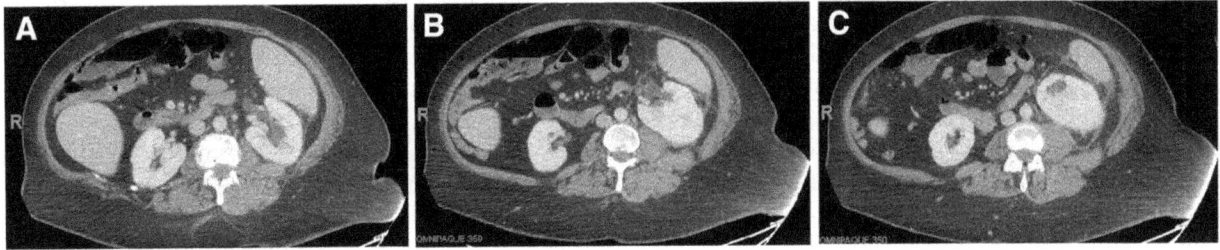

Fig. 1 Axial CT scan demonstrating left renal hydronephrosis **a** and a non enhancing lesion of the left kidney **c** (arrowhead). Asymmetric psosas muscle **b** is identified and noticeable fat stranding along the posterior peritoneal wall (arrowhead). Ureteral calyces identified and demostrate distention possibly hemorrhaging

thickening involving the anterior and posterior left renal fascia. Based on these findings, hemorrhagic angiomyolipoma was felt to be the most likely condition. Past medical history was significant for bipolar disorder and chronic right foot wounds associated with contiguous spread of chronic osteomyelitis of the 5th metatarsal.

Physical exam was remarkable for enlarged body habitus (BMI 34.7), limited ROM in right shoulder, arm, and neck. Laboratory abnormalities included an elevated glucose (186 mg/dl) and calcium (6.9 mg/dl). White cell count, BUN, and creatinine levels were within normal limits. Urine culture demonstrated no growth in 18–24 h and showed < 10,000 col./ml.

The decision was made to treat the patient with open left partial nephrectomy. Intraoperatively, the mass was easily found along the inferior portion of the kidney. The mass had a large desmoplastic reaction surround it from a prior bleeding episode. Adhesions surrounding the vascular pedicle were released. The pedicle was then clamped and cold ischemia was induced after mannitol injection. Resection of the mass was performed by scoring the mass with Bovie electrocautery and carefully dissecting the mass from the normal parenchyma by blunt

dissection with a Penfield nerve retractor. All bleeding vessels were ligated. There was 36 min of cold ischemia time and 200 ml of estimated blood loss. After appropriate closure of the surgical sites, the mass was sent to pathology and because of considerable need for pyelocaliceal closure a double J ureteral stent and foley were placed. Postoperatively, the patient experienced urinary retention after foley catheter removal. Once stable, she was discharged back to skilled nursing facility with a catheter in place that was later removed.

At 10 day postoperative outpatient follow up, the patient was doing well and asymptomatic. BUN and creatinine levels were within normal limits but calcium remained low. Ureteral stent was easily removed during office cystoscopy. Eight months later the patient reported no signs of flank pain or hematuria and has remained at her pre-operative baseline.

Discussion

XGP is well known for its capacity to mimic many other disorders, most notably renal neoplasms [5, 6]. Previously published case series have shown a higher incidence of disease in older women, patients obstructed

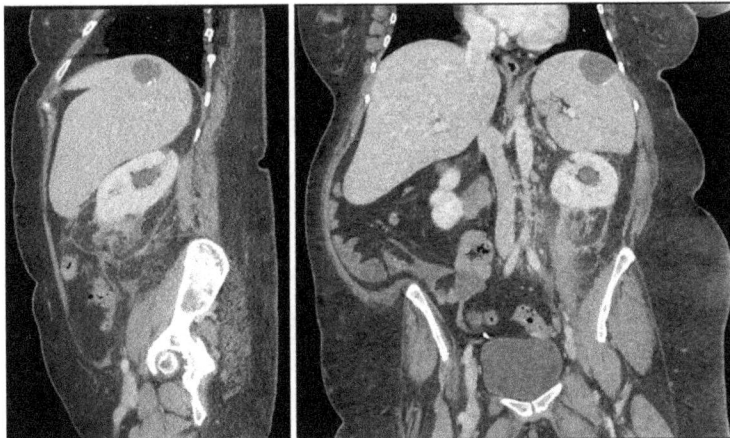

Fig. 2 Coronal and sagittal CT scan demonstrating abnormal mass of left kidney, fat stranding, and hepatospenomegaly. There is a 3.5 cm round low attenuated area with peripheral calcifications in the spleen. Likely relates to prior trauma or infection

from nephrolithiasis, and infection by *Escherichia coli* or *Proteus mirabilis*. [7–9]. XGP is classified into either the more prominent diffuse form or a focal entity [10]. It is further subdivided into 3 stages (nephric, perinephric, and paranephric) on the basis of the extent of inflammatory response. In part due to the rarity of XGP, preoperative diagnosis is difficult with most cases diagnosed post-operatively on pathological examination. Clinical diagnosis is hampered by non-specific symptoms, and pre-operative radiologic imaging has been found to be of only moderate assistance in diagnosis [11]. While the classic "bear's paw" sign is reasonably diagnostic of XGP, further radiologic specificity is limited by the heterogenous nature of the disease. One study of 11 patients with XGP found that 91% of patients demonstrated extrarenal extension of inflammatory changes and 82% had multiple dilated calyces and abnormal parenchyma, but 27% had focal fat deposits and a separate 27% had extensive retroperitoneal inflammation up to and including inflammation of the abdominal wall [12].

SRH, also known as Wunderlich Syndrome, is another uncommon urologic condition. The etiology of SRH is most frequently due to renal neoplasm but has also been known to arise due to vascular disease or infection [13]. While the infectious etiologies of SRH are known to include emphysematous pyelonephritis, to the best of our knowledge this is only the 5th case in the literature of XGP presenting with Wunderlich syndrome, although this is difficult to assess due to the many different terms applied to the condition [14–17]. SRH may classically present with "Lenk's triad" (acute flank pain, abdominal tenderness, and symptoms of internal bleeding), but the disease is also known to present similarly to other abdominal conditions such as appendicitis or dissecting abdominal aortic aneurysm [13, 18]. Unlike XGP, CT imaging of SRH patients is able to identify 100% of patients suffering from the disease, though it lacks sensitivity for the etiology of SRH. Ultrasound has also been used for the detection of SRH but was not shown to be as reliable.

Three of 4 XGP cases presenting with Wunderlich syndrome are summarised and can be reviewed in Table 1. Canale et al., in a letter to the editor, presents a

case of retroperitoneal hemorrhage with hemorrhagic shock [15]. Briefly, a 36 year old woman presented with right lower abdominal pain with palpable mass over right pelvic area. Laboratory findings included microcytic anemia and elevated white blood cell count (12,000 per mm^3). Urinalysis (UA) was positive for leukocytes and pyuria. Urine culture was negative.

CT scan demonstrated bilateral central staghorn calculi with replacement of renal parenchyma with low attenuated collections in a hydronephrotic pattern. CT also showed a lower pole mass in the right kidney consistent with perinephric inflammatory changes. T1 and T2 weighted MRI images of the mass showed multiple enhancing septa.

Two days following the initial presentation the patient was seen again for acute abdominal pain with a red cell count of 6 g/dl, blood pressure of 80/60, and was transferred to the intensive care unit for hemorrhagic shock. CT scan now showed an interval increase in the size of the renal mass and hemoperitoneum. After right nephrectomy pathological examination of the mass revealed abundant foamy macrophage aggregates, neutrophils, fibrosis, and inflammatory cell infiltrations, confirming the diagnosis of XGP [15].

Altinoluk et al., describe a case of XGP with spontaneous kidney rupture in a young female [16]. A 25 year old woman presented with sudden onset right flank pain associated with fever and nausea. She was previously treated for UTI the week prior. Her blood pressure was 90/55 mmHg, hemoglobin 6.3 g/dl, white blood cell count was 16,700 per mm^3. UA revealed hematuria only. Abdominal ultrasound and computed tomography displayed a large hypoechoic mass (12 X 7 cm) around the right kidney which extended into the pelvis and paravertebral space. Exploration of the mass revealed a large perirenal hematoma, abscess, and renal rupture. Culture of the abscess grew *Proteus mirabilis*. Histopathological examination following right nephrectomy revealed foamy, lipid laden macrophages, giant cells, polymorphonuclear cells, granulomatous reaction and fibrosis. A diagnosis of XGP was made [16].

Lastly, Sharma et al., reported a case of a 60 year old male who presented with left sided flank pain,

Table 1 Summary of XGP cases presenting as Wunderlich syndrome

Case	Presentation	CBC	UA	Culture (urine or site)	Surgery	Pathology
Canle et al. [15], 2007	Right lower abdominal pain and asthenia	Hgb 8 9/dl WBC 12000/mm^3	+leukocyte +Pyuria	*Streptococcus anginosus*	Right total nephrectomy	Foamy macrophages aggregates, neutrophils, fibrosis. Inflammatory cell infiltrate
Altinoluk et al. [17], 2012	Right flank pain, fever, nausea	Hgb 6.3 g/dl WBC 16.7/ uL	Hematuria only	*Proteus mirabilis*	Right total nephrectomy	Foamy, lipid laden macrophages, giant cells, granulomatous reaction and fibrosis
Sharma et al. [16], 2013	Left flank pain, intermittent fever, weakness x15days	Hgb 9 g/dl WBC 13500/mm3	–	*Klebsiella*	Left total nephrectomy	Chronic granulomatous pyelonephritis. With dilated vascular channels

intermittent fever, and weakness for 15 days [17]. A known diabetic, the patient was anemic (Hgb 9.0) with an elevated white blood cell count (13,500 per mm^3). Urine culture was positive for *Klebsiella* and the patient was subsequently started on IV antibiotics. MRI abdomen demonstrated a hydronephrotic left kidney with an ill-defined mass of the lower pole suggestive of perinephric hematoma. Further, the patient was suspected to have a hemorrhagic angiomyolipoma and was thus surgically explored. During exploration, the kidney was noted to be hydronephrotic with thinned out parenchyma and palpable thickening of the lower pole which warranted nephrectomy. Unlike the previous cases, lipid-laden macrophage aggregates were not seen though further histopathological examination of the mass revealed chronic granulomatous pyelonephritis with dilated vascular channels and no evidence of neoplasia [17].

Management

The traditional approach to XGP has been radical nephrectomy, though a nephron-sparing approach has been reported in the management of focal cases of XGP [19–21]. Conservative management of XGP has been achieved with parenteral antibiotic therapy or a combination of oral and parenteral therapy which may be supplemented with drainage of the urinary tract and/or abscesses [22–24]. Conservative management has even proven successful in renal allograft patients with XGP [25]. However, conservative management is inappropriate for patients with stage III or diffuse XGP, as may be seen in many patients at the time of diagnosis. Nephron-sparing management has been successfully attempted in cases of multifocal XGP, a distinct entity from diffuse XGP. As XGP is often diagnosed first at pathological specimen, the decision for treatment is usually based on a presumptive diagnosis in which radical nephrectomy may be more appropriate.

Management of SRH is first pursued through conservative or minimally invasive approaches. As the underlying cause of SRH may be focally identified by renal arteriography, embolization is an important therapeutic treatment that may preclude the need for surgery. In cases of iatrogenic renal hemorrhage, the combined use of urokinase injections and external drainage has been reported as an effective strategy in patients with large hematomas who nonetheless had stable vital signs [26]. This approach could also prove useful in SRH though we can find no explicit report of this in the literature. In the case of the unstable patient, surgical exploration is necessary if angioembolization is not available or is unsuccessful. Surgical exploration can be especially important if the source of the bleeding is found to be a renal neoplasm. Even in cases where bleeding can be managed conservatively, surgical evacuation of the clot may be required in instances of hypertension secondary to Page kidney.

All four previous reports of XGP presenting with SRH were managed by radical nephrectomy. We report the first case of nephron-sparing surgery for XGP presenting with SRH. Our management decision was facilitated by a pre-operative differential heavily weighted towards AML as the etiology of SRH. Prior to this procedure our approach to cases involving a large XGP lesion would have been unlikely to include a nephron-sparing approach, though we are happy to report that such an approach is certainly technically feasible.

Conclusion

This report describes a rare presentation of an uncommon infectious disease. Our review of the literature confirms the rarity of XGP presenting with SRH. The importance of a broad differential diagnosis for this condition cannot be overlooked. Nephron-sparing surgery should always be considered as a possibility even in these difficult cases.

Abbreviations

CT: Computed tomography; Hgb: Hemoglobin; SRH: Spontaneous renal hemorrhage; UA: Urinalysis; WBC: White blood cell count; XGP: Xanthogranulomatous Pyelonephritis

Acknowledgments

We would like to thank Dr. Ray Dyer for his assistance in interpreting radiological images used in the study and for his guidance in drafting and editing this manuscript.

Authors' contributions

MM was the responsible urologist for the patient and performed the surgery. WB, FV, & MM contributed to the concept and design of the study. WB & FV both contributed to the acquisition of data, analysis and interpretation of data, as well as the drafting of the manuscript. MM & RD participated in the critical revision of the manuscript for important intellectual content, material support, and supervision. RD & MM also contributed to the acquisition of valuable data, analysis and interpretation of data, and final approval of the manuscript. All authors read and approved the final manuscript.

Competing interests

The authors declare that they have no competing interests.

Author details

[1]Department of Urology, Wake Forest Baptist Health, Medical Center Blvd, Winston-Salem, NC 27157, USA. [2]Wake Forest School of Medicine, Winston-Salem, NC 27157, USA. [3]Department of Radiology, Wake Forest Baptist Health, Winston-Salem, NC 27157, USA.

References

1. Schlagenhaufer F. Uber eigentumlich staphylomykosender neiven und des pararenalen bindegewebes. Frankfurt Z Pathol. 1916(19):139–48.

2.   Yoshino T, Moriyama H. Case of the diffuse form of Xanthogranulomatous
     pyelonephritis. Case Rep Urol. 2013; ID 936035: 3 pages.
3.   Bonet T. Sepulchretum, sive anatomiapractica ex cadaverbius
     morbobdenatis. Geneva: L Chouet; 1679.
4.   Wunderlich CR. Handbuck der Pathologie und Therapie. In: ed 2nd, editor.
     Polkey Vynalek. Stuttgart: Ebner and Seubert; 1856.
5.   Zoros I, Moutzouris V, Petraki C, et al. Xanthogranulomatous pyelonephritis –
     the "great imitator" justifies its name. Scand J Urol Nephrol. 2002;36:74–6.
6.   Gerber WL, Catalona WJ, Fair WR, et al. Xanthogranulomatous pyelonephritis
     masquerading as occult malignancy. Urology. 1978;11:466–71.
7.   Addison B, Zargar H, Lilic N, Merrilees D, Rice M. Analysis of 35 cases of
     Xanthogranulomatous pyelonephritis. ANZ J Surg. 2015;85:150–3.
8.   Korkes F, Favoretto RL, Bróglio M, Silva CA, Castro MG, Perez MD.
     Xanthogranulomatous pyelonephritis: clinical experience with 41 cases.
     Urology. 2008;71:178–80.
9.   Kim SW, Yoon BI, Ha US, Sohn DW, Cho YH. Xanthogranulomatous pyelonephritis:
     clinical experience with 21 cases. J Infect Chemother. 2013;19(6):1221–4.
10. Samuel M, Duffy P, Capps S, Mouriquand P, Williams D, Ransley P.
     Xanthogranulomatous pyelonephritis in childhood. J Pediatr Surg.
     2001;36:598–601.
11. Malek RS, Elder JS. Xanthogranulomatous pyelonephritis: a critical analysis of
     26 cases and of the literature. J Urol. 1978;119:589–93.
12. Rajesh A, Jakanani G, Mayer N, Mulcahy K. Computed tomography findings
     in xanthogranulomatous pyelonephritis. J Clin Imaging Sci. 2011;1:45.
13. Zhang JQ, Fielding JR, Zou KH. Etiology of spontaneous perirenal
     hemorrhage: a meta-analysis. J Urol. 2002;167:1593–6.
14. Wakasugi E, Kato Y, Yano H, Kanbara N, Kurita T. Spontaneous renal rupture
     due to xanthogranulomatous pyelonephritis; a case report. Hinyokika Kiyo.
     1996;42:47–50. Japanese
15. Canale S, Deux JF, De la Taille A, Bouanane M, Luciani A, Rahmouni A. Acute
     retroperitoneal hemorrhage complicating a xanthogranulomatous
     pyelonephritis. Eur Radiol. 2007;17:1128–9.
16. Altinoluk B, Sayar H, Özkaya M, Sahinkanat T, Malkoc O.
     Xanthogranulomatous pyelonephritis presented with spontaneous kidney
     rupture in a young woman. Eur J Gen Med. 2012;9:138–41.
17. Sharma A, Rehan F, Sanjay RP, Ratkal CS, Kamath AJ, Venkatesh GK. An unusual
     presentation of chronic granulomatous pyelonephritis presenting as an acute
     spontaneous retroperitoneal Hemmorhage. J Case Rep. 2013;3:114–6.
18. Albi G, del Campo L, Tagarro D. Wünderlich's syndrome: causes, diagnosis
     and radiological management. Clin Radiol. 2002;57:840–5.
19. Osca JM, Peiro MJ, Rodrigo M, Martinez-Jabaloyas JM, Jimenez-Cruz JF. Focal
     xanthogranulomatous pyelonephritis: partial nephrectomy as definitive
     treatment. Eur Urol. 1997;32:375–9.
20. Shinde S, Kandpal DK, Chowdhary SK. Focal xanthogranulomatous
     pyelonephritis presenting as renal tumor. Indian J Nephrol. 2013;23:76–7.
21. Peréz LM, Thrasher JB, Anderson EE. Successful management of bilateral
     xanthogranulomatous pyelonephritis by bilateral partial nephrectomy.
     J Urol. 1993;149:100–2.
22. Chlif M, Chakroun M, Ben Rhouma S, Ben Chehida MA, Sellami A, Gargouri MM,
     Nouira Y. Xanthogranulomatous pyelonephritis presenting as a pseudotumour.
     Can Urol Assoc J. 2016;10:E36–40.
23. Friedl A, Tuerk C, Schima W, Broessner C. Xanthogranulomatous
     pyelonephritis with staghorn Calculus, acute gangrenous appendicitis and
     enterocolitis: a multidisciplinary challenge of kidney-preserving conservative
     therapy. Curr Urol. 2015;8:162–5.
24. Brown PS, Dodson M, Weintrub PS. Xanthogranulomatous pyelonephritis:
     report of non surgical management of a case and review of the literature.
     Clin Infect Dis. 1996;22:308–14.
25. Elkhammas EA, Mutabagani KH, Sedmak DD, Tesi RJ, Henry ML, Fergu-son RM.
     Xanthogranulomatous pyelonephritis in renal allografts: report of 2 cases.
     J Urol. 1994;151:127–8.
26. Shen Z, He W, Liu D, Pan F, Li W, Han X, Li B. Novel technique for the treatment
     of large subcapsular renal hematoma: combined use of percutaneous drainage
     and urokinase injection. Int Urol Nephrol. 2014;46:1751–5.

22

Involvement of the bone morphogenic protein/SMAD signaling pathway in the etiology of congenital anomalies of the kidney and urinary tract accompanied by cryptorchidism

Kentaro Mizuno[1], Akihiro Nakane[1], Hidenori Nishio[1], Yoshinobu Moritoki[1], Hideyuki Kamisawa[1], Satoshi Kurokawa[1], Taiki Kato[1], Ryosuke Ando[1], Tetsuji Maruyama[1], Takahiro Yasui[1] and Yutaro Hayashi[2]*

Abstract

Background: Congenital anomalies of the kidney and urinary tract (CAKUT), such as renal dysplasia, hydronephrosis, or vesicoureteral reflux, are the most common causes of end-stage renal disease. However, the genetic etiology of CAKUT remains unclear. In this study, we performed whole exome sequencing (WES) to elucidate the genetic etiology of symptomatic CAKUT and CAKUT accompanied by cryptorchidism.

Methods: Three patients with unilateral renal dysplasia accompanied by ipsilateral cryptorchidism were included in this analysis. Genomic DNA was extracted from peripheral blood, and WES was performed. Disease-specific single nucleotide polymorphisms (SNPs) were determined by comparison with the human genome reference sequence (hg19). Additionally, we searched for SNPs that were common to all three patients, with a particular focus on the coding regions of the target genes.

Results: In total, 8710 SNPs were detected. Of the genes harboring these SNPs, 32 associated with renal or testicular development were selected for further analyses. Of these, eight genes (i.e., *SMAD4*, *ITGA8*, *GRIP1*, *FREM1*, *FREM2*, *TNXB*, *BMP8B*, and *SALL1*) carried a single amino acid substitution that was common to all three patients. In particular, SNPs in *SMAD4* (His290Pro and His291Pro) have not been reported previously in patients with symptomatic CAKUT. Of the candidate genes, four genes (i.e., *ITGA8*, *GRIP1*, *FREM1*, and *FREM2*) were Fraser syndrome-related genes, encoding proteins that functionally converged on the glial cell-derived neurotrophic factor/RET/bone morphogenic protein (BMP) signaling pathways. As another candidate gene, the protein encoded by *BMP8B* activates the nuclear translocation of SMAD4, which regulates the expression of genes associated with the differentiation of primordial germ cells or testicular development. Additionally, BMP4, a member of the BMP family, regulates the interaction between metanephric mesenchyme and ureteric buds by suppressing GDNF.

Conclusions: Taken together, our findings suggested that the development of the kidney and urinary tract is intimately linked with that of male reproductive organs via BMP/SMAD signaling pathways.

Keywords: Congenital anomalies of the kidney and urinary tract, Cryptorchidism, Exome sequencing, Renal development

* Correspondence: yutaro@med.nagoya-cu.ac.jp
[2]Department of Pediatric urology, Nagoya City University Graduate School of Medical Sciences, 1 Kawasumi, Mizuho-cho, Mizuho-ku, Nagoya, Japan
Full list of author information is available at the end of the article

Background

Congenital anomalies of the kidney and urinary tract (CAKUT) account for approximately 40–50% cases of end-stage renal disease in children [1]. CAKUT is a comprehensive disease concept, including renal hypoplasia, dysplasia, hydronephrosis (ureteropelvic junction obstruction or ureterovesical junction obstruction), ureter duplex, vesicoureteral reflux, and posterior urethral valves [2]. The incidence of CAKUT is estimated to be 3–6 per 1000 live births [3]. In general, the structural anomalies found in patients with CAKUT are often related because impaired codevelopment of nephrogenic tissues derived from the metanephric mesenchyme and ureteric bud is thought to contribute to the pathogenesis of CAKUT [4]. Thus, the etiology of CAKUT is heterogeneous and includes mutations in genes involved in the embryonic development of the kidneys [2]. A previous study showed that monogenic causes could be detected in about 12% of patients [5]. Thus, elucidating the genetic etiology of CAKUT is important for the diagnosis of asymptomatic renal disease, advanced diagnosis of inheritance patterns, and referral to genetic counseling in the clinical setting [2].

While CAKUT most frequently occurs as an isolated case and without renal or urinary tract structural anomalies or symptoms, it may also appear with other systemic disorders, such as Fraser syndrome [1], Hirchsprung disease [6], or vertebral defects, anal atresia, cardiac defects, tracheo-esophageal fistula, renal anomalies, and limb abnormalities (VACTERL association) [7]. Notably, anomalies in the epididymis are sometimes encountered during surgery for cryptorchidism. Although the complete mechanism of testicular descent remains unclear, a recent study revealed that maldevelopment of the epididymis is associated with problems in testicular descent [8]. Because both the epididymis and ureteric bud are embryologically derived from the mesonephric duct, we hypothesized that a common mechanism may be responsible for the maldevelopment of the ureteric bud and impaired testicular descent. A previous study demonstrated that the pathogenesis of CAKUT is associated with mutations in several genes, including HNF1B, PAX2, or SALL1 [9]. In contrast, studies in knockout mice [10, 11] and genome-wide association studies [12] have shown that INSL3 and TGFBR3 are involved in the onset of cryptorchidism. However, few reports have described the genetic etiology of CAKUT accompanied by cryptorchidism [13].

Thus, in the present study, whole-exome sequencing (WES) was used to elucidate the genetic etiology of "symptomatic CAKUT," i.e., CAKUT accompanied by cryptorchidism. We identified single nucleotide polymorphisms (SNPs) common to all patients and detected 10 non-synonymous SNPs from eight genes known to be associated with CAKUT or testicular development, including BMP8B and SMAD4, whose gene products function in the same signaling pathway. Our findings provide important insights into the relationship between renal and testicular development and these signaling pathways.

Methods

Patients and sample preparation

From patients who were treated or followed-up at Nagoya City University Hospital from July 2011 to January 2015, three patients with CAKUT complicated by ipsilateral cryptorchidism were enrolled in this study. Patient characteristics are shown in Table 1. At the initial visit, every patient was referred to our hospital because scrotal contents were absent and abdominal ultrasonography, computed tomography (CT) scanning, or magnetic resonance imaging (MRI) examinations revealed renal aplasia or multicystic dysplastic kidney. Case 3 had a pelvic dysplastic kidney and underwent ipsilateral nephrectomy simultaneously with orchiectomy for abdominal testis. Chromosome analysis was performed for all patients; case 3 showed chromosomal abnormality (46,Y, add (X) (p22.3)). Genomic DNA was extracted from the peripheral blood of the patients using a Wizard genomic DNA purification kit, according to the manufacturer's instructions, as previously reported [14]. The purity of the extracted DNA was determined by measuring the absorbance and visually by gel electrophoresis.

WES analysis

Whole exons were purified from genomic DNA using a SureSelevtXT Human All Exon v5 Kit (Agilent Technologies, Santa Clara, CA, USA). After ligation of specific adaptors for exon fragments, paired-end sequencing was performed on a Hiseq 2500 instrument (Illumina Inc., San Diego, CA, USA). Raw sequence data in fastq format were uploaded to the DNAnexus platform server (DNAnexus Inc., San Francisco, CA, USA) and aligned to the human reference genome (hg19). After all data were exported to Microsoft Excel and Access, we searched for SNPs that were common to all three patients, with a particular focus on the coding region.

Table 1 Patient characteristics

Case No.	Diagnosis	Age	G-banding	Treatment
1	Right renal aplasia, Right abdominal testis, Agenesis of right vas deferens and seminal vesicle	31 y	46,XY	Laparoscopic right orchiopexy
2	Left multicystic dysplastic kidney, Bil. cryptorchidism, Micropenis	1 y	46,XY	Laparoscopic bilateral orchiopexy
3	Left multicystic dysplastic kidney (pelvis), Left abdominal testis, Agenesis of left vas deferens	2 y	46,Y, add(X) (p22.3)	Laparoscopic left nephrectomy left orchiectomy

SNP analysis at specific gene loci

Next, we selected 32 genes that have been reported to be associated with CAKUT or testicular development: *BMP7, CDC5L, CHD1L, GATA3, HNF1B, PAX2, RET, ROBO2, SALL1, SIX2, SIX5, EYA2* [9], *FRAS1, FREM2, GRIP1, FREM1, ITGA8, GREM1, ILK, LIN7C, DACT1* [1], *TNXB* [15], *DSTYK* [16], *WNT4, WT1, PAX7* [17], *SALL4* [18, 19], *BMP4, SMAD4* [20], *BMP8B* [21], *GDNF,* and *GFRA1* [13]. From the WES data, we evaluated SNPs in these 32 genes. We further examined the shared SNPs among 3 cases using by subsequent filtering of variants based on their frequencies (minor allele frequency (MAF)) in databases including Exome Aggregation Consortium (ExAC), 1000 Genome Project, Exome Variant Server (ESP).

Ethics statement

Studies using human genomic material were performed only after obtaining written informed consent from the patient (case 1) and the families of the patients and approval from the Nagoya City University Hospital review board (approval no. 184).

Results

The total number of sequencing reads for all exons of the three patients (cases 1, 2, and 3) were 55,657,960, 50,214,710, and 55,301,946, respectively. To improve the accuracy of the SNP data, raw data were filtered using the DNAnexus platform server under the following conditions: variant score > 30, iRef >30, and coverage >30. Subsequently, the numbers of SNPs in cases 1, 2, and 3 were decreased to 84,810, 76,182, and 82,791, respectively. In total, 8710 SNPs were common to all three patients (Fig. 1). The chromosomal locations of these SNPs were determined; chromosomes 1, 11, 12, 17, and 19 showed the highest number of SNPs. Chromosome Y harbored only two SNPs (Fig. 2).

We further investigated the SNPs within 32 specific gene loci and detected 10 non-synonymous SNPs within eight genes (Table 2). Of these SNPs, two in *SMAD4* had not been reported previously, suggesting that these may be novel variants in patients with CAKUT. *SMAD4* is a central mediator of the transforming growth factor (TGF)-β/bone morphogenic protein (BMP) signaling pathway and promotes transcriptional activation of target genes [22]. We also detected an SNP in *BMP8B* (rs179472; Ser276Thr). *BMP8B* belongs to the TGF-β superfamily and triggers the phosphorylation of intracellular receptor-regulated SMADs (R-SMADs), which function as transcription factors. Phosphorylated R-SMAD interacts with SMAD4 and translocates to the nucleus, where it regulates the transcription of over 500 target genes [23]. SNPs in *ITGA8, GRIP1, FREM1,* and *FREM2* have been reported in a WES study of patients with isolated CAKUT [1]; however, these findings were not

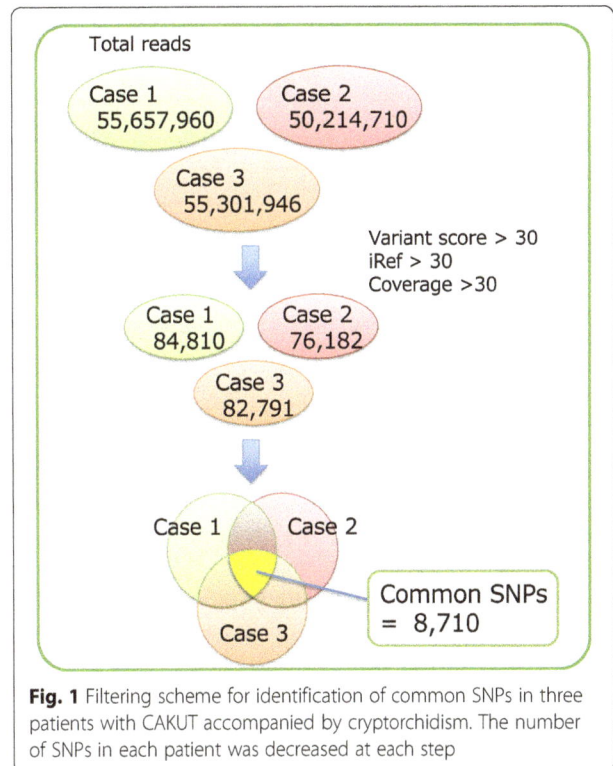

Fig. 1 Filtering scheme for identification of common SNPs in three patients with CAKUT accompanied by cryptorchidism. The number of SNPs in each patient was decreased at each step

consistent with our results. In addition, although a deleterious heterozygous mutation in *TNXB* (Thr3257Ile) has been shown to cause hereditary vesicoureteral reflux (VUR) [15], this was not true for the SNP detected in the present study (rs6457477; Arg504His). Moreover, the SNP identified in *SALL1* (rs4614723; Val1178Ile) was different from that reported in a WES study for familial CAKUT [9]; however, the same SNP was reported in a previous case report [24]. MAF of SNPs in *SMAD4* and *FREM2* (rs2496423) is lower than 1%, and remaining 7 SNPs in 7 genes are more common in the general population.

Discussion

In the present study, we performed WES of samples from three patients with CAKUT accompanied by cryptorchidism to elucidate the genetic etiology of the disease. We detected 10 non-synonymous SNPs in the coding regions of eight genes. In particular, we identified two novel SNPs in *SMAD4* (His290Pro and His291Pro) and one SNP in *BMP8B* (rs179472; Ser276Thr). Both *BMP8B* and *SMAD4* function in the same signaling pathway, and it is likely that this pathway is involved in the etiology in CAKUT accompanied by cryptorchidism. The other candidate SNPs (*ITGA8, GRIP1, FREM1, FREM2, TNXB,* and *SALL1*) identified in this study were consistent with previous WES studies examining isolated or familial CAKUT [1, 9, 15, 24]. In particular, four of these genes (i.e., *ITGA8, GRIP1, FREM1,* and *FREM2*) were Fraser syndrome-related genes reported previously by Kohl et al. [1]. Fraser syndrome is a rare

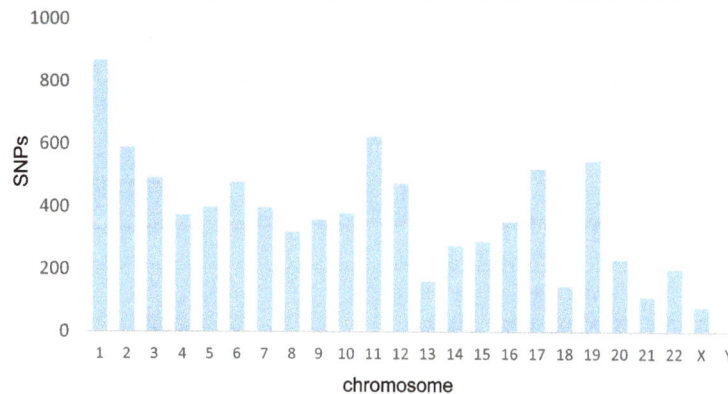

Fig. 2 Graphical view of the number of SNPs in each chromosome. The number of SNPs was greater in chromosomes 1, 11, 12, 17, and 19 than in the other chromosomes. Chromosome Y had only two SNPs

autosomal-recessive disorder with features of cryptophthalmos, syndactyly, ambiguous genitalia, laryngeal and genitourinary malformations, oral clefting, and mental retardation [25]. Because such mutated Fraser syndrome-related genes encode proteins that functionally converge on the glial cell-derived neutotrophic factor (GDNF)-RET/BMP signaling pathways at the interface of the ureteric bud and metanephric mesenchyme [1], these results also supported our hypothesis that alterations in the BMP/SMAD signaling pathway may cause renal maldevelopment with ipsilateral cryptorchidism. In case 3 patient, he has chromosomal abnormality (46,Y, add(X)(p22.3)). This chromosomal abnormality means addition of unknown fragment to terminal end of the short arm of X chromosome. Although there is the possibility that this chromosomal abnormality provide cause of his phenotype, there are no common SNPs in X chromosome among 3 cases.

In humans, the metanephros is the structure that develops into the kidneys. This structure begins to form as the ureteric bud at about 4 weeks of gestation [26]. The ureteric bud invades the metanephric mesenchyme and undergoes recursive branching to form the collecting system of the urinary tract [13]. The key regulators of primary ureteric bud outgrowth and branching are GDNF, which is secreted by the metanephric mesenchyme, and its receptor RET, which is expressed on the ureteric bud [27]. Following the binding of RET, a receptor tyrosine kinase, to the GDNF coreceptor GDNF family receptor α-1 (GFRA1), GDNF activates the RET/GFRA1 receptor tyrosine kinase and thereby triggers a signaling cascade that includes the extracellular signal-regulated kinase (ERK), phosphoinositol 3-kinase (PI3K), and phospholipase (PLC) ζ pathways [13]. Activation of these pathways eventually leads to the outgrowth of the ureteric bud and subsequent renal development [27]. As an upstream regulator of the GDNF-RET/GFRA1 signaling pathway, BMP4 acts as a negative regulator [28]. Moreover, as members of the TGF-β superfamily, BMPs regulate gene expression by receptor-mediated activation of SMAD transcription factors [23]. Therefore, the BMP/SMAD and GDNF-RET/GFRA1 signaling pathways are intimately involved in the development of the ureteric bud, which is derived from the metanephric duct, during the early phase of renal development.

Several studies have reported the role of the BMP/SMAD signaling pathway in testicular development.

Table 2 Genes and SNPs common to patients with CAKUT accompanied by cryptorchidism

Gene Symbol	Gene Name	Gene ID	Chromosomal location	RefSeq	SNPs	SNP ID	Amino acid replacement
SMAD4	SMAD family member 4	4089	chr18: 48584791	A	C	–	His290Pro
			chr18: 48584794	A	C	–	His291Pro
ITGA8	Integrin a8	8516	chr10: 15573050	A	G	rs1041135	Val979Ala
GRIP1	Glutamate receptor interacting protein 1	23426	chr12: 66786091	G	C	rs7970387	Gln822Glu
FREM2	FRAS1 related extracellular matrix protein 2	341640	chr13: 39263714	T	C	rs2496423	Ser745Pro
			chr13: 39,430,314	C	T	rs9548509	Thr2326Ile
FREM1	FRAS1 related extracellular matrix protein 1	158326	chr9: 14737506	T	G	rs10961689	Gln2143Pro
TNXB	Tenascin XB	7148	chr6: 31977391	C	T	rs6457477	Arg504His
BMP8B	Bone morphogenetic protein 8b	656	chr1: 40230336	C	G	rs179472	Ser276Thr
SALL1	Spalt-like transcription factor 1	6299	chr16: 51171175	C	T	rs4614723	Val1178Ile

BMP4 and *BMP8B* are important for the specification of primordial germ cells during fetal development [29], and *SMAD4* and *SMAD3* are necessary for the proliferation and maturation of fetal Sertoli cells [29]. The GDNF-RET/GFRA1 signaling pathway is also associated with spermatogenesis, and GDNF is essential for the self-renewal and differentiation of spermatogonial stem cells [30]. Cryptorchidism is a multifactorial disease, and its etiology is linked to multiple genomic loci as well as maternal and/or environmental factors. The genomic loci and pathways involved in its etiology remain unclear; however, Barthold et al. recently reported a phenotype-specific association of the *TGFBR3* locus with nonsyndromic cryptorchidism [12]. Furthermore, *SMAD4* mutations have been identified in patients with Myhre syndrome, which features cryptorchidism [31].

In the present study, non-synonymous SNPs in both *BMP8B* and *SMAD4* loci were found to be common to all patients with CAKUT accompanied by cryptorchidism, suggesting that impairment of the BMP/SMAD signaling pathway was likely involved in the pathogenesis of this condition. Furthermore, because renal anomalies and cryptorchidism were ipsilateral in all our patients, it is likely that development of the ipsilateral metanephric duct was impaired in these patients. CAKUT is a comprehensive disease concept that encompasses a wide array of phenotypes. To elucidate the genetic etiology of CAKUT, it will be necessary to analyze a greater number of cases. Indeed, several studies on isolated or familial CAKUT have been planned and reported [1, 2, 5, 9, 13]; however, narrowing down the patient setting can reduce the number of cases that need to be studied in order to determine the associated gene loci.

To date, several WES studies have been reported, with the aim of elucidating the genetic cause of CAKUT [5, 32–34]. Consequently, mutations in the *ZBTB24*, *WFS1*, *HPSE2*, *ATRX*, *ASPH*, *AGXT*, *AQP2*, *CTNS*, *PKHD1* [5], *TBX18* [32], *SLIT2*, *SRGAP1* [33], and *TBC1D1* genes [34] have been identified. Although these results did not include our candidate SNPs, we assumed that this discrepancy was related to our focus on cases of CAKUT accompanied by cryptorchidism. Genome-wide analyses have made it possible to investigate multiple gene loci simultaneously. Chatterjee et al. investigated mutations in several genes involved in the GDNF-RET signaling pathway and subsequently detected double non-synonymous variants of RET (G691S/R982C) in a patient with complex CAKUT and cryptorchidism [13]. They also reported that the CAKUT and cryptorchidism phenotypes could be explained by the occurrence of a combination of rare, novel, and common deleterious variants affecting the RET pathway. However, the complete pathological mechanism can only be explained by genome-wide analyses because monogenic causes are detected in only 5–12% of patients [5, 13]. Exons account for only 2% of the whole genome, and the roles of noncoding regions or epigenetics in CAKUT remain unclear. Indeed, we have previously demonstrated that copy number variations in the region upstream of *SOX3*, suspected to act as a promoter or enhancer, are associated with testicular differentiation [14].

The present study had several limitations. First, the sample size used in the study was too small to investigate a specific phenotype. Moreover, we did not determine whether genetic variations in these eight genes resulted in a dysfunction at the protein level. We investigated the effects of the identified amino acid substitutions on protein function using the SIFT platform (http://sift.jcvi.org/). All 10 SNPs detected in the present study were predicted to be tolerant in the in silico analysis (data not shown). Besides, MAF of SNPs in *SMAD4* and *FREM2* (rs2496423) is lower than 1%, suggesting that these rare variants is possibly pathogenic for CAKUT accompanied with by cryptorchidism. Further investigations are needed to determine whether other factors associated with the BMP/SMAD signaling pathway are involved in the onset of CAKUT with cryptorchidism.

Conclusions

We detected 10 non-synonymous SNPs in eight genes in patients with CAKUT accompanied by cryptorchidism. These SNPs were candidate polymorphisms associated with the development of the kidney, urinary tract, and testis. BMP8B is known to activate the nuclear translocation of SMAD4, which regulates the expression of genes associated with the differentiation of primordial germ cells or testicular development. Additionally, BMP4, a member of the BMP family, regulates the interaction between the metanephric mesenchyme and ureteric bud by suppressing GDNF. Taken together, these findings suggested that the developmental mechanisms of the kidneys and urinary tract were intimately linked with that of the male reproductive organs through genetic alterations.

Abbreviations
CAKUT: Congenital anomalies of kidney and urinary tract; SNP: Single nucleotide polymorphism; WES: Whole exome sequencing

Acknowledgements
The authors are grateful to the laboratory technician, Ms. Kasuga, Ms. Noda, and Ms. Ando who provided preservation and preparation of samples. And the 261st JUA Tokai Divisional Meeting Best Presentation Award was given for the case of this manuscript.

Funding
This work was supported by JSPS KAKENHI Grant Number 26462421.

Authors' contributions

Conception and design: KM, AN, and YH; enrollment of patients and acquisition of data: KM, HN, and TK; drafting of the manuscript: KM and YH; data mining of whole exome sequencing and statistical analysis: KM, YM, HK, SK, and TM; analysis and interpretation of data: RA and TY; supervision: YH. We confirm that all authors read and approved the final manuscript.

Competing interests

The authors declare that they have no competing interests.

Author details

[1]Department of Nephro-urology, Nagoya City University Graduate School of Medical Sciences, Nagoya, Japan. [2]Department of Pediatric urology, Nagoya City University Graduate School of Medical Sciences, 1 Kawasumi, Mizuho-cho, Mizuho-ku, Nagoya, Japan.

References

1. Kohl S, Hwang DY, Dworschak GC, Hilger AC, Saisawat P, Vivante A, et al. Mild recessive mutations in six Fraser syndrome-related genes cause isolated congenital anomalies of the kidney and urinary tract. J Am Soc Nephrol. 2014;25:1917–22.
2. Vivante A, Kohl S, Hwang DY, Dworschak GC, Hildebrandt F. Single-gene causes of congenital anomalies of the kidney and urinary tract (CAKUT) in humans. Pediatr Nephrol. 2014;29:695–704.
3. Harambat J, van Stralen KJ, Kim JJ, Tizard EJ. Epidemiology of chronic kidney disease in children. Pediatr Nephrol. 2012;27:363–73.
4. Ichikawa I, Kuwayama F, Pope JC 4th, Stephens FD, Miyazaki Y. Paradigm shift from classic anatomic theories to contemporary cell biological views of CAKUT. Kidney Int. 2002;61:889–98.
5. Vivante A, Hwang DY, Kohl S, Chen J, Shril S, Schulz J, et al. Exome sequencing discerns syndromes in patients from consanguineous families with congenital anomalies of the kidneys and urinary tract. J Am Soc Nephrol. 2017;28:69–75.
6. Pini Prato A, Musso M, Ceccherini I, Mattioli G, Giunta C, Ghiggeri GM, et al. Hirschsprung disease and congenital anomalies of the kidney and urinary tract (CAKUT): a novel syndromic association. Medicine (Baltimore). 2009;88:83–90.
7. Saisawat P, Kohl S, Hilger AC, Hwang DY, Yung Gee H, Dworschak GC, et al. Whole-exome resequencing reveals recessive mutations in TRAP1 in individuals with CAKUT and VACTERL association. Kidney Int. 2014;85:1310–7.
8. Hadziselimovic F. Involvement of fibroblast growth factors and their receptors in epididymo-testicular descent and maldescent. Mol Syndromol. 2016;6:261–7.
9. Hwang DY, Dworschak GC, Kohl S, Saisawat P, Vivante A, Hilger AC, et al. Mutations in 12 known dominant disease-causing genes clarify many congenital anomalies of the kidney and urinary tract. Kidney Int. 2014;85: 1429–33.
10. Nef S, Parada LF. Cryptorchidism in mice mutant for Insl3. Nat Genet. 1999; 22:295–9.
11. Zimmermann S, Steding G, Emmen JM, Brinkmann AO, Nayernia K, Holstein AF, et al. Targeted disruption of the Insl3 gene causes bilateral cryptorchidism. Mol Endocrinol. 1999;13:681–91.
12. Barthold JS, Wang Y, Kolon TF, Kollin C, Nordenskjöld A, Olivant Fisher A, et al. Phenotype-specific association of the TGFBR3 locus with nonsyndromic cryptorchidism. J Urol. 2015;193:1637–45.
13. Chatterjee R, Ramos E, Hoffman M, VanWinkle J, Martin DR, Davis TK, et al. Traditional and targeted exome sequencing reveals common, rare and novel functional deleterious variants in RET-signaling complex in a cohort of living US patients with urinary tract malformations. Hum Genet. 2012;131:1725–38.
14. Mizuno K, Kojima Y, Kamisawa H, Moritoki Y, Nishio H, Nakane A, et al. Elucidation of distinctive genomic DNA structures in patients with 46,XX testicular disorders of sex development using genome-wide analyses. J Urol. 2014;192:535–41.
15. Gbadegesin RA, Brophy PD, Adeyemo A, Hall G, Gupta IR, Hains D, et al. TNXB mutations can cause vesicoureteral reflux. J Am Soc Nephrol. 2013;24:1313–22.
16. Sanna-Cherchi S, Sampogna RV, Papeta N, Burgess KE, Nees SN, Perry BJ, et al. Mutations in DSTYK and dominant urinary tract malformations. N Engl J Med. 2012;369:621–9.
17. Aloisio GM, Nakada Y, Saatcioglu HD, Peña CG, Baker MD, Tarnawa ED, et al. PAX7 expression defines germline stem cells in the adult testis. J Clin Invest. 2014;124:3929–44.
18. Yamaguchi YL, Tanaka SS, Kumagai M, Fujimoto Y, Terabayashi T, Matsui Y, et al. Sall4 is essential for mouse primordial germ cell specification by suppressing somatic cell program genes. Stem Cells. 2015;33:289–300.
19. Toyoda D, Taguchi A, Chiga M, Ohmori T, Nishinakamura R. Sall4 is transiently expressed in the caudal Wolffian duct and the ureteric bud, but dispensable for kidney development. PLoS One. 2013;8:e68508.
20. Tripathi P, Wang Y, Casey AM, Chen F. Absence of canonical Smad signaling in ureteral and bladder mesenchyme causes ureteropelvic junction obstruction. J Am Soc Nephrol. 2012;23:618–28.
21. Ciller IM, Palanisamy SK, Ciller UA, McFarlane JR. Postnatal expression of bone morphogenetic proteins and their receptors in the mouse testis. Physiol Res. 2016; [Epub ahead of print]
22. Yan J, Zhang L, Xu J, Sultana N, Hu J, Cai X, et al. Smad4 regulates ureteral smooth muscle cell differentiation during mouse embryogenesis. PLoS One. 2014;9:e104503.
23. Massagué J. TGFbeta signalling in context. Nat Rev Mol Cell Biol. 2012;13: 616–30.
24. Liang Y, Shen D, Cai W. Two coding single nucleotide polymorphisms in the SALL1 gene in Townes-brocks syndrome: a case report and review of the literature. J Pediatr Surg. 2008;43:391–3.
25. Slavotinek A, Li C, Sherr EH, Chudley AE. Mutation analysis of the FRAS1 gene demonstrates new mutations in a propositus with Fraser syndrome. Am J Med Genet A. 2006;140:1909–14.
26. Dressler GR. The cellular basis of kidney development. Annu Rev Cell Dev Biol. 2006;22:509–29.
27. Krause M, Rak-Raszewska A, Pietila I, Quaggin SE, Vainio S. Signaling during kidney development. Cell. 2015;4:112–32.
28. Davis TK, Hoshi M, Jain S. To bud or not to bud: the RET perspective in CAKUT. Pediatr Nephrol. 2014;29:597–608.
29. Itman C, Loveland KL. Smads and cell fate: distinct roles in specification, development, and tumorigenesis in the testis. IUBMB Life. 2013;65:85–97.
30. Chen LY, Willis WD, Eddy EM. Targeting the Gdnf gene in peritubular myoid cells disrupts undifferentiated spermatogonial cell development. Proc Natl Acad Sci U S A. 2016;113:1829–34.
31. Le Goff C, Mahaut C, Abhyankar A, Le Goff W, Serre V, Afenjar A, et al. Mutations at a single codon in mad homology 2 domain of SMAD4 cause Myhre syndrome. Nat Genet. 2012;44:85–8.
32. Vivante A, Kleppa MJ, Schulz J, Kohl S, Sharma A, Chen J, et al. Mutations in TBX18 cause dominant urinary tract malformations via transcriptional dysregulation of ureter development. Am J Hum Genet. 2015;97:291–301.
33. Hwang DY, Kohl S, Fan X, Vivante A, Chan S, Dworschak GC, et al. Mutations of the SLIT2-ROBO2 pathway genes SLIT2 and SRGAP1 confer risk for congenital anomalies of the kidney and urinary tract. Hum Genet. 2015;134:905–16.
34. Kosfeld A, Kreuzer M, Daniel C, Brand F, Schäfer AK, Chadt A, et al. Whole-exome sequencing identifies mutations of TBC1D1 encoding a Rab-GTPase-activating protein in patients with congenital anomalies of the kidneys and urinary tract (CAKUT). Hum Genet. 2016;135:69–87.

23

Primary synovial sarcoma of the kidney: a case report of complete pathological response at a Lebanese tertiary care center

Alissar El Chediak[1], Deborah Mukherji[1], Sally Temraz[1], Samer Nassif[2], Sara Sinno[2], Rami Mahfouz[2] and Ali Shamseddine[1]*(iD)

Abstract

Background: Primary synovial sarcoma of the kidney is a rare type of soft tissue sarcoma. Its presenting features can resemble those of other renal tumors; rendering its early diagnosis, a dilemma. Several cases of renal synovial sarcoma have been reported in the literature with varying treatment options and outcomes. This article describes a rare case of primary renal synovial sarcoma and reviews all cases in the literature.

Case presentation: A 26-year-old male presented with flank pain and hematuria. Initially diagnosed with Wilm's tumor, revision of pathology and histology, along with the immunohistochemical profile, confirmed, nevertheless, the diagnosis of primary monophasic synovial sarcoma of the kidney with the SYT-SSX2 fusion transcript. Follow-up, post nephrectomy, revealed recurrence within the lungs and at the surgical bed. Surgical resection followed by adjuvant chemotherapy regimen constituting of Doxorubicin and Ifosfamide, achieved complete pathological response.

Conclusion: In this case report, we emphasize the need for accurate diagnosis and prompt treatment. We propose multimodality treatment approach including surgery along with anthracycline-based chemotherapy to induce complete remission.

Keywords: Synovial sarcoma, SYT-SSX, Doxorubicin, Ifosfamide, Pathological response, Survival

Background

Soft tissue sarcoma (STS) is a rare malignant tumor of mesenchymal origin having an incidence of 2–3 cases per 100,000, thus contributing to less than 1% of all adult malignancies [1, 2]. Synovial sarcoma (SS), or sarcoma of tissues adjacent to joints, is a rare type of STS, and represent 5 to10% of all STSs [1]. SS is commonly found in the proximal limb of young adults and has a male predominance [3]. Other unusual sites of occurrence include the head and neck, heart, lungs, and kidneys [4]. Very few reports have tackled this tumor due to its rarity and difficulty to distinguish from other renal pathologies. The first case of primary SS of the kidney has been reported by Faria et al. in 1999 [5]. We present a case of primary synovial sarcoma of the kidney, initially thought to be a

* Correspondence: as04@aub.edu.lb
[1]Department of Internal Medicine, Division of Hematology/Oncology, American University of Beirut - Medical Center, P.o.Box: 11-0236, Riad El Solh, Beirut 110 72020, Lebanon
Full list of author information is available at the end of the article

Wilm's tumor, along with patient follow-up, showing complete pathological response to treatment, followed by a literature review of this disease entity.

Case presentation

A 26-year-old male experienced recurrent flank pain and gross hematuria over several months duration. Kidney ultrasound showed a lower pole mass concerning for renal cell carcinoma. After confirmation of a right kidney tumor, measuring 6 cm, by an enhanced CT scan, he underwent right radical nephrectomy with para-caval lymph node dissection, at another institute, with pathology there, read initially as adult type Wilm's tumor. After referral to our institute for rereading of the pathological slides, the morphological and immunostaining profiles were analyzed, and results came out to be consistent with synovial sarcoma of the right kidney. The tumor was monophasic and showed a cellular spindle cell proliferation with a prominent perivascular growth pattern and partial necrosis. It was positive for vimentin, BCL-2, CD56, MCK (partial), and negative for CD10, 31, 34, 99, 117, CK7, Desmin, SMA, MyoD1, EMA, WT-1, S100, RCC, PAX8, GATA-3, and Synaptophysin (Fig. 1).

Molecular studies on the paraffin-embedded blocks were performed to test for the t(X; 18) SYT/SSX fusion transcript, using RT-PCR, at the University of Michigan Health System. RT-PCR amplification was performed using fluorescent dye-labeled primers, specific for the SYT-SS18 and SYT-SSX genes. The PCR products were then detected and sized by capillary electrophoresis to identify the presence of chimeric transcripts. A concurrent internal control was run to ensure the integrity of the mRNA. FISH analysis was also performed using a break-apart style probe. The results were unfortunately negative due to the low quality samples.

According to these findings, a diagnosis of primary monophasic SS of the kidney was made. It was elected for serial follow up and no adjuvant treatment, thereafter. Six months later, a follow up CT scan detected a 1.5cmx1.7 cm left lower lobe lung nodule suggestive of metastasis. Consequently, he underwent a smooth left lower lobe wedge resection. Fusion gene product analysis on the resected lung tissue, via FISH, revealed SYT-SSX 2 gene rearrangement confirming the SS diagnosis. Three months afterwards, CT scan of the chest, abdomen, and pelvis revealed another disease recurrence in the nephrectomy surgical bed, with tumor invasion of the inferior vena cava and the presence of conglomerate suspicious aorto-iliac lymph nodes. A multidisciplinary team approach decided to start the patient on Doxorubicin 50 g/m^2 and Ifosfamide 5 g/m^2 chemotherapeutic

regimen. Following the third cycle, CT scan and MRI showed a 30 to 50% interval decrease in size of tumor masses in the right nephrectomy bed and adjacent retroperitoneum, IVC tumor, and distal aortocaval lymph nodes, indicating partial treatment response. The patient were received a total of 5 cycles, with no adjunct side effects.

A follow-up MRI, several months later, showed continued decrease in the size of 3 masses at the previous surgical site, IVC tumor invasion, and aortocaval lymph nodes, indicating continued response to treatment. One of the small masses in the nephrectomy bed almost completely resolved, on imaging, with no new progression. It was then decided to have the patient undergo surgical resection of the residual masses at the previous surgical bed with removal of the aorto-caval lymph nodes, thrombectomy with vena caval repair. All surgical margins were negative. Final pathology came out to be necrosis, with no viable tumor identified. Thus, a complete pathological response was achieved using the Adriamycin/Ifosfamide regimen, a year after the initial nephrectomy. A sample of the kidney lysate was again tested for the (X; 18) SYT/SSX fusion transcript via RT-PCR and FISH, and results were negative, suggestive of complete treatment response.

Discussion

Synovial sarcoma is a mesenchymal spindle cell tumor which displays variable epithelial differentiation and has a specific chromosomal translocation t(X; 18) (p11; q11), which results from the fusion of the SYT gene on chromosome 18 to exon 5 of either SSX1 or SSX2 genes

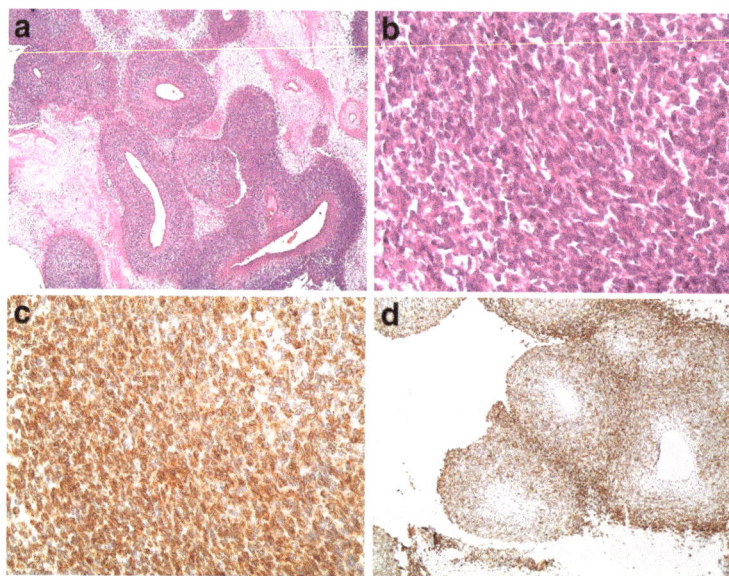

Fig. 1 Partially necrotic, densely cellular proliferation with a prominent perivascular growth pattern (**a**, H&E stain, 40×). Tumor cells are essentially spindle in appearance (**b**, H&E stain, 400×), and express vimentin (not shown), focal keratin (not shown), BCL-2 (**c**, 400×), and CD56 (**d**, 100×)

on chromosome X [6]. It was recently reported that the SSX4 gene is also involved in such a translocation [6, 7]. Nonetheless, SS of the kidney can be first misdiagnosed as a renal cell carcinoma due to similar clinical presentation [3]. The identification of the monophasic type of renal SS is also controversial as it has similar microscopic features to other spindle cell tumors, such as fibrosarcoma, leiomyosarcoma, malignant peripheral nerve sheath tumors, adult Wilm's tumor, spindle cell carcinoma and spindle cell melanoma [3]. While monophasic SS of the kidney is made up exclusively of monomorphic spindle cells, the biphasic type is a mixture of both spindle-shaped cells and epithelial cells. SS of the kidney is a rare disease such as 64 cases have been reported since the Faria et al. cases up to 2012 [6]. We conducted a literature review using Embase and PubMed databases and included all cases (even those published in languages other than English) till the year 2016. This yielded a total of 114 cases (Table 1) constituting the largest series of renal SS cases to be reported. Noteworthy, our case is the first to be reported from the Middle East.

The median age of patients with renal SS was 40.5 (15–78) years, which is half the median age for diagnosis of renal cell carcinoma [7]. The female to male ratio was 1:1. Regarding the predominant presentation symptoms, data was only available for 82 cases. The most frequently reported symptom on presentation was isolated flank/lumbar pain which was found in 20 patients (24.4%).This is in concordance with a review conducted on older data where this same predominant symptom occurred in 55.5% of cases [8]. Hematuria was present in 37 patients (44%) upon presentation. Kohle et al. reported similar data, albeit smaller sample size, where 98% of their patients were symptomatic at the time of presentation, with 67% having pain and 38% having hematuria [6]. These figures are in concordance with our analysis of the world literature.

According to our analysis, the leading fusion variant was the SYT-SSX 2, detected in 42 (36.8%) patients, as opposed to the SYT-SSX 1 variant, detected in 23 (20.2%) patients, in total (Table 1).

Data on metastasis and disease recurrence was available for 70 and 57 patients, respectively. 19 (27.1%) patients had metastasis, whereas 14 (24.6%) patients had tumor recurrence on follow-up. These numbers are similar to what was published in previous series [9].

A 30 to 50% of the patients who underwent surgical resection of their primary tumor were reported to witness metastasis to the lungs or liver [10]. Our patient is of no exception. In terms of median survival for patients with localized disease, size represents an important prognostic factor [10]. A retrospective analysis was done on 135 consecutive patients with extremity and truncal variant of synovial sarcomas, seen at three institutions in

Boston, between years 1961 and 1996. Patients with localized synovial sarcomas, less than 5 cm in longest diameter, had a survival at 10 years equivalent to 88%, compared with a 10-year survival of 38 and 8% for 5 to 10 cm and greater than 10 cm sarcomas, respectively [10]. Similar results were reported by Singer et al. on 48 consecutive patients with extremity and truncal synovial sarcomas, seen between years 1966 and 1994 [11].

SS of the kidneys presents a diagnostic dilemma, as it resembles renal cell carcinoma amongst other tumors. Diagnosis can be based on morphological (spindle cell) and immunological tumor profile. It can also be established by genetic analysis via FISH and RT-PCR, demonstrating the SYT18-SSX gene translocation. Demonstrating which translocation, the tumor possesses, has been a delicate matter. For instance, a SS case that was previously shown to be negative for SYT/SSX1 and SYT/SSX2 gene expression by conventional RT-PCR, was instead found to be SYT/SSX4 positive, as the sole fusion transcript expressed in this tumor sample, when the RT-PCR was redesigned [6]. This might have explained our negative results, when trying to identify the translocations, since our RT-PCR was only designed to detect SYT/SSX1 and SYT/SSX2 fusion gene variants.

Moreover, the value of TLE1 antibody in the diagnosis of SS has also been examined. TLE1 was found to be an excellent discriminator of SS from other sarcomas, in a study by Terry et al. [12]. They reported that TLE1 monoclonal and polyclonal antibodies gave intense and/or diffuse nuclear staining in 91 out of 94 molecularly confirmed synovial sarcoma patients. In contrast, TLE1 staining has been detected much less frequently and at lower levels, if et al.l, in 40 other mesenchymal tumors; thereby making this a robust immunohistochemical marker for SS. Jagdis et al. also supported this view as their findings confirmed that TLE1 was more sensitive and specific for synovial sarcoma, than any other currently available immunohistochemical kits [13]. Kosemehmetoglu et al. confirmed the sensitivity, but not the specificity, of TLE1 antibodies in diagnosing synovial sarcomas [14].

The prognostic implication of SYT-SSX fusion type in synovial sarcomas is still under debate. The SYT-SSX fusion type and the presence of metastasis, at diagnosis, were both proven to be important prognostic indicators [15]. Kawai et al. analyzed SYT–SSX fusion transcripts in 45 synovial sarcomas by reverse-transcriptase polymerase chain reaction, and compared the results with relevant clinical and pathological data [16]. SYT- SSX2 fusion type carried a significant positive prognosis for overall survival [16]. This was thought to be due to an association with a lower prevalence of metastatic disease at diagnosis, in patients having this rearrangement [16]. In another study by Ladanyi et al., the SYT–SSX2 fusion

Table 1 List of 114 cases of renal SS published in the literature

Case Report/ Series	Author/ Year of publication	No of cases	Age(Y)/Gender (M/F)	Presenting symptoms	Fusion gene Variant	Treatment	Outcome
1	Argani P et al.; 2000 [5]	17	10 M 7 F Median age: 35	Abdominal pain; hematuria; incidental finding for hypertension workup; other data not available	1: SYT-SSX1; 4: SYT-SSX2	Radical nephrectomy	N/A
2	Kim DH et al.; 2000 [17]	2	53/M 47/M	Rt flank pain Rt flank pain, gross hematuria	SYT-SSX2;	Rt radical nephrectomy; Rt radical nephrectomy with IVC thrombectomy	No recurrence 6 mons later; lung mets 5 mons later, death 10mons post-op
3	Chen S et al.; 2001 [18]	1	48/M	Hematuria	SYT-SSX 2	Lt radical nephroureterectomy; Radiation to surgical bed; 4 cycles of ifosfamide and Doxorubicin	N/A
4	Koyama S et al.; 2001 [8]	1	47/F	Right back pain	SYT-SSX 2	Rt radical nephrectomy	No recurrence 17 mons later
5	Bella AJ et al.; 2002 [25]	1	24/M	Gross hematuria	SYT-SSX t(X;18)	Rt radical nephrectomy, adjuvant Actinomycin + Vincristine	No clinical evidence of disease 18 mons after nephrectomy
6	Dai YC et al.; 2002 [26]	1	19/F	Abdominal Pain, 3 mons of amenorrhea	SYT-SSX t(X;18)	Rt nephrectomy	Recurrence of tumor in retroperitoneum and abdominal wall 9 mons after surgery
7	Vesoulis Z et al.; 2003 [27]	1	38/M	Acute abdominal pain	SST-SSX1	Lt radical nephrectomy	N/A
8	Moch H et al.; 2003 [28]	2	47/M 56/F	Renal mass	SST-SSX1/ SYT-SSX2	Nephrectomy/ Rt nephrectomy	Local recurrence 11 years later/ N/A
9	Chen PC et al.; 2003 [29]	1	19/M	left flank pain and intermittent hematuria	N/A	Lt radical nephrectomy + IVC thrombectomy; adjuvant Ifosfamide + Etoposide	died of sepsis 1 month after surgery
10	Park SJ et al.; 2004 [9]	1	32/F	Intermittent abdominal pain	N/A	Lt radical nephrectomy + thormbectomy; 6 cycles Ifosfamide + Doxorubicin	Metastasis to lung 4 mons post-op, complete remission after chemotherapy
11	Jun SY t al; 2004 [30]	3	27, 35/F 26/M	Rt flank pain	SYT-SSX2	Rt radical nephrectomies	1F: disease free 5 mons post-op; 2F: lumbar vertebral mets 5 mons post-op, 6 mons disease free post-resection; 3 M: bilateral hemothorax; death 34 days post-op
12	Tornkvist M et al.; 2004 [24]	1	34/F	N/A	SYT-SSX 2	Rt nephrectomy, chemotherapy	Visceral recurrence; lung metastases
13	Schaal CH et al.; 2004 [14]	1	27/M	Hematuria and large abdominal mass	N/A	Ifosfamide and Adriamycin, followed by Rt Radical nephrectomy	No recurrence after one year
14	Shao L et al.; 2004 [31]	4	N/A	N/A	N/A	N/A	N/A

Table 1 List of 114 cases of renal SS published in the literature *(Continued)*

Case Report/ Series	Author/ Year of publication	No of cases	Age(Y)/Gender (M/F)	Presenting symptoms	Fusion gene Variant	Treatment	Outcome
15	Shannon BA et al.; 2005 [32]	1	60/M	Hematuria	SYT-SSX 2	Rt radical nephrectomy, Imatinib, 5 cycles of adjuvant chemotherapy	Pulmonary metastasis 6 mons after surgery; death 12 mons later
16	Perlmutter AE et al.; 2005 [33]	1	61/F	Right flank pain and gross hematuria	SYT-SSX 2	Rt nephrectomy, refused adjuvant chemotherapy	No recurrence 5 mons post-surgery
17	Stage et al.; 2005 [34]	1	51/F	Renal masses incidentally found	N/A	N/A	N/A
18	Paláu L MA et al.; 2007 [35]	1	71/F	Flank pain and gross hematuria	SYT-SSX 2	Lt nephrectomy	Recovery in 22 mons after surgery
19	Drozenova et al.; 2008 [36]	2	33/M 57/F	Rt flank pain Lt flank pain	SYT-SSX1/ SYT-SSX1	Rt Radical nephrectomy/ Lt Radical nephrectomy	Local recurrence and lung mets; death 6 mons later/ N/A
20	Mirza M et al.; 2008 [37]	1	17/M	Flank pain and gross hematuria	SYT-SSX 2	Lt radical nephrectomy	No recurrence 1 year later
21	Gabilondo F et al.; 2008 [38]	1	32/F	Mild abdominal pain; gross hematuria	SYT-SSX t(X;18)	Rt radical nephrectomy	N/A
22	Zakhary MM et al.; 2008 [39]	1	52/F	Right flank pain	N/A	Rt nephrectomy	N/A
23	Chung SD et al.; 2008 [40]	2	30/F 49/F	Rt flank pain Lt loin pain	SYT-SSX1	Rt radical nephrectomy/ Lt radical nephrectomy	No recurrence 15 mons post-op/ No recurrence 27 mons post-op
24	Erturhan S et al.; 2008 [41]	1	59/M	Right lumbar pain and palpable mass	N/A	N/A	N/A
25	Divetia M et al.; 2008 [42]	7	2-M 5-F (15–46 years)	Abdominal lump, hematuria	3 SYT-SSX1/ 1 SYT-SSX2	Radical nephrectomy	Lung mets in 2 patients; death at 6 and 12 mons, respectively
26	Dassi V et al.; 2009 [43]	1	20/F	Flank pain	SYT-SSX t(X;18)	Lt radical nephrectomy	N/A
28	Kawahara et al.; 2009 [44]	1	40/F	Abdominal pain	SYT-SSX 1	Radical nephrectomy	N/A
29	Long JA et al.; 2009 [45]	3	(Age range: 27–33 years)	Back pain and spontaneous rupture	SYT-SSX t(X;18)	2 Rt radical nephrectomy; 1 Lt radical nephrectomy	2 patients: total remission 25 mons post-op; 1 patient: death 24 mons post-op
30	Wezel F et al.; 2010 [46]	1	47/M	Hematuria, abdominal pain, weight loss	SYT-SSX t(X;18)	Nephrectomy	No recurrence 18 weeks after surgery
31	Wang Z-H et al.; 2009 [47]	4	2/F 2/M 32 to 48 years	Low back pain, hematuria	SYT-SSX1	Radical nephrectomy; 3 Lt side, 1 Rt side	Liver + lung metastasis; death at 5, 8, 18, and 21 mons post-op, respectively
32	Kageyama S et al.; 2010 [48]	1	67/M	Gross hematuria and right flank pain	SYT-SSX 2	Rt nephroureterectomy; Ifosfamide and Etoposide regimen	Tumor recurrence 33 mons post nephrectomy; Liver mets; death 4 years later
33	Tan YS et al.; 2010 [49]	4	N/A	N/A	N/A	N/A	N/A
34	Romero-Rojas AE et al.; 2013 [50]	1	15/M	Lt abdominal pain; weight loss	N/A	Neoadjuvant chemotherapy followed by Lt radical nephrectomy	Death 1.8 years later
35	Lakshmaiah KC et al.; 2010 [51]	2	50/F 45/M	Rt flank pain/ Lt flank pain, hematuria	SYT-SSX2/ NOT DONE	Radical nephrectomy	No recurrence 2 years post-op/ lost to follow-up

Table 1 List of 114 cases of renal SS published in the literature *(Continued)*

Case Report/ Series	Author/ Year of publication	No of cases	Age(Y)/Gender (M/F)	Presenting symptoms	Fusion gene Variant	Treatment	Outcome
36	Kataria et al.; 2010 [52]	1	52/F	Renal mass	SYT-SSX 2	Radical nephrectomy IVC thrombectomy; adjuvant chemo-radiation	Mets to lung
37	Grampurohit VU et al.; 2011 [53]	1	21/F	Fever, hematuria; right flank pain	SYT-SSX t(X;18)	Rt nephrectomy	No recurrence 6 mons post-surgery
38	Ozkan EE et al.; 2011 [20]	1	68/F	Right flank pain and abdominal distention	N/A	Rt nephroureterectomy, 4 cycles Ifosfamide and Doxorubicin	No recurrence one year later
39	Karafin M et al.; 2011 [54]	3	39/F 41/M 53/M	N/A	SYT-SSX2 SYT-SSX2 N/A	N/A	N/A
40	Nishida T et al.; 2011 [55]	1	63/F	Dysuria, hematuria	SYT-SSX 1 & 2	Rt Radical nephrectomy	No recurrence one year postop
41	Pitino A et al.; 2011 [8]	1	67/M	Lumbar pain, gross hematuria	SYT-SSX 2	Lt Nephroureterectomy; adjuvant Epirubicin post-op	Local recurrence of disease 24 mons post- surgery
42	Bakhshi et al.; 2012 [56]	1	33/F	Abdominal pain and gross hematuria	SYT-SSX 2	Lt radical nephrectomy; external radiotherapy	No recurrence at 2 years
43	Lopes et al.; 2013 [3]	1	19/M	Lumbar pain, gross hematuria	Negative translocation	Lt nephrectomy, thrombectomy; 5 cycles of doxorubicin	Lung mets several mons post-op
44	Pereira E Silva R et al.; 2013 [57]	1	17/M	Incidental large renal mass after workup for secondary hypertension	Negative translocation	Radical nephrectomy followed by ifosfamide	No recurrence 29 mons later
45	Marković-Lipkovski J et al.; 2013 [12]	1	38/M	Rt flank pain; fever; hematuria	SYT-SSX2	Rt radical nephrectomy	Died three mons later
46	Moorthy et al.; 2014 [58]	1	46/M	Flank pain	SYT-SSX 2	Lt radical nephrectomy	N/A
47	Majumber et al.; 2014 [59]	1	46/F	Flank pain, hematuria	N/A	Rt radical nephrectomy	No evidence of disease after 2 mons follow up
48	Schoolmeester JK et al.; 2014 [60]	16	9M/7F 17-78 yrs.; Median: 46 yrs	N/A; Rt: 10; Lt: 6;	SYT-SSX2: 10; SYT-SSX1: 5; 1: failed	14: Radical nephrectomy; 1: partial nephrectomy; 1: needle biopsy	6: death within 1–58 mons (mean 31mons); 5: no recurrence 12–77 mons (39 mons); 1: alive with spine mets 11mons later
49	Kim MS et al.; 2014 [61]	1	38/F	Lt flank pain	SYT-SSX2	Lap Lt radical nephrectomy followed by radiation to surgical bed	Recurrence at the distal ureter and uretero-vesical junction 6 mons post- surgery
50	Ozkanli SS et al.; 2014 [62]	1	45/M	Flank pain; macroscopic hematuria	SYT-SSX t(X;18)	Lt radical nephrectomy	N/A
51	Mishra S et al.; 2015 [13]	1	60/M	Flank pain, hematuria	SYT-SSX t(X;18)	Radical nephrectomy	N/A
52	Wang Z et al.; 2015 [61]	1	54/F	Flank pain, hematuria	SYT-SSX 1	Radical nephrectomy	No recurrence 12 mons post-surgery
53	Vedana M et al.; 2015 [63]	1	76/F	Flank pain; hematuria	SYT-SSX t(X;18)	Rt radical nephro-ureterectomy	No recurrence 20 mons post-surgery

Table 1 List of 114 cases of renal SS published in the literature *(Continued)*

Case Report/ Series	Author/ Year of publication	No of cases	Age(Y)/Gender (M/F)	Presenting symptoms	Fusion gene Variant	Treatment	Outcome
54	Lv X-F et al.; 2015 [64]	5	2F/3M (15–43 yrs.; Median: 27.4 yrs)	N/A	N/A	N/A	N/A
55	Present case El Chediak A. et al.; 2016	1	26/M	Rt flank pain; hematuria	SYT-SSX2	Rt radical nephrectomy, Doxorubicin Ifosfamide	Lung metastasis 6 mons post nephrectomy; no recurrence one year post chemotherapy

M Males, *F* Females, *Yrs* Years, *Rt* Right, *Lt* Left, *Mets* Metastasis, *Mons* Months, *IVC* Inferior vena cava, *N/A* Not Applicable

transcript had a significantly longer metastasis-free survival [15]. On the contrary, Japanese patients, with synovial sarcoma, having positive SYT-SSX fusion transcript, were retrospectively analyzed [17]. They concluded that *SYT-SSX* fusion type was not found to be a significant prognostic factor, unlike tumor size and histological grading, for patients with localized synovial sarcoma [17]. Another study by Guillou et al. also confirmed that histologic grading, and not SYT-SSX fusion type, was a stronger predictor of survival, by collecting retrospective data on 165 SS patients [18].

In our sample, staging information was available for 46 patients, based on the 7th edition TNM staging for soft tissue sarcomas. Among the patients having the SYT-SSX2 fusion protein. 53.8% were stage II and 34.6% were of stage III. 33 and 25% of patients with SYT-SSX1 transcript were stage II and III, respectively. 25% of patients with SYT-SSX1 were of stage IV, versus only 7.7% for SYT-SSX2 patients.

Lungs were the most common metastatic site, regardless of the fusion type. However, 50% of patients with SYT-SSX2 fusion type had metastasis to the liver. Although lungs and liver are common sites for metastasis for renal SS [19, 20], it was not reported before whether there is a relation between the site of metastasis and the type of fusion transcript. From the above, it appears that SYT-SSX 1 behaves more aggressively. However, studies with a larger number of patients and longer follow-up periods are needed to verify these observations, especially in the light of the contradicting data, presenting on the prognostic value of the SYT-SSX fusion protein.

Although SS is considered an aggressive form of STS where metastasis can occur in 50% of the cases, it was found to be sensitive to Anthracycline based chemotherapy [21]. However, due to the rarity of the tumor, a standard therapy has not been established. Treatment modalities include surgical resection and chemotherapy. A combination of chemotherapy (Ifosfamide and Doxorubicin) and surgery has yielded positive results [6, 9, 12, 13]. Based on our review of the literature, 10 patients took Ifosfamide and Doxorubicin, either together or in combination with other chemotherapeutic agents. 5 out of 10 cases were reported to have complete remission. This further corroborates the effectiveness of giving Ifosfamide and Doxorubicin as a regimen to treat primary renal SS. The basis for chemotherapy was tumor volume reduction, mainly attributed to Ifosfamide. In one case report, the combination of Ifosfamide and Doxorubicin lead to a 50% reduction of the tumor before consequent resection [14]. The controversy of the impact of adjuvant chemotherapy on overall survival, in SS patients, is limited by randomized clinical trials'(RCTs) sample size and varied chemotherapy regimens with discrepant results [22]. The Sarcoma Meta-analysis Collaboration (SMAC) group performed a meta-analysis of all known randomized clinical trials in 1997. Their results indicated that doxorubicin-based chemotherapy served to significantly improve time to local and distant recurrence, as well as overall recurrence-free survival in comparison to patients who were just observed [23]. An increase in overall survival was not statistically significant [23]. Another meta-Analysis of RCTs of adjuvant chemotherapy for localized resectable STS was conducted by Pervais et al. where they built on the results of the SMAC study and narrowed the confidence intervals [24]. This meta-analysis demonstrated marginal efficacy of doxorubicin based chemotherapy with respect to local recurrence, distant recurrence, overall recurrence, and overall survival, in comparison to those who did not receive adjuvant chemotherapy [22].

Conclusion

In conclusion, primary SS of the kidney is an aggressive rare disease that can be mistaken for other types of renal cell carcinomas. Its diagnosis is based on morphological and molecular studies demonstrating spindle cells and the SYT-SSX translocation. However, establishing a correct diagnosis may be difficult. Prognosis can be enhanced by use of anthracycline based chemotherapy. Moreover, the combination of surgery and chemotherapy has shown positive results. Particularly, we propose the use of Ifosfamide and Doxorubicin as a standard chemotherapy to induce complete remission. Since the disease may have rapid course with unfavorable outcomes, clinicians need to be aware of the existence of this rare entity, so that timely and appropriate therapy can be initiated.

Abbreviations

CT: Computer tomography; FISH: fluorescence in situ hybridization; IVC: Inferior vena cava; MRI: Magnetic resonance imaging; N/A: Not available; RCT: Randomized clinical trials; RT-PCR: reverse transcriptase-polymerase chain reaction; SS: Synovial sarcoma; STS: Soft tissue sarcoma

Funding

No funding from an external party was received. Genetic testing was conducted using the corresponding author's research fund.

Authors' contributions

EA was involved in acquisition, analysis, and interpretation of data (literature), and manuscript writing. SN and SS performed histological examination of the resected tumor and provided the pathological images in our manuscript. MR performed molecular analysis of the tumor sample. Both MD and TS were involved in manuscript writing and editing. SA was involved in data analysis, interpretation of data (literature), and revising the manuscript. He also gave final approval of the version prior to submission. All authors read and approved the final manuscript.

Competing interests

The authors declare that they have no competing interests.

Author details

[1]Department of Internal Medicine, Division of Hematology/Oncology, American University of Beirut - Medical Center, P.o.Box: 11-0236, Riad El Solh, Beirut 110 72020, Lebanon. [2]Department of Pathology and Laboratory Medicine, American University of Beirut - Medical Center, Beirut, Lebanon.

References

1. Fletcher CD. The evolving classification of soft tissue tumours - an update based on the new 2013 WHO classification. Histopathology. 2014;64(1):2–11.
2. Goldblum JR, Weiss SW, Andrew L. Folpe Enzinger and Weiss's soft tissue tumors. sixth ed. St Louis, Missouri: Saunders; 2001. 1176.
3. Lopes H, et al. Primary monophasic synovial sarcoma of the kidney: a case report and review of literature. Clin Med Insights Oncol. 2013;7:257–62.
4. Spillane AJ, et al. Synovial sarcoma: a clinicopathologic, staging, and prognostic assessment. J Clin Oncol. 2000;18(22):3794–803.
5. Argani P, et al. Primary renal synovial sarcoma: molecular and morphologic delineation of an entity previously included among embryonal sarcomas of the kidney. Am J Surg Pathol. 2000;24(8):1087–96.
6. Kohle O, et al. Soft tissue sarcomas of the kidney. Rare Tumors. 2015;7(1):5635.
7. Namita Chittoria, B.I.R. Renal Cell Carcinoma. 2013 [cited 2016; Available from: http://www.clevelandclinicmeded.com/medicalpubs/diseasemanagement/nephrology/renal-cell-carcinoma/#top. Accessed 25 May 2017.
8. Pitino A, et al. Primary synovial sarcoma of the kidney. A case report with pathological appraisal investigation and literature review. Pathologica. 2011; 103(5):271–8.
9. Park SJ, et al. A case of renal synovial sarcoma: complete remission was induced by chemotherapy with doxorubicin and ifosfamide. Korean J Intern Med. 2004;19(1):62–5.
10. Deshmukh R, Mankin HJ, Singer S. Synovial sarcoma: the importance of size and location for survival. Clin Orthop Relat Res. 2004;419:155–61.
11. Singer S, et al. Synovial sarcoma: prognostic significance of tumor size, margin of resection, and mitotic activity for survival. J Clin Oncol. 1996;14(4): 1201–8.
12. Markovic-Lipkovski J, et al. Rapidly progressive course of primary renal synovial sarcoma–case report. Srp Arh Celok Lek. 2013;141(11–12):814–8.
13. Mishra S, et al. Primary synovial sarcoma of the kidney. Saudi J Kidney Dis Transpl. 2015;26(5):996–9.
14. Schaal CH, Navarro FC, Moraes Neto FA. Primary renal sarcoma with morphologic and immunohistochemical aspects compatible with synovial sarcoma. Int Braz J Urol. 2004;30(3):210–3.
15. Ladanyi M. Fusions of the SYT and SSX genes in synovial sarcoma. Oncogene. 2001;20(40):5755–62.
16. Kawai A, et al. SYT-SSX gene fusion as a determinant of morphology and prognosis in synovial sarcoma. N Engl J Med. 1998;338(3):153–60.
17. Kim DH, et al. Primary synovial sarcoma of the kidney. Am J Surg Pathol. 2000;24(8):1097–104.
18. Chen S, et al. Primary synovial sarcoma of the kidney: a case report with literature review. Int J Surg Pathol. 2001;9(4):335–9.
19. Iacovelli R, et al. Clinical and pathological features of primary renal synovial sarcoma: analysis of 64 cases from 11 years of medical literature. BJU Int. 2012;110(10):1449–54.
20. Ozkan EE, Mertsoylu H, Ozardali HI. A case of renal synovial sarcoma treated with adjuvant ifosfamide and doxorubicin. Intern Med. 2011;50(15):1575–80.
21. Karavasilis V, Seddon BM, Ashley S, Al-Muderis O, Fisher C, Judson I. Significant clinical benefit of first-line palliative chemotherapy in advanced soft-tissue sarcoma: retrospective analysis and identification of prognostic factors in 488 patients. Cancer. 2008;112(7):1585–91. https://www.ncbi.nlm.nih.gov/pubmed/18278813.
22. Pervaiz N, et al. A systematic meta-analysis of randomized controlled trials of adjuvant chemotherapy for localized resectable soft-tissue sarcoma. Cancer. 2008;113(3):573–81.
23. Adjuvant chemotherapy for localised resectable soft tissue sarcoma in adults. Cochrane Database Syst Rev, 2000(4): p. Cd001419.
24. Tornkvist M, et al. A novel case of synovial sarcoma of the kidney: impact of SS18/SSX analysis of renal hemangiopericytoma-like tumors. Diagn Mol Pathol. 2004;13(1):47–51.
25. Bella AJ, Winquist EW, Perlman EJ. Primary synovial sarcoma of the kidney diagnosed by molecular detection of SYT-SSX fusion transcripts. J Urol. 2002;168(3):1092–3.
26. Dai YC, et al. A rare synovial sarcoma of the kidney exhibiting translocation (X;18) and SYT-SSX2 fusion gene. Zhonghua Yi Xue Za Zhi (Taipei). 2002; 65(6):293–7.
27. Vesoulis Z, et al. Fine needle aspiration biopsy of primary renal synovial sarcoma. A case report. Acta Cytol. 2003;47(4):668–72.
28. Moch H, et al. Primary renal synovial sarcoma. A new entity in the morphological spectrum of spindle cell renal tumors. Pathologe. 2003;24(6): 466–72.
29. Chen PC, et al. Primary renal synovial sarcoma with inferior vena cava and right atrium invasion. Int J Urol. 2003;10(12):657–60.
30. Jun SY, et al. Synovial sarcoma of the kidney with rhabdoid features: report of three cases. Am J Surg Pathol. 2004;28(5):634–7.
31. Shao L, Hill DA, Perlman EJ. Expression of WT-1, Bcl-2, and CD34 by primary renal spindle cell tumors in children. Pediatr Dev Pathol. 2004;7(6):577–82.
32. Shannon BA, Murch A, Cohen RJ. Primary renal synovial sarcoma confirmed by cytogenetic analysis: a lesion distinct from sarcomatoid renal cell carcinoma. Arch Pathol Lab Med. 2005;129(2):238–40.
33. Perlmutter AE, et al. Primary synovial sarcoma of the kidney. Int J Urol. 2005; 12(8):760–2.
34. Stage AC, Pollock RE, Matin SF. Bilateral metastatic renal synovial sarcoma. Urology. 2005;65(2):389.
35. Palau LM, et al. Primary synovial sarcoma of the kidney with rhabdoid features. Int J Surg Pathol. 2007;15(4):421–8.
36. Drozenova J, et al. Primary synovial sarcoma of the kidney. Cesk Patol. 2008; 44(1):20–2.
37. Mirza M, Zamilpa I, Bunning J. Primary renal synovial sarcoma. Urology. 2008;72(3):716. e11-2
38. Gabilondo F, et al. Primary synovial sarcoma of the kidney: corroboration with in situ polymerase chain reaction. Ann Diagn Pathol. 2008;12(2):134–7.
39. Zakhary MM, et al. Magnetic resonance imaging features of renal synovial sarcoma: a case report. Cancer Imaging. 2008;8:45–7.
40. Chung, S.D., et al., Primary synovial sarcoma of the kidney. J Formos Med Assoc, 2008. 107(4): 344–347.
41. Erturhan S, et al. Primary synovial sarcoma of the kidney: use of PET/CT in diagnosis and follow-up. Ann Nucl Med. 2008;22(3):225–9.
42. Divetia M, et al. Synovial sarcoma of the kidney. Ann Diagn Pathol. 2008; 12(5):333–9.

43. Dassi V, et al. Primary synovial sarcoma of kidney: a rare tumor with an atypical presentation. Indian J Urol. 2009;25(2):269–71.

44. Kawahara T, et al. Primary synovial sarcoma of the kidney. Case Rep Oncol. 2009;2(3):189–93.

45. Long JA, et al. Primitive renal synovial sarcoma: a cystic tumor in young patients. Prog Urol. 2009;19(7):474–8.

46. Wezel F, et al. Primary biphasic synovial sarcoma of the kidney. Urologe A. 2010;49(3):411–4.

47. Wang ZH, Wang XC, Xue M. Clinicopathologic analysis of 4 cases of primary renal synovial sarcoma. Chin J Cancer. 2010;29(2):212–6.

48. Kageyama S, et al. Primary synovial sarcoma arising from a crossed ectopic kidney with fusion. Int J Urol. 2010;17(1):96–8.

49. Tan YS, et al. Synovial sarcoma of the kidney: a report of 4 cases with pathologic appraisal and differential diagnostic review. Anal Quant Cytol Histol. 2010;32(4):239–45.

50. Romero-Rojas AE, et al. Early age renal synovial sarcoma. Arch Esp Urol. 2010;63(6):464–71.

51. Lakshmaiah KC, et al. Primary synovial sarcoma of kidney-a report of 2 cases and review of literature. J Egypt Natl Canc Inst. 2010;22(3):149–53.

52. Kataria T, et al. Pulmonary metastasis from renal synovial sarcoma treated by stereotactic body radiotherapy: a case report and review of the literature. J Cancer Res Ther. 2010;6(1):75–9.

53. Grampurohit VU, Myageri A, Rao RV. Primary renal synovial sarcoma. Urol Ann. 2011;3(2):110–3.

54. Karafin M, et al. Diffuse expression of PAX2 and PAX8 in the cystic epithelium of mixed epithelial stromal tumor, angiomyolipoma with epithelial cysts, and primary renal synovial sarcoma: evidence supporting renal tubular differentiation. Am J Surg Pathol. 2011;35(9):1264–73.

55. Nishida T, et al. Monophasic primary renal synovial sarcoma accompanied with a hemorrhagic cyst. Urol J. 2011;8(3):244–7.

56. Bakhshi GD, et al. Primary renal synovial sarcoma. Clin Pract. 2012;2(2):e44.

57. Pereira ESR, et al. Primary synovial sarcoma of the kidney with unusual follow up findings. Can J Urol. 2013;20(2):6734–6.

58. Moorthy HK, Pillai BS, Varghese J. Primary renal synovial sarcoma: an oncologic surprise. Urol Case Rep. 2014;2(5):152–3.

59. Majumder A, et al. Primary renal synovial sarcoma: a rare tumor with an atypical presentation. Arch Iran Med. 2014;17(10):726–8.

60. Schoolmeester JK, Cheville JC, Folpe AL. Synovial sarcoma of the kidney: a clinicopathologic, immunohistochemical, and molecular genetic study of 16 cases. Am J Surg Pathol. 2014;38(1):60–5.

61. Wang Z, et al. Primary synovial sarcoma of the kidney: a case report. Oncol Lett. 2015;10(6):3542–4.

62. Ozkanli SS, et al. Primary synovial sarcoma of the kidney. Urol Int. 2014;92(3): 369–72.

63. Vedana M, et al. Primary synovial cell sarcoma of the kidney: case report and review of the literature. Case Reports in Oncology. 2015;8(1):128–32.

64. Lv XF, et al. Primary renal synovial sarcoma: computed tomography imaging findings. Acta Radiol. 2015;56(4):493–9.

24

BAP1 and PBRM1 in metastatic clear cell renal cell carcinoma: tumor heterogeneity and concordance with paired primary tumor

Jeanette E. Eckel-Passow[1], Daniel J. Serie[2], John C. Cheville[3], Thai H. Ho[4], Payal Kapur[5], James Brugarolas[6,7], R. Houston Thompson[8], Bradley C. Leibovich[8], Eugene D. Kwon[8], Richard W. Joseph[9] and Alexander S. Parker[2]*

Abstract

Background: BAP1 and PBRM1 are frequently mutated in primary clear cell renal cell carcinoma (ccRCC) tumors; however, the frequency and clinical relevance of these mutations in metastatic ccRCC tumors is unknown. Additionally, while intra-tumor heterogeneity has been shown to be common in primary ccRCC, little is known regarding heterogeneity in metastatic ccRCC tumors.

Materials and methods: We analyzed BAP1 and PBRM1 loss of protein expression in patient-matched primary and metastatic tumors from 97 patients. Expression was determined using a validated immunohistochemistry assay, which has been shown to be correlated with mutation status.

Results: Of the 97 patients evaluated, 20 and 57% showed loss of BAP1 and PBRM1 in their primary tumors, respectively. Comparing expression across patient-matched primary-metastatic tumor pairs, 98 and 90% had concordant BAP1 and PBRM1 expression, respectively. Both patients who demonstrated discordant BAP1 expression showed loss of BAP1 expression during progression to metastatic ccRCC. Similarly, seven of the ten patients that demonstrated discordant PBRM1 expression showed loss of PBRM1 expression during progression to metastatic ccRCC. We evaluated intra-metastatic tumor heterogeneity using 12 patients who had multiple blocks available from the same tumor with representative pathology; 100 and 92% showed concordant BAP1 and PBRM1 expression, respectively. Amongst 32 patients who had serial metastatic tumors available, both BAP1 and PBRM1 had 97% concordant expression.

Conclusions: We observed minimal intra- and inter- tumor heterogeneity in metastatic ccRCC tumors. Patients with discordant BAP1 or PBRM1 expression across their matched primary and metastatic tumors usually showed loss of expression during progression to metastatic ccRCC.

Keywords: Clonal, Prognostic, Immunohistochemistry

* Correspondence: parker.alexander@mayo.edu
[2]Department of Health Sciences Research, Mayo Clinic, 4500 San Pablo Road, Jacksonville, FL 32224, USA
Full list of author information is available at the end of the article

Background

Mutations that cause loss of expression of BAP1 and PBRM1 are two of the most frequently occurring molecular events in primary clear cell renal cell carcinoma (ccRCC) with a prevalence of approximately 10 and 40%, respectively [1–3]. Both of these genes are located on chromosome arm 3p, which is deleted in approximately 90% of ccRCC patients. While mutations in BAP1 and PBRM1 have been shown to be associated with poor cancer-specific survival [1, 4, 5], the frequency of these mutations (and their clinical relevance) in metastatic ccRCC tumors is unknown. Related to this, Gerlinger and colleagues compared mutations from patient-matched primary and metastatic tumors in four patients; all four were BAP1 wild type and two had PBRM1 mutations [6, 7]. One of the two patients with a PBRM1 mutation (EV002) had a PBRM1 mutation in all six biopsies from the primary tumor as well as in a biopsy from a metastasis obtained at the time of disease progression on everolimus treatment. The other patient with a PBRM1 mutation (RMH004) had a mutation in three of the five biopsies from the primary tumor and a different PBRM1 mutation in a tumor thrombus from the renal vein. The value of this initial exploration notwithstanding, investigations focused on larger cohorts of patients with matched primary and metastatic ccRCC tumors are necessary to obtain estimates of the prevalence of BAP1 and PBRM1 mutations in metastatic ccRCC tumors and to better inform the potential value of these alterations as potential biomarkers for response to therapy.

When evaluating candidate tumor-based biomarkers for metastatic ccRCC, it is important to acknowledge that previous investigators have reported evidence of intra-tumor molecular heterogeneity in primary ccRCC. Specifically, authors of two studies evaluated molecular heterogeneity by performing DNA sequencing on serial biopsies taken from multiple regions of primary ccRCC tumors [6, 7]. In doing so, they observed spatial heterogeneity in every tumor evaluated and thus concluded that a single tumor biopsy gives only a small glimpse into the molecular profile of a primary ccRCC tumor. Of note, the authors in each study did not account for tumor grade and presence of necrosis in evaluating intra-tumor heterogeneity, two features that are well reported to be prognostic indicators for patients with ccRCC. Thus, their observation of intra-tumor molecular heterogeneity is not surprising given that the multiple biopsies could represent areas of the tumor with varying tumor purity as well as different aggressive pathological features. In fact, ccRCC biomarkers have been shown to be associated with pathological features of aggressiveness [8–11]. Thus, with respect to the aforementioned need to evaluate BAP1 and PBRM1 in metastatic ccRCC, these efforts should account for key underlying pathologic features of the tumor.

Motivated by gaps in the literature on BAP1 and PBRM1 in metastatic ccRCC, our objective was four-fold. First, we evaluated whether loss of expression of BAP1 and PBRM1 is a molecular homogenous or heterogeneous event within metastatic ccRCC tumors. Second, we determined the prevalence of loss of BAP1 and PBRM1 expression in metastatic ccRCC. Third, we assessed whether loss of BAP1 and PBRM1 expression in metastatic tumors is associated with cancer-specific outcome. Lastly, we evaluated the concordance of loss of BAP1 and PBRM1 expression across patient-matched primary and metastatic tumors in a large cohort of ccRCC patients.

Methods

Patient selection and pathology review

We identified 111 patients at Mayo Clinic Rochester who were treated surgically for ccRCC between 1990 and 2005, had synchronous (M1) or metachronous (M0 at presentation) ccRCC metastases, underwent metastasectomy for at least one of their metastatic tumors and had formalin-fixed, paraffin-embedded (FFPE) tissue available from their primary tumor and at least one metastatic tumor. For the purposes of this study, multifocal renal tumors and contralateral renal tumors were not considered as metastatic. A single pathologist (JCC) comprehensively reviewed all tumors to confirm histological subtype (1997 AJCC/UICC classification), 2010 tumor stage, 2012 ISUP tumor grade, tumor size, and presence of coagulative tumor necrosis and sarcomatoid differentiation. The FFPE block(s) that was most representative of the tumor (highest grade and presence of necrosis) was identified. If multiple blocks were identified as representative of the tumor, then all blocks were analyzed in order to evaluate intra-tumor heterogeneity across regions of the metastatic tumor that have equivalent pathological features. This study was approved by the Mayo Clinic IRB.

BAP1 and PBRM1

Five-μm thick FFPE sections were stained using a validated and published immunohistochemical (IHC) method [2]. Blinded to the paired nature of the samples, each stained slide was reviewed to determine loss of expression of BAP1 and PBRM1. As described previously [1, 4, 5], positive staining in the background stromal cells and intratumoral lymphocytes was used as a positive internal control. Tumors were categorized as PBRM1 (BAP1) positive when tumors expressed strong diffuse nuclear staining and PBRM1 (BAP1) negative when tumor cells showed a diffuse lack of nuclear staining. In a small number of tumors only a distinct tumor nodule or area showed absent nuclear staining; these focal negative areas were thought to represent subclones of the tumor. Since some tumor cells showed lack of nuclear staining, they were deemed to be PBRM1 (BAP1) negative. Additionally, a small number of tumors showed weak nuclear staining and these weak positive cases were deemed PBRM1 (BAP1) positive. The IHC assays for BAP1 and PBRM1 have been validated and have been shown to be correlated with mutation status [2, 4].

Statistical methods
Protein expression of PBRM1 and BAP1 were dichotomized as positive or negative, as described above. Concordance between patient-matched primary and metastatic tumors was calculated as the percentage of pairs where the primary and patient-matched metastatic tumor had the same designation. Cox proportional hazards regression was used to determine if expression in metastatic tumors was associated with ccRCC-specific survival adjusting for age at diagnosis; dichotomized expression was modeled as a time-dependent covariate. If a patient had multiple simultaneous metastases with discordant PBRM1 (BAP1) status, then the tumor with loss of expression was used in the Cox model [12]. For patients that had multiple blocks from the same metastatic tumor stained for BAP1 and PBRM1 (to estimate intra-metastatic tumor heterogeneity; each replicate block had the same tumor grade and necrosis status) we randomly chose one block to represent the metastatic tumor in the Cox model. P-values (p) <0.05 were considered statistically significant.

Results
Patient characteristics
Our cohort entailed 111 patients who had a primary ccRCC tumor and at least one ccRCC metastatic tumor available for molecular staining (Table 1). A total of 158 patient-matched metastases were available for these 111 patients (Table 2 and Table 3). The median time from nephrectomy to first metachronous metastasis was 1.80 years (min = 31 days, max = 10.73 years). Pulmonary metastases were the most common, accounting for 38% of all metastases (Table 2).

Concordance across patient-matched primary and metastatic ccRCC tumors
BAP1
Of the available 111 patients, 97 (87%) primary ccRCC tumors successfully stained for BAP1 (Table 1) and 20% showed loss of BAP1 expression (IHC negative). We analyzed a total of 138 metastatic tumors from these 97 patients. Overall concordance between patient-matched primary and metastatic tumors from the 97 patients was 98%: 100% in metachronous and 96% in synchronous metastatic tumors (Table 4). With respect to the two patients with discordant primary-metastatic tumor pairs, one patient had a synchronous pulmonary metastasis and one patient

had a synchronous bone metastasis. The primary tumor for both patients was IHC positive and the metastatic tumors were IHC negative.

PBRM1
Ninety-seven (87%) primary tumors successfully stained for PBRM1 (Table 1) and 57% showed loss of PBRM1 (IHC negative). Ninety-six of these 97 patients also had BAP1 status available: 6 (6%) had loss of both BAP1 and PBRM1, 49 (51%) had loss of PBRM1 only, 13 (14%) had loss of BAP1 only and 28 (29%) lost neither BAP1 nor PBRM1. For the 97 patients with staining of PBRM1 in the primary tumor, we analyzed a total of 138 patient-matched metastatic tumors. Overall concordance between patient-matched primary and metastatic tumors from the 97 patients was 90%: 89% in metachronous and 90% in synchronous metastatic tumors (Table 4). Discordance was observed across metastatic sites. Of the 10 patients that had at least one discordant primary-metastatic tumor pair, five had synchronous metastatic tumors and five had metachronous metastatic tumors. Among these 10 patients, seven (70%) demonstrated loss of PBRM1 during progression to metastatic ccRCC.

Intra-metastatic tumor heterogeneity
Replicate blocks were analyzed for BAP1 and PBRM1 expression in 12 metastatic tumors in order to investigate intra-tumor heterogeneity (median = 2, max = 5 replicate blocks per metastatic tumor). Of these, we observed 100% concordance in BAP1 status and 92% concordance in PBRM1 status.

Concordance across longitudinal metastatic ccRCC tumors
BAP1 and PBRM1 staining was performed on longitudinal metastatic tumors for 32 patients (median = 2, max = 4 metastatic tumors per patient). We observed inter-metastatic tumor heterogeneity of BAP1 in one (3%) patient. The primary tumor for this patient was BAP1 IHC positive, the first bone metastasis (synchronous) was IHC negative and the second bone metastasis (diagnosed approximately 9 months later) was IHC positive. Similarly, we observed inter-metastatic tumor heterogeneity of PBRM1 in one (3%) patient. This patient had two available synchronous pulmonary metastases (i.e., at the time of surgery, these two metastases were determined to be different pulmonary nodules): the primary tumor was PBRM1 IHC positive, one pulmonary nodule was IHC negative and the other pulmonary nodule was IHC positive.

Associations of metastatic tumor expression with RCC-specific survival
We did not observe a statistically significantly association with ccRCC-specific survival for either metastatic

Table 1 Clinical characteristics of the primary-metastatic cohort and pathological information associated with the primary ccRCC tumor

	M0 at presentation (N = 57)	M1 (N = 54)	Total (N = 111)
Gender			
No	15 (26.3%)	14 (25.9%)	29 (26.1%)
Yes	42 (73.7%)	40 (74.1%)	82 (73.9%)
Age at Surgery (years)			
Mean	62.0	58.5	60.3
Median	63.6	59.1	61.4
Range	(34.9–78.8)	(38.2–73.7)	(34.9–78.8)
Max Tumor Size (cm)			
Mean	9.6	10.9	10.2
Median	9.0	10.0	9.5
Range	(2.5–18.0)	(2.1–23.0)	(2.1–23.0)
2010 pT			
Missing	0	1	1
1A	3 (5.3%)	1 (1.9%)	4 (3.6%)
1B	8 (14.0%)	8 (15.1%)	16 (14.5%)
2A	14 (24.6%)	6 (11.3%)	20 (18.2%)
2B	4 (7.0%)	5 (9.4%)	9 (8.2%)
3A	17 (29.8%)	20 (37.7%)	37 (33.6%)
3B	7 (12.3%)	4 (7.5%)	11 (10.0%)
3C	2 (3.5%)	1 (1.9%)	3 (2.7%)
4	2 (3.5%)	8 (15.1%)	10 (9.1%)
2010 pN			
0	18 (31.6%)	20 (37.0%)	38 (34.2%)
1	4 (7.0%)	9 (16.7%)	13 (11.7%)
X	35 (61.4%)	25 (46.3%)	60 (54.1%)
TNM Stage			
I	11 (19.3%)	0 (0.0%)	11 (9.9%)
II	18 (31.6%)	0 (0.0%)	18 (16.2%)
III	26 (45.6%)	0 (0.0%)	26 (23.4%)
IV	2 (3.5%)	54 (100.0%)	56 (50.5%)
Grade			
1	1 (1.8%)	1 (1.9%)	2 (1.8%)
2	14 (24.6%)	5 (9.3%)	19 (17.1%)
3	32 (56.1%)	31 (57.4%)	63 (56.8%)
4	10 (17.5%)	17 (31.5%)	27 (24.3%)
BAP1 IHC in Primary Tumor			
Negative	13 (27.7%)	6 (12.0%)	19 (19.6%)
Positive	34 (72.3%)	44 (88.0%)	78 (80.4%)
NA[a]			14
PBRM1 IHC in Primary Tumor			
Negative	28 (60.9%)	27 (52.9%)	55 (56.7%)
Positive	18 (39.1%)	24 (47.1%)	42 (43.2%)
NA[a]			14
Number of Longitudinal Metastases			
1	34 (59.6%)	41 (75.9%)	75 (67.6%)
2	15 (26.3%)	12 (22.2%)	27 (24.3%)
3	6 (10.5%)	1 (1.9%)	7 (6.3%)
4	2 (3.5%)	0 (0.0%)	2 (1.8%)

Table 1 Clinical characteristics of the primary-metastatic cohort and pathological information associated with the primary ccRCC tumor (Continued)

[a]Denotes that the IHC stain was unsuccessful

expression of BAP1 (HR = 1.29, 95% confidence interval (CI): 0.76–2.19, $p = 0.34$) or PBRM1 (HR = 0.92, 95% CI: 0.55–1.52, $p = 0.79$).

Discussion

Chromosome arm 3p loss is a common event in primary ccRCC tumors and four of the most commonly mutated genes are all located on 3p: VHL, BAP1, PBRM1 and SETD2. We evaluated BAP1 and PBRM1 loss of protein expression in a large cohort of patient-matched primary and metastatic ccRCC tumors. Additionally, we examined molecular heterogeneity in metastatic ccRCC tumors.

While previous investigators have reported evidence of intra-tumor molecular heterogeneity in primary ccRCC [6, 7], little is known regarding heterogeneity in metastatic ccRCC tumors. The current research evaluating intra-tumor heterogeneity in primary ccRCC tumors has been performed comparing multiple biopsy samples derived from the same tumor. Such analyses provide important information to determine if biopsy samples can be used for selecting biomarker-based neoadjuvant systemic therapy. Our objective herein was to determine if intra-tumor molecular heterogeneity exists across multiple samples from the same surgically-resected tumor that all have similar pathological feature. It is well known that the drivers, in terms of behavior based on conventional morphology, are tumor grade and necrosis and the areas of a tumor with the highest grade and presence of necrosis are likely enriched for the molecular drivers of metastasis. In fact, for studies evaluating candidate tumor biomarkers, it has been suggested that areas of high nuclear grade should be analyzed [12]. Indeed, the concordance in morphology between patient-matched primary and metastatic tumors supports this recommendation [13]. Thus, we evaluated if intra-tumor heterogeneity exists across samples from the same tumor with similar pathological features. Similar analyses have been performed comparing ccA/ccB ccRCC gene expression subtypes for this cohort of patient-matched

Table 2 Clinical and pathological features associated with the metastatic tumors

	M0 at presentation (N = 90)	M1 (N = 68)	Total (N = 158)
Year of Metastasectomy			
Median	1999	1998	1999
Range	(1991–2005)	(1990–2004)	(1990–2000)
Metastatic Site			
BONE	9 (10.0%)	10 (14.7%)	19 (12.0%)
BOWEL	1 (1.1%)	0 (0.0%)	1 (0.6%)
BRAIN	7 (7.8%)	4 (5.9%)	11 (7.0%)
CONTRALATERAL ADRENAL	3 (3.3%)	5 (7.4%)	8 (5.1%)
HEART	0 (0.0%)	1 (1.5%)	1 (0.6%)
IPSILATERAL ADRENAL	2 (2.2%)	8 (11.8%)	10 (6.3%)
LIVER	4 (4.4%)	5 (7.4%)	9 (5.7%)
MUSCLE	0 (0.0%)	1 (1.5%)	1 (0.6%)
NON-REGIONAL NODES	9 (10.0%)	1 (1.5%)	10 (6.3%)
OMENTUM	0 (0.0%)	1 (1.5%)	1 (0.6%)
OTHER	6 (6.7%)	8 (11.8%)	14 (8.9%)
PANCREAS	5 (5.6%)	2 (2.9%)	7 (4.4%)
PULMONARY	40 (44.4%)	20 (29.4%)	60 (38.0%)
SKIN	2 (2.2%)	2 (2.9%)	4 (2.5%)
SPLEEN	1 (1.1%)	0 (0.0%)	1 (0.6%)
THYROID	1 (1.1%)	0 (0.0%)	1 (0.6%)
Metastatic Grade			
2	16 (17.8%)	13 (19.1%)	29 (18.4%)
3	60 (66.7%)	36 (52.9%)	96 (60.8%)
4	14 (15.6%)	19 (27.9%)	33 (20.9%)
Metastatic Necrosis			
No	57 (63.3%)	38 (55.9%)	95 (60.1%)
Yes	33 (36.7%)	30 (44.1%)	63 (39.9%)
Metastatic Sarcomatoid			
No	86 (95.6%)	62 (91.2%)	148 (93.7%)
Yes	4 (4.4%)	6 (8.8%)	10 (6.3%)

primary and metastatic tumors [14]. Herein, we observed minimal intra- and inter-tumor heterogeneity of BAP1 and PBRM1 loss of expression in metastatic ccRCC tumors. Together, these results suggest that multiple samples from the same metastatic tumor may not be necessary if stringent pathological review is incorporated. However, similar analyses should be performed on additional molecular markers to verify that the results are concordant for other markers.

Previous investigators have reported that BAP1 mutations occur in approximately 10% of ccRCC tumors [1, 2, 4] and loss of BAP1 expression is associated with reduced survival [1]. The higher prevalence of loss of BAP1 expression observed herein is likely due to our high-risk (metastatic) cohort. We observed that loss of BAP1 protein expression

was nearly 100% concordant between patient-matched primary and metastatic tumors. This further underscores that BAP1 is likely a truncal mutation and essential to both ccRCC development and pathogenesis [7, 15]. The two patients that were discordant demonstrated loss of BAP1 during progression to metastatic ccRCC, which suggests the presence of a clone in the primary tumor that had lost BAP1. While loss of BAP1 expression in primary ccRCC tumors has been shown to be prognostic [1, 16], we did not observe a statistically significant association in metastatic ccRCC tumors. However, due to the low prevalence of loss of BAP1 expression, associations with outcome should be examined in larger cohorts of metastatic ccRCC tumors.

PBRM1 mutations have been shown to be prevalent in approximately 40% of ccRCC tumors [1, 3, 4] and loss of

Table 3 Comparison of primary tumor with a total of 158 patient-matched metastatic tumors

	Primary Tumor	Metastatic Tumor	N (%)
Grade	1	2	2 (1.3)
	1	3	1 (0.6)
	2	2	11 (7.0)
	2	3	17 (10.8)
	3	2	14 (8.9)
	3	3	64 (40.5)
	3	4	12 (7.6)
	4	2	2 (1.3)
	4	3	14 (8.9)
	4	4	21 (13.3)
Necrosis	No	No	52 (32.9)
	No	Yes	16 (10.1)
	Yes	No	43 (27.2)
	Yes	Yes	47 (29.7)
Sarcomatoid	No	No	136 (86.1)
	No	Yes	4 (2.5)
	Yes	No	12 (7.6)
	Yes	Yes	6 (3.8)

PBRM1 expression has been shown to be associated with overall survival [4]. The higher prevalence of loss of PBRM1 expression observed herein is likely due to the cohort of high-risk patients. We observed a negative genetic interaction between BAP1 and PBRM1, confirming a result that was reported previously [5]. Under independence we would have expected 11% of the primary tumors to show loss of both BAP1 and PBRM1; however, 6% of our primary tumors had loss of expression for both genes. We observed high concordance of loss of PBRM1 expression between patient-matched primary and metastatic tumors. Of the 10 patients that

Table 4 Percent (%) concordance across primary-metastatic tumor pairs for 97 patients

	% Concordant	
	PBRM1	BAP1
Overall	89.7	97.9
M0 at presentation	89.1	100
M1	90.2	96.0
Pulmonary	85.3	97.1
M0 at presentation	82.4	100
M1	88.2	94.1
Non-pulmonary	92.1	98.4
M0 at presentation	93.1	100
M1	91.2	97.0

demonstrated discordance, 70% had primary tumors that were IHC positive and subsequently the metastatic tumors demonstrated PBRM1 loss of expression. This corroborates our findings that when patient-matched primary and metastatic tumors had discordant ccA/ccB molecular subtype, 80% of these discordant patients progressed from having a primary tumor classified as ccA and a metastatic tumor classified as ccB [14]. Furthermore, when evaluating pathological characteristics across patient-matched primary and metastatic RCC tumors, trends for higher grade and tumor necrosis in the metastatic tumor have been observed [13]. Overall, our results suggest that there may be a clone in the primary tumor that had lost PBRM1. Discordance was observed across multiple metastatic sites, and thus, does not appear to be site specific. Additionally, we did not observe an association between metastatic PBRM1 expression and ccRCC-specific survival.

We acknowledge that there may be systematic differences between subjects who underwent metastasectomy and subjects with distant metastases that were not treated surgically. However, tissue will only be available from patients undergoing metastasectomy, so this limitation is unavoidable. We used IHC to measure BAP1 and PBRM1 protein loss instead of directly determining BAP1 and PBRM1 mutation status. Thus, even though the IHC assays for BAP1 and PBRM1 have been validated and shown to be correlated with mutation status in previous studies [2, 4], the impact of mutations in these proteins could not be determined. IHC is both more cost effective and easily applied to formalin-fixed paraffin-embedded specimens, which are both important considerations when attempting to analyze hundreds of clinically-stored tissue specimens. We only analyzed metastatic tumors from patients whom we also had a patient-matched surgically-resected primary ccRCC tumor available for analysis. Because we ignored metastatic tumors from patients who did not have a nephrectomy at our institution, we may have a biased sample of metastatic tumors. Thus, future studies examining the molecular characteristics of metastatic tumors and identification of prognostic markers should evaluate all available metastatic tumors.

Conclusions

We observed minimal molecular heterogeneity across sections from the same metastatic tumor that had similar pathological features. With respect to progression from primary-to-metastatic ccRCC, loss of BAP1 and PBRM1 expression demonstrated minimal heterogeneity. Thus, BAP1 and PBRM1 are likely key events in both ccRCC development and progression to metastasis. Currently, the presence or absence of either of these mutations does not guide clinical decision making, especially in regards to choosing therapy for metastatic disease. However, there are multiple potential therapeutic targets where these mutations could be clinically relevant in the future. And, given the high concordance of these mutations between primary and metastatic tumors, testing the more readily-available primary tumor might be sufficient. Going forward, analyzing serial samples from the same patient and mapping the clonal evolution of ccRCC will aid in understanding the molecular alterations that underlie ccRCC pathogenesis [6, 7, 17–22]. As demonstrated herein, this approach needs to be taken using larger cohorts and associations with pathological features and outcome should be conducted.

Abbreviations
ccRCC: clear cell renal cell carcinoma; CI: Confidence interval; FFPE: Formalin-fixed, paraffin-embedded; HR: Hazard ratio; IHC: Immunohistochemical; P: p-value; RCC: Renal cell carcinoma

Acknowledgements
The authors acknowledge the Mayo Clinic Comprehensive Cancer Center Biospecimens Accessioning and Processing Shared Resource and the Pathology Research Core Shared Resource. The authors also acknowledge Sue Harrington, Tracy Hilton, Christine Lohse and Amanda Shreders for reviewing earlier versions of the manuscript.

Funding
This work was supported by National Institutes of Health: R21CA176422 (JEEP), R01CA134466 (ASP), R01CA134345 (EDK) and R01CA175754 (JB). JB is also supported by grants from the Cancer Prevention and Research Institute of Texas (RP130603).

Authors' contributions
JEEP, THH, EDK, RWJ, and ASP designed the study. PK and JB performed the experiments and collected the data. JEEP and DJS analyzed the data. JEEP, DJS, JCC, PK, JB, THH, RHT, BCL, RWJ and ASP interpreted the data. All authors were involved in writing the paper and had final approval of the submitted manuscript.

Competing interests
James Brugarolas is on Bethyl's advisory board.

Author details
[1]Division of Biomedical Statistics and Informatics, Mayo Clinic, Rochester, MN, USA. [2]Department of Health Sciences Research, Mayo Clinic, 4500 San Pablo Road, Jacksonville, FL 32224, USA. [3]Laboratory Medicine and Pathology, Mayo Clinic, Rochester, MN, USA. [4]Division of Hematology and Medical Oncology, Mayo Clinic, Scottsdale, AZ, USA. [5]Department of Pathology, University of Texas Southwestern Medical Center, Dallas, TX, USA. [6]Kidney Cancer Program, Simmons Comprehensive Cancer Center, University of Texas Southwestern Medical Center, Dallas, TX, USA. [7]Division of Hematology-Oncology, University of Texas Southwestern Medical Center, Dallas, TX, USA. [8]Department of Urology, Mayo Clinic, Rochester, MN, USA. [9]Division of Hematology/Oncology, Mayo Clinic, Jacksonville, FL, USA.

References
1. TCGA TCGA. Comprehensive molecular characterization of clear cell renal cell carcinoma. Nature. 2013;499:43–9.
2. Pena-Llopis S, Vega-Rubin-de-Celis S, Liao A, et al. BAP1 loss defines a new class of renal cell carcinoma. Nat Genet. 2012;44:751–9.
3. Varela I, Tarpey P, Raine K, et al. Exome sequencing identifies frequent mutation of the SWI/SNF complex gene PBRM1 in renal carcinoma. Nature. 2011;469:539–42.
4. Kapur P, Pena-Llopis S, Christie A, et al. Effects on survival of BAP1 and PBRM1 mutations in sporadic clear-cell renal-cell carcinoma: a retrospective analysis with independent validation. Lancet Oncol. 2013;14:159–67.
5. Joseph RW, Kapur P, Serie DJ, et al. Clear cell renal cell carcinoma subtypes identified by BAP1 and PBRM1 expression. J Urol. 2016;195:180–7.
6. Gerlinger M, Rowan AJ, Horswell S, et al. Intratumor heterogeneity and branched evolution revealed by multiregion sequencing. N Engl J Med. 2012;366:883–92.
7. Gerlinger M, Horswell S, Larkin J, et al. Genomic architecture and evolution of clear cell renal cell carcinomas defined by multiregion sequencing. Nat Genet. 2014;46:225–33.
8. Parker AS, Eckel-Passow JE, Serie D, et al. Higher expression of topoisomerase II alpha is an independent marker of increased risk of cancer-specific death in patients with clear cell renal cell carcinoma. Eur Urol. 2014;66:929–35.
9. Thompson RH, Kuntz SM, Leibovich BC, et al. Tumor B7-H1 is associated with poor prognosis in renal cell carcinoma patients with long-term follow-up. Cancer Res. 2006;66:3381–5.
10. Tollefson MK, Thompson RH, Sheinin Y, et al. Ki-67 and coagulative tumor necrosis are independent predictors of poor outcome for patients with clear cell renal cell carcinoma and not surrogates for each other. Cancer. 2007;110:783–90.
11. Parker AS, Kosari F, Lohse CM, et al. High expression levels of survivin protein independently predict a poor outcome for patients who undergo surgery for clear cell renal cell carcinoma. Cancer. 2006;107:37–45.
12. Callea M, Albiges L, Gupta M, et al. Differential expression of PD-L1 between primary and metastatic sites in clear-cell renal cell carcinoma. Cancer Immunol Res. 2015;3:1158–64.
13. Psutka SP, Cheville JC, Costello BA, et al. Concordance of pathologic features between metastatic sites and the primary tumor in surgically resected metastatic renal cell carcinoma. Urology. 2016;96:106–13.
14. Serie DJ, Joseph RW, Cheville JC, et al. Clear Cell Type A and B Molecular Subtypes in Metastatic Clear Cell Renal Cell Carcinoma: Tumor Heterogeneity and Aggressiveness. Eur Urol. 2016. http://dx.doi.org/10.1016/j.eururo.2016.11.018.
15. Gerlinger M, Catto JW, Orntoft TF, et al. Intratumour heterogeneity in urologic cancers: from molecular evidence to clinical implications. Eur Urol. 2015;67:729–37.
16. Joseph RW, Kapur P, Serie DJ, et al. Loss of BAP1 protein expression is an independent marker of poor prognosis in patients with low-risk clear cell renal cell carcinoma. Cancer. 2014;120:1059–67.
17. Gulati S, Martinez P, Joshi T, et al. Systematic evaluation of the prognostic impact and intratumour heterogeneity of clear cell renal cell carcinoma biomarkers. Eur Urol. 2014;66:936–48.
18. Yachida S, Jones S, Bozic I, et al. Distant metastasis occurs late during the genetic evolution of pancreatic cancer. Nature. 2010;467:1114–7.
19. Ding L, Ley TJ, Larson DE, et al. Clonal evolution in relapsed acute myeloid leukaemia revealed by whole-genome sequencing. Nature. 2012;481:506–10.
20. Wu X, Northcott PA, Dubuc A, et al. Clonal selection drives genetic divergence of metastatic medulloblastoma. Nature. 2012;482:529–33.
21. Landau DA, Carter SL, Stojanov P, et al. Evolution and impact of subclonal mutations in chronic lymphocytic leukemia. Cell. 2013;152:714–26.
22. Johnson BE, Mazor T, Hong C, et al. Mutational analysis reveals the origin and therapy-driven evolution of recurrent glioma. Science. 2014;343:189–93.

25

Clinical characteristics of XP11.2 translocation/TFE3 gene fusion renal cell carcinoma

Xiangming Cheng, Weidong Gan*, Gutian Zhang, Xiaogong Li and Hongqian Guo

Abstract

Background: Renal cell carcinoma (RCC) associated with Xp11.2 translocation/TFE3 gene fusion (Xp11.2 RCC) is a rare subtype of RCC which is firstly described as a distinct entity in 2004 so that clinical characteristics of Xp11.2 RCC in different gender and age are unknown. The purpose of systematic review and meta-analysis is to provide a comprehensive assessment on them.

Methods: MEDLINE, EMBASE and Cochrane databases were searched for studies which evaluate the clinical characteristics of Xp11.2 RCC. The literature published between July 2004 and May 2014 was searched.

Results: A total of 15 studies with 147 participants were included. The meta-analysis demonstrated that number of patients of all age in female was higher than in male with pooled OR of 3.93(95 % CI = 1.66–9.34). However, incidence of distant metastases (OR = 0.34, 95 % CI = 0.12–1.57) and lymphatic metastases (OR = 0.51, 95 % CI = 0.14–1.91), tumor stage (OR = 0.85, 95 % CI = 0.34–2.15) and overall survival (OS) (OR = 0.46, 95 % CI = 0.05–4.34) between male and female were comparable. Incidence in female was higher than in male with pooled OR of 5.13(95 % CI = 1.67–15.72) in adults, while in children no gender-related predominance (OR = 1.19, 95 % CI = 0.38–3.72) was observed. In addition, incidence of distant metastases (OR = 1.00, 95 % CI = 0.13–7.84) and lymphatic metastases (OR = 1.00, 95 % CI = 0.07–13.67) and tumor stage (OR = 1.94, 95 % CI = 0.20–19.03) between children and adults were comparable. Survival curves presented comparable outcomes between male and female (P = 0.707) as well as between children and adults (P = 0.383).

Conclusions: Female patients with Xp11.2 RCC in adults exhibit a high incidence compared to male, but not in children. Comparable clinical characteristics including incidence of distant and lymphatic metastases, tumor stage and prognosis is presented between male and female as well as between children and adults.

Keywords: Age groups, Carcinoma, Gender identity, Renal cell, Xp11.2 translocation

Background

Renal cell carcinoma (RCC) associated with Xp11.2 translocation/TFE3 gene fusion (Xp11.2 RCC) is a rare subtype of RCC which is delineated as a distinct entity in the 2004 World Health Organization renal tumor classification [1]. This subtype affects primarily children more than adults, accounts for 20–40 % of pediatric RCC and 1–1.6 % of

RCC in adults [2]. In addition, Xp11.2 RCC were reported more aggressive than other subtypes of RCC and associated with a poorer prognosis [3].

Xp11.2 RCCs are generally characterized by several translocations on chromosome Xp11.2 resulting in a gene fusion between TFE3 and at least 6 possible partners [4]. Since these translocations are located on the X chromosome, it seems reasonable to suggest that there are gender differences in the clinical characteristics of Xp11.2 RCC. However, comparative analysis regarding the clinical course of Xp11.2 RCC between male and

* Correspondence: gwd@nju.edu.cn; dr.gwd@yeah.net
Department of Urology, Nanjing Drum Tower Hospital, the Affiliated Hospital of Nanjing University Medical School, No. 321 Zhongshan Road, Nanjing 210008, Jiangsu Province, China

female remains controversial due to relatively rare incidence [5–8]. In addition, as Xp11.2 RCC predominantly among children and associated with a poorer prognosis, the comparison of the prognosis between children and adults exists as well [9]. Due to such controversy in gender and age of Xp11.2 RCC, in this systematic review and meta-analysis, we studied the clinical characteristics of Xp11.2 RCC regarding patient demographics, incidence of distant and lymphatic metastases, tumor stage and prognosis in order to better define the difference of Xp11.2 RCC between male and female as well as between children and adults.

Methods
Literature search
The present meta-analysis was conducted following the Preferred Reporting Items for Systematic Reviews and Meta-Analyses (PRISMA) statement (accessible at http://www.prisma-statement.org/). A computer-aided literature search was performed in May 2014 with usage of the Cochrane, MEDLINE, EMBASE and Science Citation Index. An initial search strategy use keywords describing TFE3, Xp11.2 renal cell carcinoma. The literature published between July 2004 and May 2014 was searched since Xp11.2 RCC was first definitely diagnosed as a distinct entity in 2004. Additional studies were searched by reference lists from primary studies to identify any studies missed by the electronic search strategies.

Study selection
Two authors reviewed abstracts of all candidate articles independently and read full-text review if articles could not be categorized based on title and abstract alone. All articles were checked for unified inclusion criteria. Discrepancies were resolved by consensus with a third author. Authors of included studies were not contacted for additional, unreported data.

Study inclusion/exclusion criteria
Studies were included if they fulfilled the following criteria: (1) Studies reported clinical parameters of patients with Xp11.2 RCC including gender and age. (2) The diagnosis of all patients with Xp11.2 RCC was confirmed by immunohistochemical (IHC) assay for TFE3 combined with fluorescence in-situ hybridization polyclonal (FISH) assay or other strict criteria. When the results of FISH assay and other molecular biology such as Reverse Transcription - Polymerase Chain Reaction (RT-PCR) were contradicted with IHC assay, definite diagnosis of Xp11.2 RCC was made by genetic analysis including FISH assay and other molecular biology. Inclusion was not limited to randomized controlled trials (RCTs). Studies were excluded if they were (1) performed in the lab with animal or cell models; (2) reviews and case

reports with only one case due to one case was not enough to compare the gender and age diference; (3) molecular or mechanism researches. When duplicate patient populations were published from on institution, the most recent data were used.

Quality assessment of primary
Quality of primary articles was assessed in duplicate by independent authors. Issues such as number of case, manner of diagnosis and study design were analyzed. Any disagreement was dealt with consensus and discussion with a third author.

Data extraction
Data extraction fields for each study included the following: (1) demographic data concerning patient gender, age, treatment and condition during follow-up period; (2) tumor data for different gender and age including stage, lymphatic and distant metastases. For age, patients was divided into children (≤ 14 years) and adults (> 14 years). When gender-related incidences in children and adults were studied, reference would be excluded if only 1 patient was presented in the study. The cases of Xp11.2 RCC would be excluded if the lymphatic and distant metastases of tumor cannot be determined when we studied tumor metastases and stage. If journal articles contained insufficient information, we attempted to contact authors to obtain missing details. If failed, we could just present out the existing results.

Data synthesis and analysis
The clinical data included number of Xp11.2 RCC in different gender and age for which tumor stage, lymphatic metastases, distant metastases and prognosis such as overall survival (OS) were analyzed. All above data were recorded from original articles. The statistical software Review Manager (Version 5.0 for Windows) was applied to carry out all the analysis. Data regarding incidence of Xp11.2 RCC, tumor stage, metastases and overall survival were dichotomous data which was shown as odds ratios (ORs). For dichotomous data, when no statistically significant heterogeneity was detected, Mantel-Haenszel fixed-effect model was used to pool ORs with 95 % confidence intervals (CIs). The heterogeneity across the studies was investigated using a $\chi 2$-based test of homogeneity and evaluation of the inconsistency index (I^2) statistic. The p value less than 0.1 was considered as statistically significant heterogeneity. An I^2 value > 50 % was considered to represent substantial heterogeneity across studies, which was the symbol of applying random- effect model. Publication bias for each of the pooled study groups was assessed by funnel plot if the number of studies in group was ≥ 10.

We also estimated the survival curves in different gender and age, all of whom were treated by surgical procedure such as nephron sparing surgery (NSS) and radical nephrectomy (RN). The probability of survival was analyzed by the Kaplan-Meier methods within the log-rank test. Reported p values were statistical significance set at $p < 0.05$.

Results

Literature and study characteristics

As shown in Fig. 1, 15 studies [4, 10–23] with 147 subjects met the inclusion criteria. All of the enrolled studies were retrospective, in which 2 of them provided all the clinical parameters in different gender while the other gave part of these parameters, as shown in Table 1. None of study provided detailed information about OS in comparison of different age while other clinical parameters were shown in Table 2. The number of studies in the pooled group of gender-related incidence in adults were ≥ 10, as well as patients of all ages, publication bias of the groups were described as visual assessment of a funnel plot in Fig. 2.

Primary outcomes

The forest plots about gender-related differences and age-related differences were shown in Figs. 3 and 4. In study of gender-related difference in incidence of Xp11.2, subgroup analysis was made to learn gender-related incidence in children and adults.

Gender

Totally, the number of included patients was 147 ($n = 98$ for women and $n = 49$ for men). We observed that I^2 value was > 50 % in the group of incidence of patients of all age in different gender (I^2 statistic = 55 %, $P = 0.005$). Therefore we applied random- effect model in meta-analysis of this data. Meanwhile, no evidence for significant publication bias was observed in this pooled group. For other group, there was no evidence for heterogeneity about incidence of distant (I^2 statistic = 0 %, $P = 0.81$) and lymphatic metastases (I^2 statistic = 0 %, $P = 0.83$), tumor stage (I^2 statistic = 0 %, $P = 0.57$) and OS (I^2 statistic = 0 %, $P = 0.51$). Results of meta-analysis demonstrated that the incidence of Xp11.2 in female was significantly higher than in male with pooled OR of 3.93(95 % CI = 1.66–9.34). However, incidence of distant

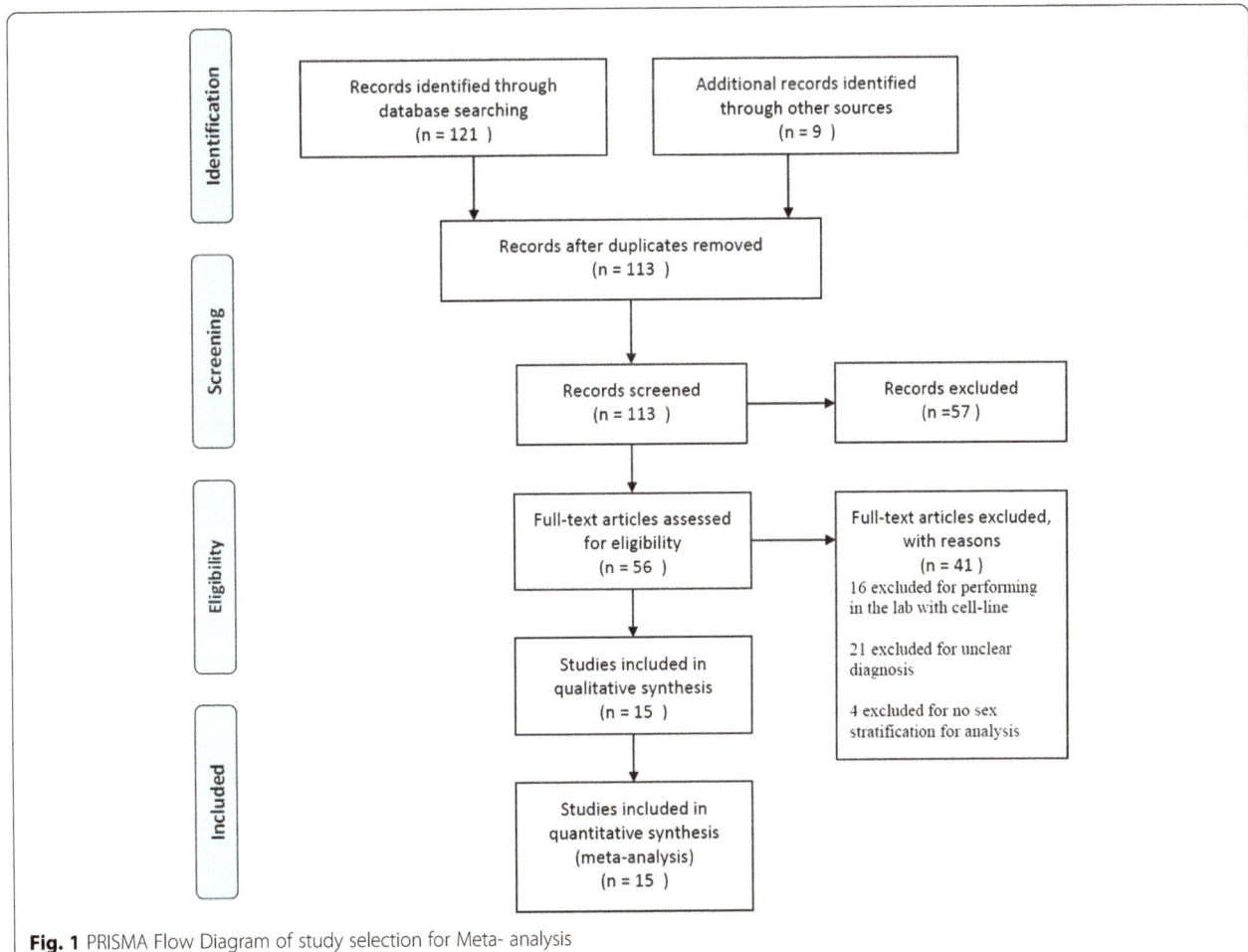

Fig. 1 PRISMA Flow Diagram of study selection for Meta- analysis

Table 1 Clinical characteristics of included studies between male and female

Reference	Number of patients		Incidence of lymphatic metastases		Incidence of distant metastases		Stage I/II (III/IV)		Overall survival	
	Male	Female	Male	Female	Male	Female	Male	Female	Male	Female
Rao et al. [20]	9	8	1/3	0/4	1/1	0/1	2/7	4/4	–	–
Hodge et al. [21]	7	12	–	–	–	–	–	–	–	–
Altinok et al. [10]	3	3	2/3	1/3	–	–	1/2	2/3	0/3	0/3
Zou et al. [22]	5	4	2/5	1/4	1/5	0/4	3/2	1/3	3/4	3/4
Hung et al. [13]	1	7	0/1	2/7	0/1	2/7	1/0	3/4	–	–
Green et al. [18]	10	21	0/0	4/5	1/1	3/4	4/6	9/12	–	–
Zhong et al. [16]	0	6	–	–	–	5/6	–	–	–	–
Choueiri et al. [11]	3	12	–	–	–	–	–	–	–	–
Pflueger et al. [19]	4	12	1/2	3/4	1/1	0/3	–	1/3	–	–
Gaillot-Durand et al. [17]	0	2	–	–	–	–	–	–	–	–
Zhong et al. [12]	0	4	–	–	–	–	–	–	–	–
Klatte et al. [4]	1	1	1/1	0/1	1/1	0/1	0/1	1/0	0/1	0/1
Sukov et al. [15]	2	4	–	1/2	0/2	1/4	–	–	2/2	2/4
Kim et al. [14]	4	0	–	–	–	–	–	–	–	–
Argani et al. [23]	0	2	–	–	–	–	–	–	–	–

metastases (OR = 0.43, 95 % CI = 0.12–1.57) and lymphatic metastases (OR = 0.51, 95 % CI = 0.14–1.91, tumor stage (OR = 0.85, 95 % CI = 0.34–2.15) and overall survival (OS) (OR = 0.46, 95 % CI = 0.05–4.34) between male and female were comparable. The result of OS consistent with analysis for clinical characteristics of Xp11.2 RCC was confirmed by survival function (P = 0.707), as shown in Fig. 5a.

Age

A total of 132 cases of Xp11.2 from 13 studies including 23 children (≤ 14 years) and 109 adults (> 14 years) were pooled for analyzing the clinical characteristics between adults and children. I^2 value was > 50 % in the group of gender-related incidence in adults (I^2 statistic = 61 %, P = 0.003) so that random- effect model was applied. According to funnel plot, there was no significant

Table 2 Clinical characteristics of included studies between children and adults

Reference	Gender		Incidence of lymphatic metastases		Incidence of distant metastases		Stage I/II (III/IV)	
	Children (Male/Female)	Adults (Male/Female)	Children	Adults	Children	Adults	Children	Adults
Rao et al. [20]	3/3	6/5	0/5	1/2	0/1	1/1	0/1	0/1
Hodge et al. [21]	1/1	6/11	–	–	–	–	–	–
Altinok et al. [10]	3/3	–	–	–	–	–	–	–
Zou et al. [22]	–	5/4	–	–	–	–	–	–
Hung et al. [13]	–	1/7	–	–	–	–	–	–
Green et al. [18]	0/2	10/19	–	4/5	1/1	4/5	1/1	14/14
Zhong et al. [16]	–	0/6	–	–	–	5/6	–	–
Pflueger et al. [19]	3/2	1/10	1/1	3/5	–	0/2	–	1/1
Gaillot-Durand et al. [17]	–	0/2	–	–	–	–	–	–
Zhong et al. [12]	–	0/4	–	–	–	–	–	–
Klatte et al. [4]	1/0	0/1	1/1	0/1	1/1	0/1	0/1	1/0
Sukov et al. [15]	–	2/4	–	–	–	–	–	–
Kim et al. [14]	1/0	3/0	–	–	–	–	–	–
Argani et al. [23]	–	0/2	–	–	–	–	–	–

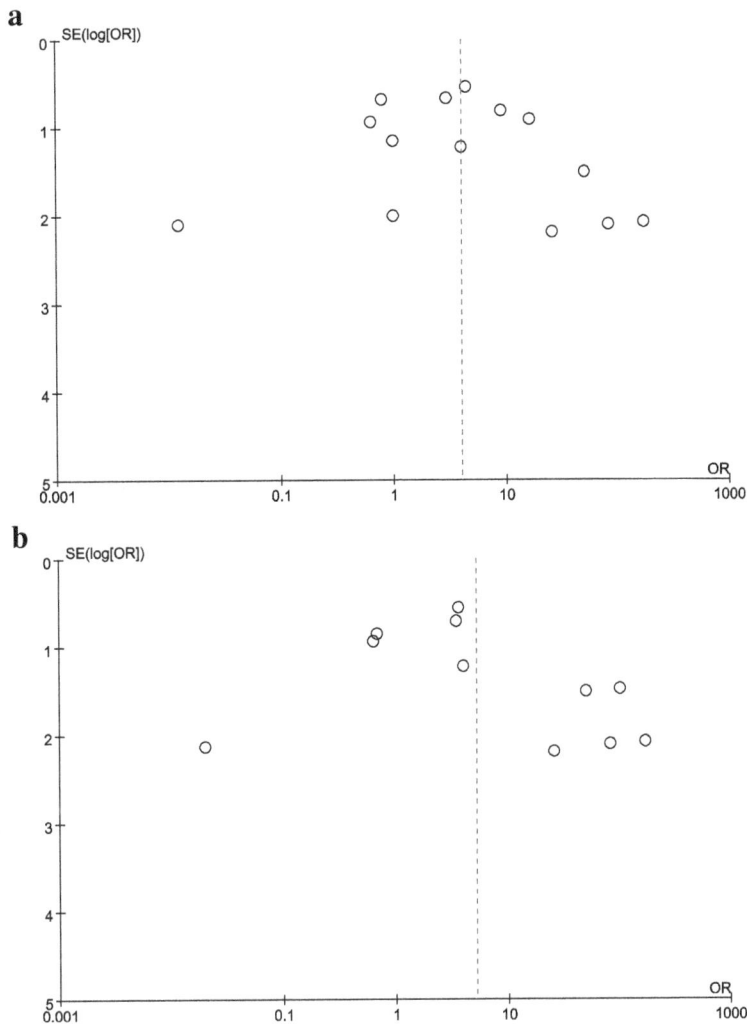

Fig. 2 Publication bias assessment for study of distribution of Xp11.2 RCC in male and female. Funnel plots show that there was no evidence for significant publication bias in any of the 2 pooled groups. **a** patients of all ages; **b** patients older than 14

publication bias in this study. P value was > 0.10 in group of gender-related incidence in children (I^2 statistic = 0 %, $P = 0.63$) and incidence of distant (I^2 statistic = 0 %, $P = 0.40$) and lymphatic metastases (I^2 statistic = 26 %, $P = 0.26$) between children and adults as well as in tumor stage (I^2 statistic = 0 %, $P = 0.42$). Results of meta-analysis demonstrated that the incidence of patients in female was significantly higher than in male with pooled OR of 5.13(95 % CI = 1.67–15.72) in adults while in children no gender-related predominance (OR = 1.19, 95 % CI = 0.38–3.72) was observed. In addition, incidence of distant metastases (OR = 1.00, 95 % CI = 0.13–7.84) and lymphatic metastases (OR = 1.00, 95 % CI = 0.07–13.67) and tumor stage (OR = 1.94, 95 % CI = 0.20–19.03) between children and adults were comparable. The result of clinical characteristics of Xp11.2 RCC was confirmed by survival function ($P = 0.383$), as shown in Fig. 5b.

Discussion

Xp11.2 RCC is a rare subtype of RCC which results from gene fusions between the transcription factor E3 (TFE3) gene and at least 5 fusion partners including ASPL-TFE3, PRCC-TFE3, PSF-TFE3, CLTC-TFE3, and Nono -TFE3, whose chromosomal rearrangement is t(X;17)(p11.2;q25), t(X;1)(p11.2;q21), t(X;1)(p11.2;p34), t(X;17)(p11.2;q23) and inv(X)(p11.2;q12), respectively [8, 24]. Due to the translocations lead to overexpression of TFE3 protein, detection of TFE3 protein by IHC assay is currently the most commonly used diagnostic technique in clinical practice [25]. Gaillot-Durand et al. showed that nuclei stained with an intensity of ++ to +++ in IHC assay was necessary to suspect the diagnosis of Xp11.2 RCC [17]. However, recent studies have found that the positive predictive value of positive TFE3 staining for Xp11.2 RCC is very low as well as highly false positive results [4, 14, 17, 18]. Definite diagnosis of Xp11.2 RCC

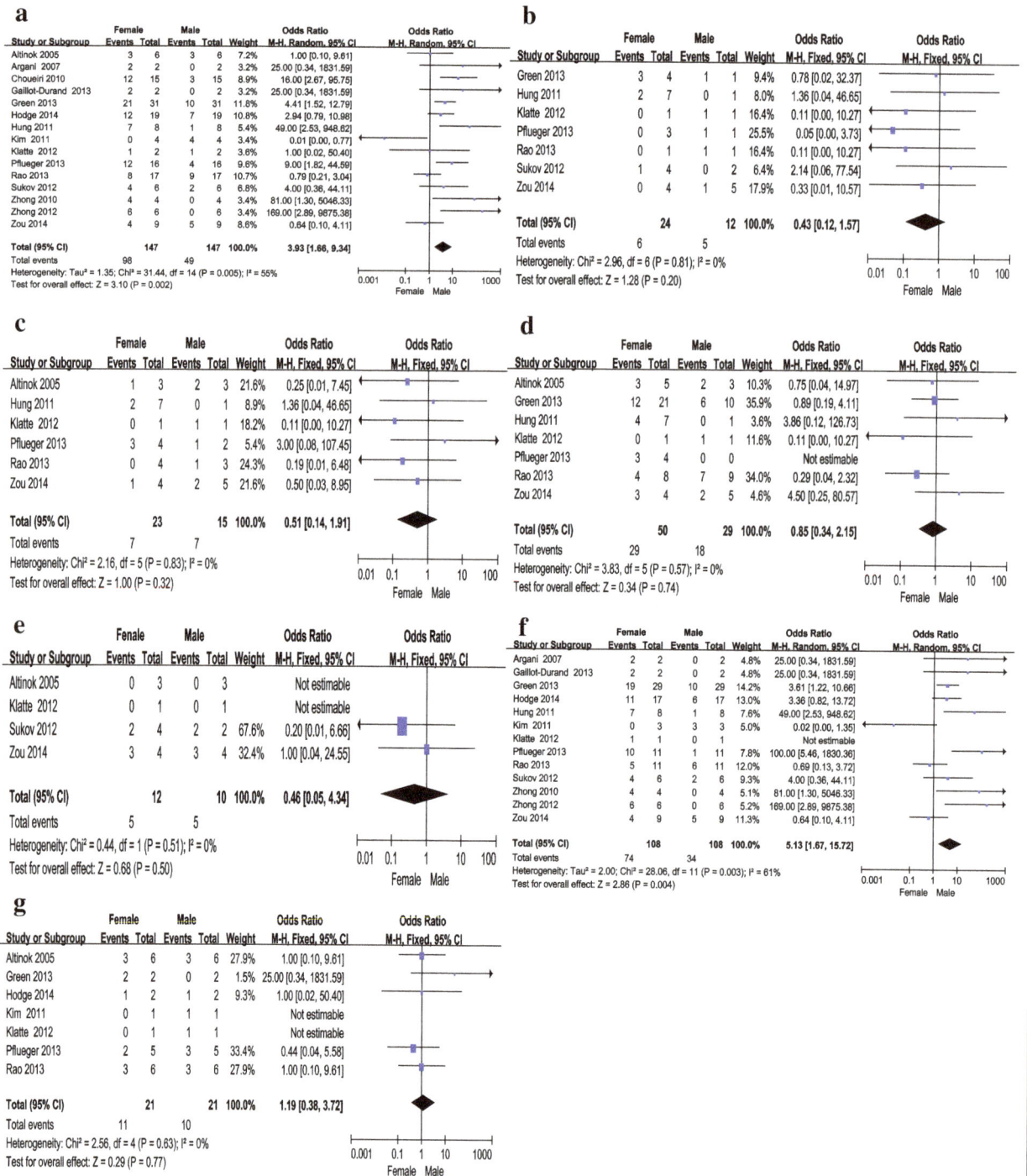

Fig. 3 Forrest plots and meta-analysis of studies showing 95 % confidence interval of male Xp11.2 RCC as compared with female Xp11.2 RCC. Clinical characteristics are reported as follows: **a** Number of patients of all ages; **b** Incidence of distant metastases; **c** Incidence of lymphatic metastases; **d** Tumor stage; **e** Overall survival (OS); **f** Different gender-related incidence in adults; **g** Different gender-related incidence in children

should be not only made by IHC assay but also by such strict criteria as FISH assay and other molecular biology [4, 17]. Thus, the strength of this study is that we first analyzed the clinical characteristics of Xp11.2 RCC with the diagnostic criteria of the combined

examination of TFE3 IHC staining and other molecular biology. In our report, 21 studies were excluded from meta-analysis because they made the diagnosis of only by IHC assay, which may be suspected to have other subtypes of RCC included.

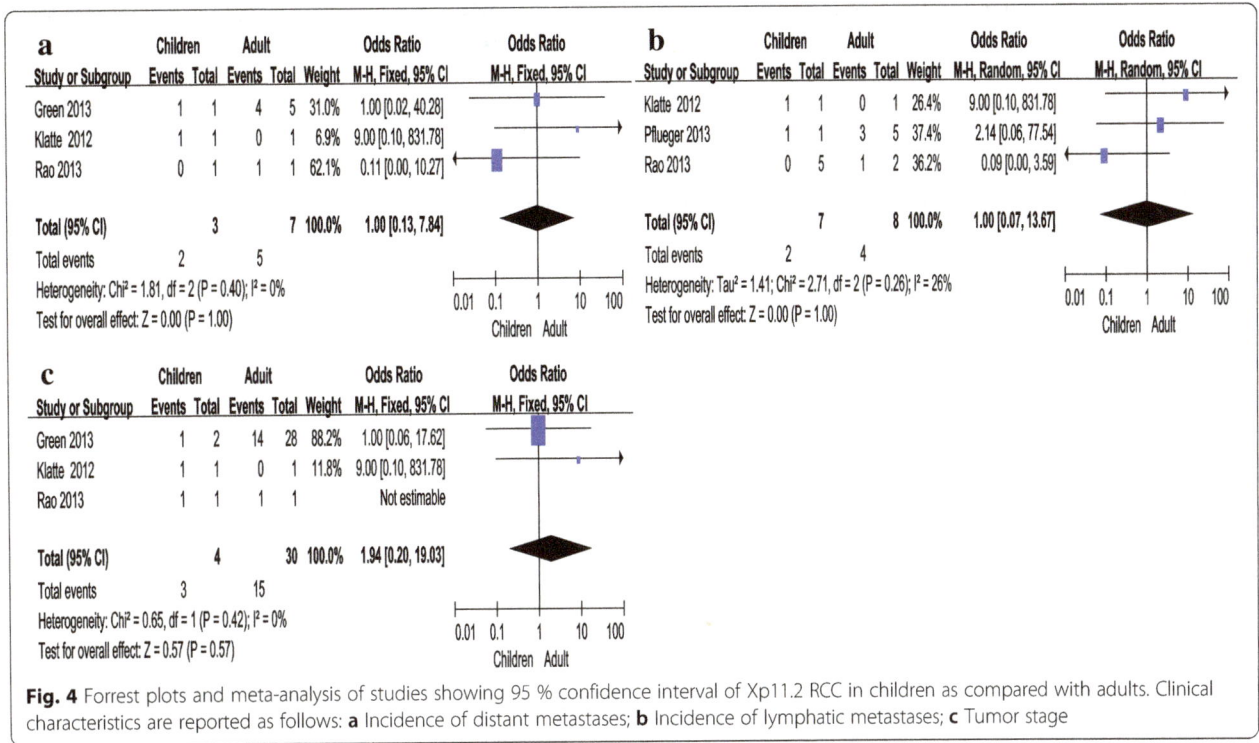

Fig. 4 Forrest plots and meta-analysis of studies showing 95 % confidence interval of Xp11.2 RCC in children as compared with adults. Clinical characteristics are reported as follows: **a** Incidence of distant metastases; **b** Incidence of lymphatic metastases; **c** Tumor stage

Gender-related difference in incidence of Xp11.2 RCC remains controversial. Several previous studies indicated a female predominance in incidence of Xp11.2 RCC [7, 8, 26], while a few reports showed a male predominance in Xp11.2 RCC [5, 22]. In addition, Altinok et al. found the male/female ratio was equal in their study of pediatric Xp11.2 RCC [10]. We gathered all references which met the inclusion criteria for meta-analysis and found that the number of patients of all ages in female was significantly higher than that in male with pooled OR of 3.93 (95 % CI = 1.66–9.34). To learn gender-related incidence of Xp11.2 RCC more comprehensively, included patients were divided into two groups as children (≤14 years, $n = 23$) and adults (>14 years, $n = 109$). We found that female predominance is seen in adults (OR = 5.13, 95 % CI = 1.67–15.72) and no gender difference in children (OR = 1.19, 95 %

CI = 0.38–3.72). Although incidence of Xp11.2 RCC in children is higher than in adults as a percentage of RCC [2], adult Xp11.2 RCC could still outnumber pediatric Xp11.2 RCC due to RCC is more common in adults (approximately 25,000 cases per year in the United States) than in children (approximately 25 cases per year in the United States) [23]. As previously mentioned, translocations are mainly located on the X chromosome. Moreover, translocations might only occur on the active X chromosome but not the Barr body (inactive X chromosome) although females have two X chromosomes. According to Sirchia [27], homozygosity (two active X chromosome) can exist in normal somatic cell due to mutations occur during mitosis. Thus, the possible explanation for gender-related difference existing in adults but not in children is that a higher level of homozygosity in adults than children

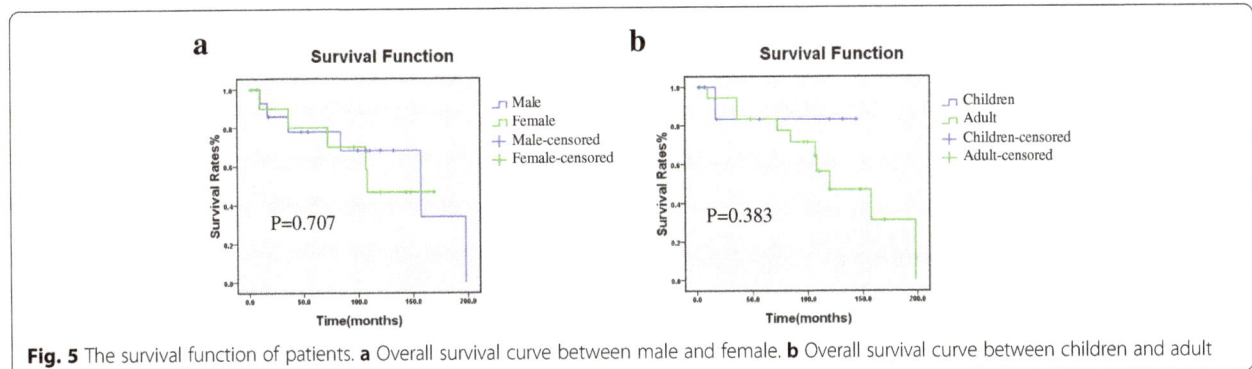

Fig. 5 The survival function of patients. **a** Overall survival curve between male and female. **b** Overall survival curve between children and adult

results from accumulation of mutations with age. Nonetheless, more comprehensive and detailed studies are required to confirm this speculation.

At diagnosis, metastases of Xp11.2 may occur in about one-third of patients [28], who were older and predominant in male [6]. Moreover, some studies showed that Xp11.2 RCC has a higher degree of invasiveness and a more rapid disease course in adult patients than children [29, 30]. Nevertheless, a study reporting contradictory data to that showed a case of children with bone metastases at diagnosis and a very aggressive course [28]. In our meta-analysis, the incidence of distant and lymphatic metastases and tumor stage between male and female were comparable as well as between children and adults. The important reason for the inconsistencies may be explained by the differences of diagnostic methods. Previously mentioned diagnosis was only based on IHC assay, while this study adopted the combined TFE3 IHC staining and FISH assay to exclude the possibility of other subtypes of RCC.

The treatment for Xp11.2 RCC is still not well defined. For Xp11.2 RCC including that with positive regional lymph nodes, surgery is the optional treatment [26] while NSS is an alternative treatment for patients with tumors measuring < 7 cm [29]. Chemotherapy such as sunitinib can be applied as well [31]. However, Xp11.2 has poorer prognosis no matter what treatment is applied [4, 32]. Recent studies reported that prognosis of pediatric Xp11.2 RCC was better than that of adult Xp11.2 RCC [30, 33, 34]. However, such conclusion was based on small sample size without strict diagnosis. In our meta-analysis, we grouped patients who have been treated by RN or NSS to analyze the prognosis of RCC. No statistically significant difference was observed in the probability of survival between children and adults. In addition, we analyzed prognosis in male and female by survival curve and OS which showed no significant difference. Thus, this meta-analysis suggested that the prognosis of Xp11.2 RCC between male and female is comparable as well as between children and adults.

There are some limitations in this meta-analysis. The sample size was still small and most of studies cannot provide completely detailed information. In addition, the number of existing high-quality studies is too small to compare parameters about prognosis such as free progress survival. Further studies are required to solve these problems.

Conclusion

This meta-analysis of the current evidence illustrate that the female patients with Xp11.2 RCC in adults exhibit a high incidence compared to the male, but not in children. Comparable clinical characteristics including incidence of distant and lymphatic metastases, tumor stage

and prognosis is presented between male and female as well as between children and adults. Based on these results, the epidemiological information about gender difference in incidence of Xp11.2 RCC in adults is provided. Further investigations on more comprehensive and heterogeneous studies should be carried out to extend our results.

Abbreviations
RCC, Renal cell carcinoma; Xp11.2 RCC, Renal cell carcinoma associated with Xp11.2 translocation/TFE3 gene fusion; OS, Overall survival; IHC, immunohistochemical; FISH, fluorescence in-situ hybridization polyclonal; RT-PCR, Reverse Transcription - Polymerase Chain Reaction; RCTs, randomized controlled rials; NSS, nephron sparing surgery; RN; radical nephrectomy; CIs, confidence intervals

Acknowledgements
This work was supported by a grant from National Natural Science Foundation of China (ID: 81572512), Natural Science Foundation of Jiangsu Province (ID: BK20131281).

Funding
None.

Authors' contribution
XC had full access to all the data in the study and takes responsibility for the integrity of the data and the accuracy of the data analysis. Conception and design was done by XL and WG. Literature review, data extraction and statistical analysis were carried out by HG and GZ. Drafting of the article was done by XC. Revision of the article was done by XL and HG. All authors read and approved the final manuscript.

Competing interests
The authors declare that they have no competing interests.

References
1. Bruder E, Passera O, Harms D, et al. Morphologic and molecular characterization of renal cell carcinoma in children and young adults. Am J Surg Pathol. 2004;28:1117–32.
2. Kmetec A, Jeruc J. Xp 11.2 translocation renal carcinoma in young adults; recently classified distinct subtype. Radiol Oncol. 2014;48:197–202.
3. Rao Q, Guan B, Zhou XJ. Xp11.2 Translocation Carcinomas Have a Poorer Prognosis Than Non-Xp11.2 Translocation Carcinomas in Children and Young Adults: A Meta-Analysis. Int J Surg Pathol. 2010;18:458–64.
4. Klatte T, Streubel B, Wrba F, et al. Renal cell carcinoma associated with transcription factor E3 expression and Xp11.2 translocation: incidence, characteristics, and prognosis. Am J Clin Pathol. 2012;137:761–8.
5. Wu A, Kunju LP, Cheng L, Shah RB. Renal cell carcinoma in children and young adults: analysis of clinicopathological, immunohistochemical and molecular characteristics with an emphasis on the spectrum of Xp11.2 translocation-associated and unusual clear cell subtypes. Histopathology. 2008;53:533–44.
6. Malouf GG, Camparo P, Molinie V, et al. Transcription factor E3 and transcription factor EB renal cell carcinomas: clinical features, biological behavior and prognostic factors. J Urol. 2011;185:24–9.
7. Su HH, Sung MT, Chiang PH, Cheng YT, Chen YT. The preliminary experiences of translocation renal cell carcinoma and literature review. Kaohsiung J Med Sci. 2014;30:402–8.

8. Wang W, Ding J, Li Y, et al. Magnetic Resonance Imaging and Computed Tomography Characteristics of Renal Cell Carcinoma Associated with Xp11.2 Translocation/TFE3 Gene Fusion. PLoS One. 2014;9:e99990.

9. Spreafico F, Collini P, Terenziani M, Marchiano A, Piva L. Renal cell carcinoma in children and adolescents. Expert Rev Anticancer Ther. 2010;10:1967–78.

10. Altinok G, Kattar MM, Mohamed A, Poulik J, Grignon D, Rabah R. Pediatric renal carcinoma associated with Xp11.2 translocations/TFE3 gene fusions and clinicopathologic associations. Pediatr Dev Pathol. 2005;8:168–80.

11. Choueiri TK, Lim ZD, Hirsch MS, et al. Vascular endothelial growth factor-targeted therapy for the treatment of adult metastatic Xp11.2 translocation renal cell carcinoma. Cancer. 2010;116:5219–25.

12. Zhong M, De Angelo P, Osborne L, et al. Dual-color, break-apart FISH assay on paraffin-embedded tissues as an adjunct to diagnosis of Xp11 translocation renal cell carcinoma and alveolar soft part sarcoma. Am J Surg Pathol. 2010;34:757–66.

13. Hung CC, Pan CC, Lin CC, Lin AT, Chen KK, Chang YH. XP11.2 translocation renal cell carcinoma: clinical experience of Taipei Veterans General Hospital. J Chin Med Assoc. 2011;74:500–4.

14. Kim SH, Choi Y, Jeong HY, Lee K, Chae JY, Moon KC. Usefulness of a break-apart FISH assay in the diagnosis of Xp11.2 translocation renal cell carcinoma. Virchows Arch. 2011;459:299–306.

15. Sukov WR, Hodge JC, Lohse CM, et al. TFE3 rearrangements in adult renal cell carcinoma: clinical and pathologic features with outcome in a large series of consecutively treated patients. Am J Surg Pathol. 2012;36:663–70.

16. Zhong M, De Angelo P, Osborne L, et al. Translocation renal cell carcinomas in adults: a single-institution experience. Am J Surg Pathol. 2012;36:654–62.

17. Gaillot-Durand L, Chevallier M, Colombel M, et al. Diagnosis of Xp11 translocation renal cell carcinomas in adult patients under 50 years: interest and pitfalls of automated immunohistochemical detection of TFE3 protein. Pathol Res Pract. 2013;209:83–9.

18. Green WM, Yonescu R, Morsberger L, et al. Utilization of a TFE3 break-apart FISH assay in a renal tumor consultation service. Am J Surg Pathol. 2013;37:1150–63.

19. Pflueger D, Sboner A, Storz M, et al. Identification of molecular tumor markers in renal cell carcinomas with TFE3 protein expression by RNA sequencing. Neoplasia. 2013;15:1231–40.

20. Rao Q, Williamson SR, Zhang S, et al. TFE3 break-apart FISH has a higher sensitivity for Xp11.2 translocation-associated renal cell carcinoma compared with TFE3 or cathepsin K immunohistochemical staining alone: expanding the morphologic spectrum. Am J Surg Pathol. 2013;34:804–15.

21. Hodge JC, Pearce KE, Wang X, Wiktor AE, Oliveira AM, Greipp PT. Molecular cytogenetic analysis for TFE3 rearrangement in Xp11.2 renal cell carcinoma and alveolar soft part sarcoma: validation and clinical experience with 75 cases. Mod Pathol. 2014;27:113–27.

22. Zou H, Kang X, Pang LJ, et al. Xp11 translocation renal cell carcinoma in adults: a clinicopathological and comparative genomic hybridization study. Int J Clin Exp Pathol. 2014;7:236–45.

23. Argani P, Olgac S, Tickoo SK, et al. Xp11 translocation renal cell carcinoma in adults: expanded clinical, pathologic, and genetic spectrum. Am J Surg Pathol. 2007;31:1149–60.

24. Liu K, Xie P, Peng W, Zhou Z. Renal carcinomas associated with Xp11.2 translocations/TFE3 gene fusions: findings on MRI and computed tomography imaging. J Magn Reson Imaging. 2014;40:440–7.

25. Komai Y, Fujiwara M, Fujii Y, et al. Adult Xp11 translocation renal cell carcinoma diagnosed by cytogenetics and immunohistochemistry. Clin Cancer Res. 2009;15:1170–6.

26. Ahluwalia P, Nair B, Kumar G. Renal Cell Carcinoma Associated with Xp11.2 Translocation/TFE3 Gene Fusion: A Rare Case Report with Review of the Literature. Case Reports Urology. 2013;2013:1–4.

27. Sirchia SM, Ramoscelli L, Grati FR, et al. Loss of the inactive X chromosome and replication of the active X in BRCA1-defective and wild-type breast cancer cells. Cancer Res. 2005;65:2139–46.

28. Sudour-Bonnange H, Leroy X, Chauvet M, Classe M, Robin PM, Leblond P. Cutaneous metastases during an aggressive course of Xp11.2 translocation renal cell carcinoma in a teenager. Pediatr Blood Cancer. 2014;61:1698–700.

29. Song HC, Sun N, Zhang WP, He L, Fu L, Huang C. Biological characteristics of pediatric renal cell carcinoma associated with Xp11.2 translocations/TFE3 gene fusions. J Pediatr Surg. 2014;49:539–42.

30. Armah HB, Parwani AV. Xp11.2 translocation renal cell carcinoma. Arch Pathol Lab Med. 2010;134:124–9.

31. Numakura K, Tsuchiya N, Yuasa T, et al. A case study of metastatic Xp11.2 translocation renal cell carcinoma effectively treated with sunitinib. Int J Clin Oncol. 2011;16:577–80.

32. Qiu R, Bing G, Zhou XJ. Xp11.2 Translocation renal cell carcinomas have a poorer prognosis than non-Xp11.2 translocation carcinomas in children and young adults: a meta-analysis. Int J Surg Pathol. 2010;18:458–64.

33. Meyer PN, Clark JI, Flanigan RC, Picken MM. Xp11.2 translocation renal cell carcinoma with very aggressive course in five adults. Am J Clin Pathol. 2007;128:70–9.

34. Koie T, Yoneyama T, Hashimoto Y, et al. An aggressive course of Xp11 translocation renal cell carcinoma in a 28-year-old man. Int J Urol. 2009;16:333–5.

26

Bilateral Xp11.2 translocation renal cell carcinoma

Takashi Karashima[1][*], Takahira Kuno[1], Naoto Kuroda[2], Hirofumi Satake[1], Satoshi Fukata[1], Masakazu Chikazawa[3], Chiaki Kawada[1], Ichiro Yamasaki[1], Taro Shuin[1], Makoto Hiroi[4] and Keiji Inoue[1]

Abstract

Background: Xp11.2 translocation renal cell carcinoma (RCC) is a rare variety of a kidney neoplasm. We report a case of bilateral Xp11.2 translocation RCC occurring metachronously and discuss this very rare entity with reference to the literature.

Case presentation: The patient was a 56-year-old woman who presented with a right renal tumor. The patient had undergone left radical nephrectomy 7 years previously, which resulted in a histopathological diagnosis of clear cell RCC. Open right partial nephrectomy was performed under the presumptive diagnosis of recurrence of clear cell RCC. The present right renal tumor was pathologically diagnosed Xp11.2 translocation RCC. More than 70% of the tumor cells in the present right tumor were strongly positive for transcription factor E3 (TFE3) expression by immunohistochemical analysis with an anti-TFE3 antibody. A break-apart of the TFE3 genes in the bilateral tumors was identified by fluorescence in situ hybridization analysis. Real time-polymerase chain reaction analysis for the alveolar soft part sarcoma locus-TFE3 fusion gene was performed, which gave a positive result in the bilateral tumors. Pathological comparison of each of the tumors might lead to a final diagnosis of Xp11.2 translocation RCC occurring metachronously.

Conclusions: We present the bilateral Xp11.2 translocation RCC. A combination of immunohistochemical, cytogenetic and molecular biological approaches allowed the final diagnosis of such a rare RCC.

Keywords: Renal cell carcinoma, Xp11.2 translocation, Bilateral, ASPL-TFE3

Background

Xp11.2 translocation renal cell carcinoma (RCC) is a rare variety of kidney neoplasm that represents approximately 1% of RCC [1]. It is a clinically identified malignant neoplasm of kidney with an advanced stage and a poorer prognosis than conventional clear cell RCC [2]. Xp11.2 translocation RCC results from gene fusions between the transcription factor E3 (TFE3) gene located on chromosome Xp11.2 and various fusion partners. These chimeric gene fusions result in overexpression of fusion proteins that contain the C-terminal portion of TFE3. The TFE3 fusion partner genes have been recently well characterized. A common fusion partner gene is alveolar soft part sarcoma critical region 1 (ASPSCR1), der(17)t(X;17)(p11.2;q25). This unbalanced translocation results in fusion of the TFE3 gene, a member of the basic-helix-loop-helix family of transcription factors, on Xp11.2, to a novel gene named alveolar soft part sarcoma locus (ASPL) on 17q25 [3]. Other common fusion genes are papillary renal cell carcinoma-TFE3 (PRCC-TFE3), t(X;1)(p11.2;q21.2) and PTB-associated splicing factor-TFE3 (PSF-TFE3), t(X;1)(p11.2;p34) [4, 5]. Less commonly observed gene fusions are NonO-TFE3 inv.(X)(p11.2;q12) and clathrin heavy chain-TFE3 (CLTC-TFE3), (X;17)(p11.2;q23) [6, 7].

In this report, we present an extremely rare case of bilateral Xp11.2 translocation RCC occurring metachronously, and discuss the uncommon features of this case as determined by histopathological, cytogenetic and molecular approaches.

Case presentation

A 56-year-old woman was introduced to Kochi Medical School from a private hospital for right renal tumor

* Correspondence: karasima@kochi-u.ac.jp
[1]Department of Urology, Kochi University, Kochi Medical School, Kohasu, Oko, Nankoku, Kochi 783-8505, Japan
Full list of author information is available at the end of the article

detected by abdominal computed tomography (CT). She had been undergone radical nephrectomy for left renal cell carcinoma (RCC) 7 years before. An abdominal CT of the present tumor revealed a right renal tumor, 5.3 cm in diameter, showing poorly-defined margins, irregular contrast and no findings of metastases (Fig. 1a, b). An abdominal CT that was performed 7 years ago revealed a left renal tumor, 7.0 cm in diameter, showing well-defined margins, irregular contrast and no findings of metastases, diagnosed clinical stage T1b N0 M0 left RCC (Fig. 1c, d). She did not have any other medical history or family history.

Open right partial nephrectomy was performed under a presumed diagnosis of clinical stage T1b N0 M0 right RCC, recurrent or due to metastasis from the previous left tumor. The tumor was a macroscopically well-circumscribed solid mass. The cross-sectional surface was lobulated and heterogenously yellow to brown with bleeding and necrosis (Fig. 2). Microscopically, the tumor showed an alveolar growth pattern admixed with eosinophilic and clear cytoplasm. Papillary architecture was also focally seen. In some areas, eosinophilic coarse granules were identified in the tumor cytoplasm. Pathological stage was pT1b pN0 with negative surgical margin. Nuclear Grade corresponded to largely Fuhrman Grade 3 and partly Grade 4. Hyaline nodules and psammoma bodies were observed in the stroma. Immunohistochemically, the tumor cells showed diffuse positivity

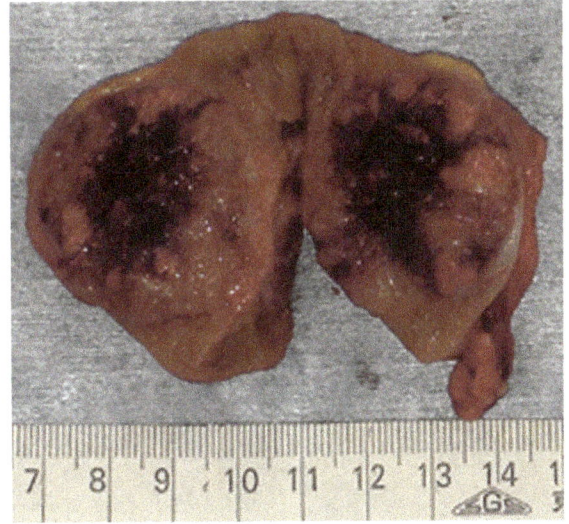

Fig. 2 Macroscopic findings of the present right tumor. The present right tumor resected by partial nephrectomy was macroscopically a well-marginated solid mass. The cross-sectional surface was lobulated and heterogenously yellow to brown with bleeding and necrosis

for renal cell carcinoma-maker (RCCMa, PN-15, 1: 100, Cell Marque, CA, USA) and cluster differentiation (CD)10 (56C16, prediluted, Novocastra Laboratories Ltd., Newcastle, UK) and negativity for Cathepsin K (3F9, Abcam, Tokyo, JP), Melanosome (Human melanoma black; HMB45, prediluted, DAKO, Glostrup, Denmark),

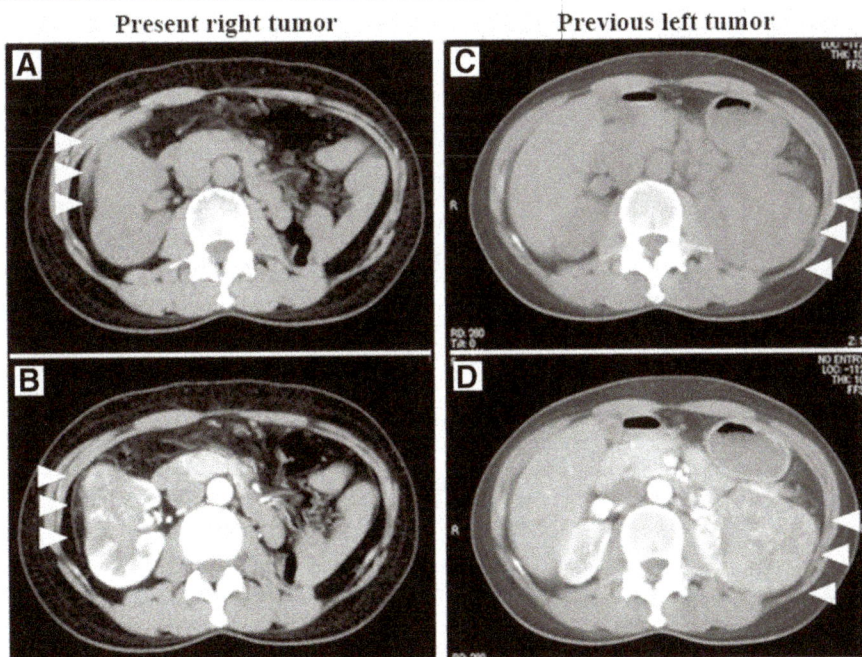

Fig. 1 Pre-operative diagnostic imaging of the present and the previous tumor. Abdominal CT images of the present right renal tumor (**a**, **b**) and the previous left renal tumor (**c**, **d**). The present right renal tumor was 5.3 cm in diameter and showed poorly-defined margins and an irregular contrast. The previous left renal tumor was 7.0 cm in diameter, and showed well-defined margins and an irregular contrast

Melan A (A103, 1: 100, Novocastra Laboratories Ltd., Newcastle, UK), and alpha smooth muscle actin (data not shown). Seventy percent of neoplastic cell nuclei stained positive for TFE3 (MRQ-37, prediluted, Ventana Medical Systems, Inc., Tucson, AZ), with a staining intensity of (moderate) 2+ to (strong) 3+ (Fig. 3). Staining for transcription factor EB (TFEB, polyclonal, V-17, 1: 400, Santa

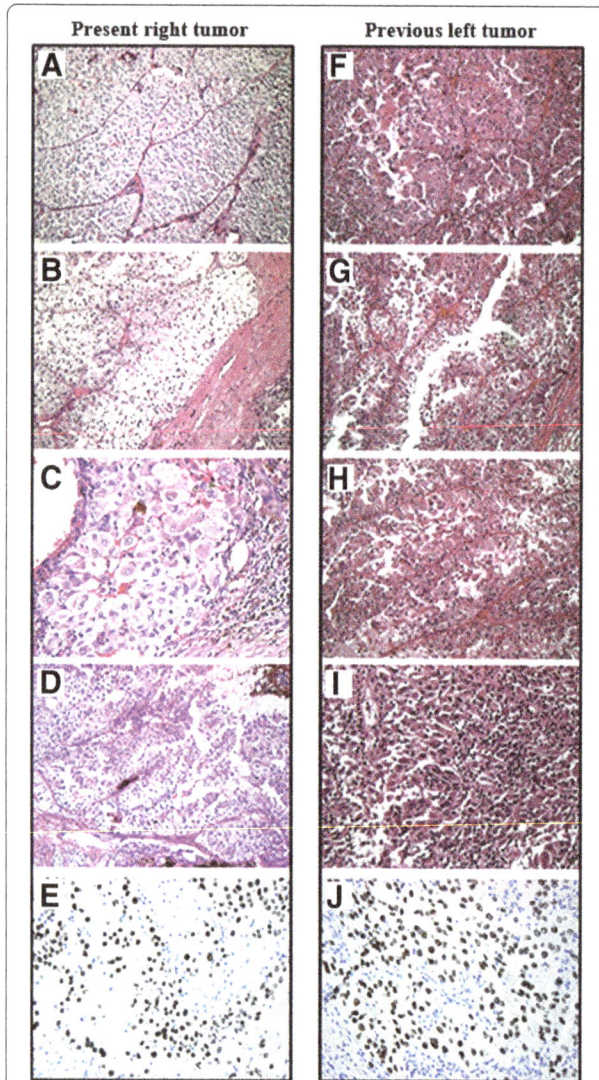

Fig. 3 Microscopic findings of the present right tumor and previous left tumor. HE staining of the present right tumor mostly showed an alveolar growth pattern (×100; **a**) with cells composed clear cytoplasm (×100; **b**). Very large tumor cells (×100; **c**) and a papillary growth pattern (×100; **d**) were focally observed. Moderate to strong immunostaining of TFE3 in the nuclei of tumor cells was seen (×200; **e**). HE staining of the previous left tumor showed an alveolar growth pattern (×100; **f**), pale eosinophilic cytoplasm (×100; **g**) and very large tumor cells (×100; **h**). Dedifferentiated sarcomatoid features were partially observed (×100; **i**). Moderate to strong immunostaining of TFE3 in the nuclei of tumor cells was seen (×200; **j**)

Cruz, Biotechnology, Inc., Dallas, TX) was generally negative (data not shown).

Hematoxylin and eosin, and immunohistochemical stains from the previous tumor were retrospectively reviewed. In H and E staining, tubular, papillary, and alveolar growth patterns were noted admixed with eosinophilic and clear cytoplasm. Additionally, very large tumor cells were seen and dedifferentiation with a discohesive area and rhabdoid features was also noted. Necrosis and hemorrhage were present. Pathological stage was pT1b pN0. Nuclear Grade corresponded to Fuhrman Grade 4. Small venous invasion by carcinoma cells was seen. Neoplastic cells showed diffuse immunohistochemical expression of RCCMa, CD10, Alpha-Methylacyl-CoA Race (AMACR; P504S, 13H4, 1: 100, DAKO, Glostrup, Denmark) and negative results for cytokeratin 7, Carbonic Anhydrase IX (CA9, D47G3, Cell Signaling, MA, USA), HMB45, Melan A and Cathepsin K (data not shown). TFE3 was positively stained in the nuclei of 5% of neoplastic cells with a staining intensity of 2+ to 3+ (Fig. 3).

We performed a dual-color, break-apart fluorescence in situ hybridization (FISH) assay to identify the chromosomal break point of TFE3 in paraffin-embedded tissue [8]. Briefly, the break-apart FISH assay with probes upstream and downstream to TFE3 showed red and green signals. A fused or closely approximated green-red signal pattern was interpreted as a normal result, whereas a TFE3 fusion resulted in a split-signal pattern. Signals were considered to be split when the green and red signals were separated by a distance of more than 2 signal diameters. For each tumor, a minimum of 100 tumor cell nuclei were examined under fluorescence microscopy at ×1000 magnification. Only nonoverlapping tumor nuclei were evaluated. Positive findings were defined as more than 10% of the tumor nuclei showing the split-signal pattern [9]. The TFE3 gene showed gene splitting in 71.55% of 130 neoplastic cells and in 76.82% of 233 neoplastic cells in the present and the previous tumor, respectively. Typical TFE3 break-apart signals of the present and previous tumors are presented in Fig. 4.

Total RNA was extracted from formalin fixed paraffin embedded tissue of the previous tumor and from frozen tissue of the present tumor using a standard organic extraction method (MACHEREY-NAGEL, Germany and QIAGEN, Germany, respectively). ASPL-TFE3 fusion transcripts were detected using an ASPL forward primer: 5'-AAAGAAGTCCAAGTCGGGCCA-3' and a TFE3 exon 4 reverse primer: 5'-CGTTTGATGTTGGGCAGCTCA-3'. Glyceraldehyde-3-phosphate dehydrogenase (GAPDH) transcripts were detected using the forward: 5'-CGGATTTGGTCGTATTGG-3' and reverse: 5'-TCCTGGAAGATGGTGATG-3' GAPDH primers [2]. The ASPL-TFE3 fusion gene was detected in the

Present right tumor **Previous left tumor**

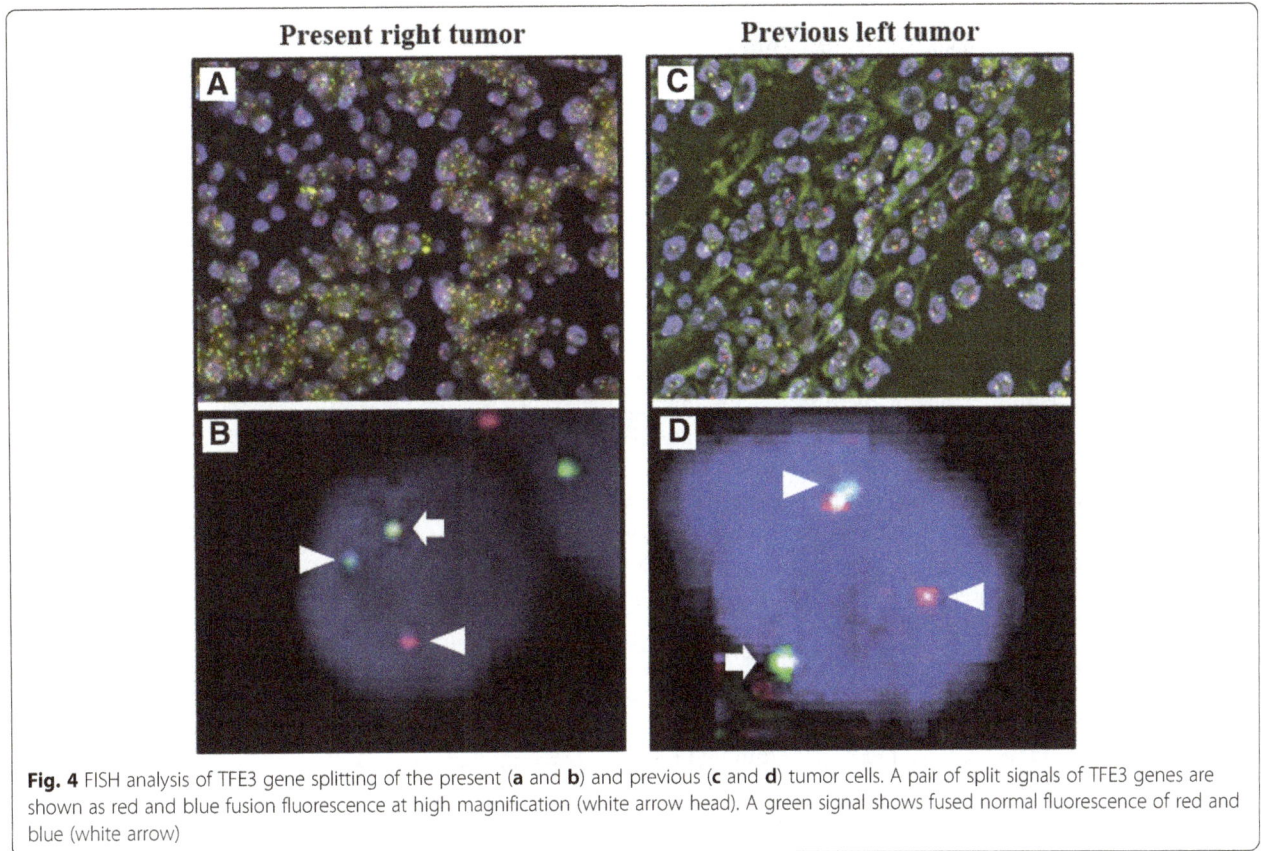

Fig. 4 FISH analysis of TFE3 gene splitting of the present (**a** and **b**) and previous (**c** and **d**) tumor cells. A pair of split signals of TFE3 genes are shown as red and blue fusion fluorescence at high magnification (white arrow head). A green signal shows fused normal fluorescence of red and blue (white arrow)

tissue from the present and the previous tumor but was not detected in the normal tissue. GAPDH that was used as a loading control was detected in each reaction (Fig. 5).

There is a no evidence of recurrence at 8 months postoperatively.

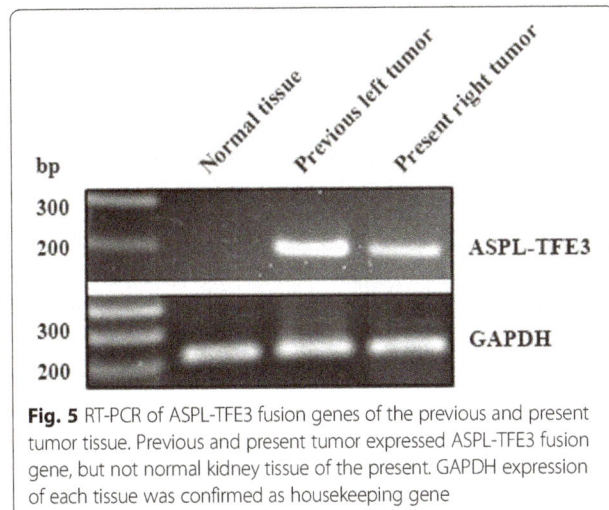

Fig. 5 RT-PCR of ASPL-TFE3 fusion genes of the previous and present tumor tissue. Previous and present tumor expressed ASPL-TFE3 fusion gene, but not normal kidney tissue of the present. GAPDH expression of each tissue was confirmed as housekeeping gene

Discussion and conclusions

Xp.11.2 translocation RCC is a rare variety of RCC that was first described in 1995 by Dijkhuizen et al [10]. It is categorized as a separate entity in the 2004 World Health Organization classification of tumors of the urinary system [11]. This type of RCC frequently affects children and adolescents. Our patient was diagnosed as Xp11.2 translocation RCC at the ages of 49 and 56 years-of age. Patients of middle age and over with Xp11.2 translocation RCC have rarely been reported [12]. There is variation in the histological features of Xp11.2 translocation RCC such as clear cell, papillary, alveolar, and nested. Seventy five percent of adult Xp11.2 translocation RCC is predominately the clear cell histological type, whereas most pediatric cases consist of papillary histological features [13]. In our present left tumor, clear cell features were the predominant type, followed by alveolar and papillary. Also, characteristic findings such as eosinophilic, voluminous and clear cytoplasm led to the diagnosis of adult Xp11.2 translocation RCC with ASPL-TFE3 fusion.

Positive immunostaining of TFE3 and negative staining of TFEB excluded 6p21 translocation RCC. The results of positive immunostaining of RCCMa and CD10, and negative staining of Cathepsin K, HMB45 or Melan A also led to a diagnosis of ASPL-TFE3 fusion. Most previous cases of Xp11.2 translocation RCC showed positive staining of

RCCMa and CD10. Negative staining of Cathepsin K supported ASPL-TFE3 fusion, while tumors with PRCC-TFE3 fusion mostly display positive staining of Cathepsin K [14]. Melanin may be upregulated in Xp11.2 translocation RCC with PSF-TFE3 and CLTC-TFE3 [7, 15]. Melanosome and Melanin A staining have not been reported in Xp11.2 translocation RCC with ASPL-TFE3 and PRCC-TFE3 fusion.

Our case is the first report of bilateral Xp11.2 translocation RCC. The next step was to consider whether the present tumor was due to metastasis from the previous tumor. Microscopic findings of the previous tumor revealed very large tumor cells, a discohesive area and rhabdoid features meaning more dedifferentiation and aggressiveness compared with the present tumor. These data suggest that these tumors occurred metachronously, and that the present tumor was not due to metastasis of the previous tumor.

We demonstrated the presence of the ASPL-TFE3 fusion gene that is the most common chimeric fusion gene resulting from the chromosome translocation that is characteristic of ASPSCR1. By using RT-PCR we also demonstrated that the tumors were negative for the PRCC-TFE3, PSF-TFE3, CLTC-TFE3 or NonO-TFE3 fusion genes. Analysis of von Hippel Lindau tumor suppressor gene mutation by direct sequencing and multiplex ligation-dependent probe amplification methods also gave a negative result (data not shown) [16]. These data supported the final diagnosis of bilateral Xp11.2 translocation RCC with ASPL-TFE3 fusion.

In conclusion, we present a case that may be diagnosed as bilateral Xp11.2 translocation RCC metachronously occurring. Immunohistochemical, cytogenetic and molecular findings allows the differential diagnosis of kidney neoplasms such as Xp11.2 translocation RCC.

Abbreviations
AMACAR: Alpha-Methylacyl-CoA Race; ASPSCR1: Alveolar soft part sarcoma critical region 1; CA9: Carbonic Anhydrase IX; CD: Cluster differentiation; CLTC: Clathrin heavy chain; CT: Computed tomography; FISH: Fluorescence in situ hybridization; GAPDH: Glyceraldehyde-3-phosphate dehydrogenase; MRI: Magnetic resonance imaging; PRCC: Papillary renal cell carcinoma; PSF: PTB-associated splicing factor; RCC: Renal cell carcinoma; RCCMa: Renal cell carcinoma maker; RT-PCR: Reverse transcription-polymerase chain reaction; TFE3: Transcription factor E3; TFEB: Transcription factor EB

Acknowledgements
None.

Funding
There are no funding sources for this study.

Authors' contributions
TK drafted the report, contributed to the concept, and cared for the patient. TK, HS, SF, MC, and IY cared for the patient. NK and MH generated the histopathological and cytogenetic results. CK generated the molecular results. TS and KI contributed to the concept and design, and approved the final version of the manuscript. All authors read and approved the final manuscript.

Competing interests
The authors declare that they have no competing interests.

Author details
[1]Department of Urology, Kochi University, Kochi Medical School, Kohasu, Oko, Nankoku, Kochi 783-8505, Japan. [2]Department of Diagnostic Pathology, Kochi Red Cross Hospital, Kochi-Shi, Kochi 780-0062, Japan. [3]Department of Urology, Izumino Hospital, Kochi-Shi, Kochi 781-0011, Japan. [4]Laboratory of Diagnostic Pathology, Kochi Medical School Hospital, Kohasu, Oko, Nankoku, Kochi 783-8505, Japan.

References
1. Macher-Goeppinger S, Roth W, Wagener N, Hohenfellner M, Penzel R, Haferkamp A, Schirmacher P, Aulmann S. Molecular heterogeneity of TFE3 activation in renal cell carcinomas. Mod Pathol. 2012;25:308–15.
2. Zhong M, De Angelo P, Osborne L, Paniz-Mondolfi AE, Geller M, Yang Y, Linehan WM, Merino MJ, Cordon-Cardo C, Cai D. Translocation renal cell carcinomas in adults: a single-institution experience. Am J Surg Pathol. 2012;36:654–62.
3. Argani P, Antonescu CR, Illei PB, Lui MY, Timmons CF, Newbury R, Reuter VE, Garvin AJ, Perez-Atayde AR, Fletcher JA, Beckwith JB, Bridge JA, Ladanyi M. Primary renal neoplasms with the ASPL-TFE3 gene fusion of alveolar soft part sarcoma: a distinctive tumor entity previously included among renal cell carcinomas of children and adolescents. Am J Pathol. 2001;159:179–92.
4. Sidhar S. The t(X;1)(p11.2;q21.2) translocation in papillary renal cell carcinoma fuses a novel gene PRCC to the TFE3 transcription factor gene. Hum Mol Genet. 1996;5:1333–8.
5. Mathur M, Das S, Samuels HH. PSF-TFE3 oncoprotein in papillary renal cell carcinoma inactivates TFE3 and p53 through cytoplasmic sequestration. Oncogene. 2003;22:5031–44.
6. Clark J, Lu YJ, Sidhar SK, Parker C, Gill S, Smedley D, Hamoudi R, Linehan WM, Shipley J, Cooper CS. Fusion of splicing factor genes PSF and NonO (p54nrb) to the TFE3 gene in papillary renal cell carcinoma. Oncogene. 1997;15:2233–9.
7. Argani P, Lui MY, Couturier J, Bouvier R, Fournet J-C, Ladanyi M. A novel CLTC-TFE3 gene fusion in pediatric renal adenocarcinoma with t(X;17)(p11.2; q23). Oncogene. 2003;22:5374–8.
8. Kim SH, Choi Y, Jeong HY, Lee K, Chae JY, Moon KC. Usefulness of a break-apart FISH assay in the diagnosis of Xp11.2 translocation renal cell carcinoma. Virchows Arch. 2011;459:299–306.
9. Rao Q, Williamson SR, Zhang S, Eble JN, Grignon DJ, Wang M, Zhou XJ, Huang W, Tan PH, Maclennan GT, Cheng L. TFE3 break-apart FISH has a higher sensitivity for Xp11.2 translocation-associated renal cell carcinoma compared with TFE3 or cathepsin K immunohistochemical staining alone: expanding the morphologic spectrum. Am J Surg Pathol. 2013;37:804–15.
10. Dijkhuizen T, van den Berg E, Wilbrink M, Weterman M, Geurts van Kessel A, Störkel S, Folkers RP, Braam A, de Jong B. Distinct Xp11.2 breakpoints in two renal cell carcinomas exhibiting X;autosome translocations. Genes Chromosomes Cancer. 1995;14:43–50.
11. Chan TY. World Health Organization classification of tumours: Pathology and Genetics of Tumours of the Urinary System and Male Genital Organs. Urology. 2005;65:214-5.
12. Argani P, Olgac S, Tickoo SK, Goldfischer M, Moch H, Chan DY, Eble JN, Bonsib SM, Jimeno M, Lloreta J, Billis A, Hicks J, De Marzo AM, Reuter VE, Ladanyi M. Xp11 translocation renal cell carcinoma in adults: expanded clinical, pathologic, and genetic spectrum. Am J Surg Pathol. 2007;31:1149–60.
13. Renshaw AA, Granter SR, Fletcher JA, Kozakewich HP, Corless CL, Perez-Atayde AR. Renal cell carcinomas in children and young adults: increased

incidence of papillary architecture and unique subtypes. Am J Surg Pathol. 1999;23:795–802.

14. Martignoni G, Gobbo S, Camparo P, Brunelli M, Munari E, Segala D, Pea M, Bonetti F, Illei PB, Netto GJ, Ladanyi M, Chilosi M, Argani P. Differential expression of cathepsin K in neoplasms harboring TFE3 gene fusions. Mod Pathol. 2011;24:1313–9.

15. Chang I-W, Huang H-Y, Sung M-T. Melanotic Xp11 translocation renal cancer: a case with PSF-TFE3 gene fusion and up-regulation of melanogenetic transcripts. Am J Surg Pathol. 2009;33:1894–901.

16. Hes FJ, van der Luijt RB, Janssen ALW, Zewald RA, De Jong GJ, Lenders JW, Links TP, Luyten GPM, Sijmons RH, Eussen HJ, Halley DJJ, Lips CJM, Pearson PL, van den Ouweland AMW, Majoor-Krakauer DF. Frequency of Von Hippel-Lindau germline mutations in classic and non-classic Von Hippel-Lindau disease identified by DNA sequencing, southern blot analysis and multiplex ligation-dependent probe amplification. Clin Genet. 2007;72:122–9.

27

Intravenous misplacement of the nephrostomy catheter following percutaneous nephrostolithotomy

Weijin Fu*, Zhanbin Yang, Zhibin Xie and Haibiao Yan

Abstract

Background: Intravenous misplacement of a nephrostomy tube after percutaneous nephrostolithotomy (PCNL) is very rare in clinical experiences. This report summarizes the characteristics and management of intravenous misplacement.

Case presentation: We present two uncommon cases of intravenous nephrostomy catheter misplacement after PCNL from among 4220 patients who underwent PCNL between January 2009 and December 2015. The tip of the tube was located in the inferior vena cava in one case and in the renal vein in the other. We preferably performed open surgery to treat the two patients, mainly to remove the residual calculi and to prepare for any possible adverse event. All patients were successfully managed and discharged uneventfully.

Conclusion: Intravenous nephrostomy tube misplacement is an uncommon PCNL complication. Furthermore, the study illustrates the importance of prompt diagnosis of renal vein perforation and its prompt management using open surgery, similar to conservative therapies.

Background

Percutaneous nephrostolithotomy (PCNL) is a minimally invasive procedure to remove kidney stones more than 2 cm in size. A nephrostomy catheter is routinely retained in the renal pelvis to compress bleeding and drain the fluid and urine from the collecting system after surgery. Although PCNL is generally safe and effective, it is occasionally associated with uncommon complications [1]. Intravenous misplacement of a urological catheter is an uncommon complication associated with PCNL.

Therefore, the mechanism and proper management of the uncommon complication should be investigated. However, few publications have reported intravenous nephrostomy tube misplacement. We researched all articles listed during the last 15 years(between January 2002 and December 2016) in the PubMed database. The search procedure was performed to identify all relevant trials retrieved using the following search terms: "intravenous misplacement or nephrostomy tube misplacement or misplacement", and "percutaneous nephrostolithotomy(PCNL)", and "inferior vena cava or vena cava or renal vein", and "Foley catheter or nephrostomy tube",with the last term being the most important.

We have retrospectively evaluated the clinical data of 4220 patients who underwent PCNL in a single institution between January 2009 and December 2015.Among the patients, 2546 were male (60.3%) and 1674 female (39.7%).Single calculi were treated in 1987 cases, there were 1012 patients of multi calculi, and 1221 patients of upper ureteral calculi. 2490 patients were treated in prone position, 1730 patients in lateral position. 2380 patients underwent by fluoroscopy-guided, 1840 patients by ultrasound-guided. 60 patients(1.4%) converted to open surgery, and 6 patients lost the diseased kidney due to refractory bleeding in the early stage. 100 (2.3%) patients received blood transfusions and 30 (0.7%) patients needed highly selective renal artery embolization.

* Correspondence: fuwj66@aliyun.com
Department of Urology, The First Affiliated Hospital of GuangXi Medical University, 6 Shuangyong Road, Nanning 530021, GuangXi Zhuang Autonomous Region, People's Republic of China

Intravenous nephrostomy tube misplacement after PCNL occurred in 1 of 4220 patients on February,2014 during mature technology phase. Another patient with intravenous misplacement of a nephrostomy tube, who underwent PCNL in another hospital, was transferred to our hospital. We have summarized our experiences with these two uncommon cases.

Case presentation

Case 1

A 68-year-old male patient underwent PCNL for a staghorn calculus in the right kidney. The PCNL was performed in the prone position. The puncture site was localized to the 11th intercostal space between the posterior axillary line and scapular line. Fluoroscopy-guided percutaneous punctures were performed with an 18-gauge needle by retrograde pyelography. A zebra guide wire was inserted into the collecting system. Access to the excretory system was achieved gradually by fascial dilators. Immediately after dilator removal, severe bleeding from the sheath led to a sudden interruption of the procedure; an 18 F nephrostomy catheter was promptly inserted and closed to control the bleeding. The blood loss was estimated 500 ml.The blood pressure had dropped. After blood transfusion, hemodynamics returned to normal.

Enhanced computed tomography scan, performed 2 days after the surgery showed that the nephrostomy catheter had traversed the lower pole of the right kidney directly into the right renal vein (Fig. 1). Exploratory laparotomy was performed under general anesthesia, in the event of massive bleeding, on the 7th postoperative day. During the operation, the appearance of renal vein was normal. No bleeding of kidney or renal vein occurred after removing the nephrostomy catheter. Simultaneously, the staghorn calculus of the right kidney was removed via anatrophic nephrolithotomy, and a double J

stent was indwelled. The patient was discharged uneventfully on the 14th postoperative day.

Case 2

A 28-year-old male patient underwent ultrasound-guided PCNL for left upper ureteral calculi, which was 1.2 cm in size, in another hospital. The procudure was performed in the prone position. Access to the excretory system was achieved by fascial dilators. A zebra guide wire was retained during the procedure. Severe venous bleeding was noted during the dilating process. The procedure was interrupted, and a nephrostomy catheter was inserted and closed to control bleeding. The nephrostomy catheter was reopened on the 7th postoperative day, and severe bleeding was observed through the drainage catheter, which was immediately closed. Subsequently, computed tomographic angiography (CTA) showed that the nephrostomy catheter had transversed the left renal parenchyma, misplaced from the left renal vein, directly into the inferior vena cava (IVC) (Fig. 2).

The patient was urgently transferred to our institution. Before we did the exploration, we consulted with vascular surgery. The vascular surgery team encouraged us to proceed safely, confirming that there would be no bleeding. Simultaneously they advised to begin anticoagulant therapy and monitoring. In the end, the patient was done as planned.

Exploratory laparotomy was performed under general anesthesia on the 14th postoperative day. Although the nephrostomy catheter was removed, a small amount of blood oozed from the rupture of the left kidney, and the patient remained hemodynamically stable. A 2-0 Vicryl suture was used to stitch up the ruptured left renal parenchyma. Simultaneously, the left upper ureteral calculus was removed by ureterolithotomy. A 4-0 Vicryl suture was used to interrupted suture the ureteral incision and a

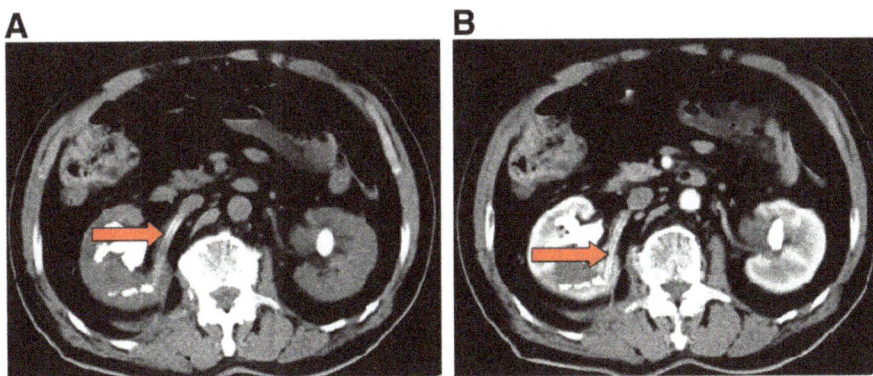

Fig. 1 CT revealed the nephrostomy tube piercing into the right renal vein. **a** Plain of CT demonstrated nephrostomy catheter (*red arrow*) had traversed the lower pole of right kidney directly into the *right* renal vein. **b** Enhanced CT scan revealed that nephrostomy catheter (*red arrow*) had transversed *left* renal vein

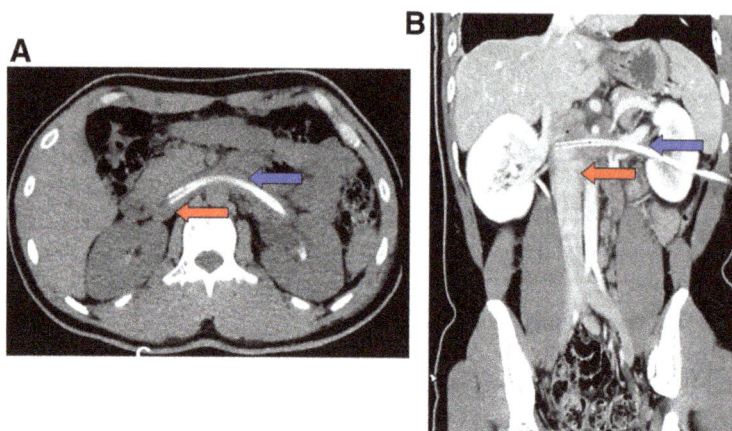

Fig. 2 CT revealed the nephrostomy tube piercing into IVC. **a** Plain of CT scan revealed that nephrostomy catheter (*blue arrow*) had transversed *left* renal vein directly into IVC (*red arrow*). **b** Enhanced CT scan demonstrated that nephrostomy catheter (*blue arrow*) had transversed *left* renal vein directly into IVC (*red arrow*)

double J stent was indwelled. The patient was discharged uneventfully on the 21st postoperative day.

Discussion

Although PCNL is an established procedure, it has been associated with some complications, including hemorrhage, sepsis, kidney or adjacent organ (such as, the liver, spleen, and bowel) injury, access lost, excretory system perforation, and so on. Hemorrhage is the most significant PCNL complication. Venous bleeding during percutaneous procedures is mild and it ceases spontaneously or detains the nephrostomy catheter into the renal pelvis [2]. Severe bleeding complications of PCNL are mainly associated with arterial injuries [3].

Placing the nephrostomy catheter into the collecting system is an effective method for compressing venous bleeding. The catheter can occasionally pierce the renal parenchyma and migrate into the renal vein and even

the IVC. Several publications have presented the rare complications with nephrostomy catheter misplacement into the vessel after PCNL [3–9] in the PubMed database. The data from these publications are summarized in Table 1.Similar to the reports of other centers, the incidence of intravenous nephrostomy tube misplacement after PCNL was 0.23% (1/4220) at our institutions.

The rare complications have been attributed to the following causes. First, the dilator sheath has likely penetrated the renal parenchyma and directly injured the renal vein. Subsequently, perforation into the renal vein by the zebra guide wire, with dilatation of the injured vein, resulted in the nephrostomy catheter migrating to the venous system. Second, the rupture in a large renal vein branch caused by the instruments used during intervention was the most likely cause of the observed bleeding. To control bleeding, the nephrostomy catheter was inadvertently inserted into the venous system, even the IVC. The two cases contributed to the former.

Table 1 Reports of intravenous misplacement of a nephrostomy tube

Author	No./sex/age	Side	Catheter	Catheter withdrawl	Operation type	Location	Subsequent treatment
Dias Filho, et al.	1/F/63	L	Foley catheter	1-step under fluoroscopy	Catheter placement	Renal vein, IVC	Second PCNL
Shaw G, et al.	2/M54	R	Nephrostomy tube	2-step under fluoroscopy	PCNL	Renal vein	Exploratory
Mazzucchi E, et al.	3/M/52	L	Nephrostomy tube	1-step under fluoroscopy	PCNL	Renal vein	No
Mazzucchi E, et al.	4/F/35	L	Nephrostomy tube	2-step under fluoroscopy	PCNL	Renal vein, IVC	No
Li, et al.	5/F/32	L	Nephrostomy tube	2-step under fluoroscopy	PCNL	Renal vein, IVC	No
CJ,Wang, et al.	6/F/66	L	Nephrostomy tube	1-step under fluoroscopy	PCNL	Renal vein	No
Kotb, et al.	7/M/50	L	Foley catheter	1-step open pyelotomy	Catheter placement	Renal vein, IVC	Open pyelotomy
XF Chen, et al.	8/M/42	L	Nephrostomy tube	2-step under CT guide	PCNL	Renal vein, IVC	Second PCNL
XF Chen, et al.	9/F/38	L	Nephrostomy tube	2-step under fluoroscopy	PCNL	Renal vein, IVC	Simultanuous PCNL
XF Chen, et al.	10/M/48	L	Nephrostomy tube	1-step under ultrasound	PCNL	Renal vein	Second PCNL

PCNL percutaneous nephrostolithotomy, *M* male, *F* female, *L* left, *R* right, *IVC* inferior vena cava

Based on previous articles, hemorrhage control could be achieved with a nephrostomy catheter, despite perforation into the major renal vein. The tract was allowed to heal with the catheter being withdrawn in stages, under fluoroscopic guidance. Similar to the other reported cases, Xiao-Feng Chen and colleagues [8] reported three cases of intravenous misplacement after PCNL. The tip of the tube was located in the IVC in two cases, and in the renal vein in one case. All cases were successfully managed with one-step (one case) or two-step (two cases) tube withdrawal, while under close monitoring.

Unlike conservative therapies, we had preferably performed open surgery under general anesthesia in two patients, mainly to remove the right renal calculi in one case and the left ureteral calculi in the other, and to be prepared for any possible adverse events. If the two patients had no residual stone, the misplaced nephrostomy tube can be successfully removed through strict bed rest, intravenous antibiotics, and under close monitoring.

Conclusions
Intravenous misplacement of a nephrostomy tube is an uncommon complication after PCNL. Although PCNL and nephrostomy catheter exchange are relatively simple procedures, they should be cautiously performed preferably under ultrasound or fluoroscopic guidance. Combined with literature, most patients may be managed conservatively with strict bed rest, intravenous antibiotics, and tube withdrawal by CT or fluoroscopy guide. Open surgery can be used as an alternative treatment.

Abbreviations
CT: Computed tomography; CTA: Computed tomographic angiography; IVC: Inferior vena cava; PCNL: Percutaneous nephrostolithotomy.

Acknowledgements
We also thank the two patients for giving us the permission to use the medical information for this publication.

Funding
This work was partially supported by Natural Science Foundation of GuangXi (No. 2015GXNSFAA139180). The funding had some roles in the manuscript writing.

Authors' contributions
WJF drafted the manuscript and was responsible for critical revision of the manuscript. HBY and ZBY performed the operation. ZBX was responsible for the conception and design of this study, interpretation of the data. All authors read and approved the final manuscript.

Competing interests
The authors declare that they have no competing interests.

References
1. Seitz C, Desai M, Hacker A, Hakenberg OW, Liatsikos E, Nagele U, et al. Incidence, prevention, and management of complications following percutaneous nephrolitholapaxy. Eur Urol. 2012;61:146–58.
2. Srivastava A, Singh KJ, Suri A, Dubey D, Kumar A, Kapoor R, et al. Vascular complications after percutaneous nephrolithotomy: are there any predictive factors? Urology. 2005;66:38–40.
3. Wang C, Chen S, Tang F, Shen B. Metachronous renal vein and artery injure after percutaneous nephrostolithotomy. BMC Urol. 2013;13:69.
4. Shaw G, Wah TM, Kellett MJ, Choong SK. Management of renal-vein perforation during a challenging percutaneous nephrolithotomy. J Endourol. 2005;19:722–3.
5. Mazzucchi E, Mitre A, Brito A, Arap M, Murta C, Srougi M. Intravenous misplacement of the nephrostomy catheter following percutaneous nephrostolithotomy: two case reports. Clinics (Sao Paulo). 2009;64:69–70.
6. Li D, Xiao L, Tang Z, Qi L, Luo K, Huang L, et al. Management of intravenous migration of urologic catheter. Urology. 2012;82:248–52.
7. Ahmed Fouad Kotb AE, Mohamed KR, Atta MA. Percutaneous silicon catheter insertion into the inferior vena cava, following percutaneous nephrostomy exchange. Can Urol Assoc J. 2013;7:e505–7.
8. Chen XF, Chen SQ, Xu LY, Gong Y, Chen ZF, Zheng SB. Intravenous misplacement of nephrostomy tube following percutaneous nephrolithotomy: three new cases and review of seven cases in the literature. Int Braz J Urol. 2014;40:690–6.
9. Dias-Filho ACCG, Borges W. Right atrial migration of nephrostomy catheter. Int Braz J Urol. 2005;31(5):470–1.

28

A Korean multi-center, real-world, retrospective study of first-line pazopanib in unselected patients with metastatic renal clear-cell carcinoma

Moon Jin Kim[4], Se Hoon Park[1*], Jae-Lyun Lee[2], Se-Hoon Lee[3], Su Jin Lee[1] and Ho Yeong Lim[1]

Abstract

Background: The efficacy and/or tolerability of pazopanib in patients with metastatic renal cell carcinoma (mRCC) have been found to differ in Western and Asian populations. This retrospective multicenter study analyzed the results of first-line pazopanib treatment in 93 consecutive patients with mRCC who were treated at the medical oncology departments of three tertiary cancer centers in Seoul, Korea.

Methods: The decision to administer pazopanib as first-line therapy was at the discretion of the treating physician in all patients with mRCC. Patients enrolled in clinical trials were excluded to ensure that the results would reflect real-world outcomes representative of daily clinical settings. All patients received 800 mg/day pazopanib. Outcomes included response rate, progression-free survival (PFS), overall survival (OS), and safety.

Results: The 93 patients included72 (77 %) male and 21 (23 %) female individuals, of median age 65 years (range, 19–84 years). The median number of metastatic sites per patient was two (range, 1–5), with the lungs being the most frequently involved site. Most patients had favorable ($n = 46$) or intermediate ($n = 36$) risk as determined by Memorial Sloan Kettering Cancer Center criteria. Pazopanib was generally welltolerated: the major hematologic adverse effect was grade 1/2 anemia (14 %); and the most frequently observed non-hematologic toxicity was grade 1/2 mucositis (22 %), followed by hair discoloration and hypertension. Of the 93 patients, three (3 %) showed complete response, 52 (56 %) showed partial response, and 21 (23 %) showed stable disease, making the objective response rate 59 % and the disease control rate 82 %. At a median follow-up of 21 months, the estimated median PFS and OS were 12.2 months (95 % confidence interval, 7.1–17.4 months) and 21.9 months (95 % confidence interval, 12.9–30.9 months), respectively.

Conclusions: In this retrospective study, first-line therapy with pazopanib demonstrated clinically relevant efficacy and tolerability in unselected real-world Korean patients with mRCC. OS and PFS of these Korean patients were similar to those reported in phase III trials.

Keywords: Clear-cell carcinoma, Renal cell carcinoma, Pazopanib, First-line

* Correspondence: hematoma@skku.edu
[1]Division of Hematology–Oncology, Department of Medicine, Samsung Medical Center, Sungkyunkwan University School of Medicine, Seoul, Korea
Full list of author information is available at the end of the article

Background

Renal cell carcinoma (RCC) is the most common type of kidney cancer [1], with clear cell carcinoma being the most common subtype. Because approximately 30 % of patients present with primary metastatic disease and one-third of patients have recurrent metastatic disease after nephrectomy with curative intent [2], over 50 % of all patients with RCC require systemic therapy during the course of their disease. RCC has been found refractory to conventional systemic chemotherapeutic agents and radiotherapy. Clear cell RCC represents a unique clinical setting for the application of antiangiogenic therapy, in that targeting of angiogenesis through pathways involving vascular endothelial growth factor receptor (VEGFR) and mammalian target of rapamycin has produced robust clinical effects and revolutionized the treatment of metastatic RCC [3]. Multi-targeted tyrosine kinase inhibitors (TKIs) against VEGFR, including sunitinib [4], sorafenib [5], and pazopanib [6], have improved progression-free survival (PFS) and/or overall survival (OS) when compared with interferon and/or supportive care in patients with metastatic RCC.

Current guidelines recommend the use of sunitinib, pazopanib, or bevacizumab plus interferon as first-line treatment for favorable- or intermediate-risk patients with metastatic, clear cell RCC [7]. Because of their oral route of administration and more favorable toxicity profiles, sunitinib and pazopanib are the most widely administered TKIs in this setting. The choice of a first-line regimen is important, because not all patients are eligible for salvage therapy, providing an obvious rationale for administering the most effective initial treatment. For example, in the large phase IIICOMPARZ (COMParing the efficacy, safety and tole Rability of paZopanib versus sunitinib) trial [8], 1,110 patients with metastatic RCC were randomly assigned to receive either sunitinib or pazopanib. Baseline patient and disease characteristics were well balanced between the two arms. Based on independent review by blinded radiologists, median PFS was 8.4 months in the pazopanib group versus 9.5 months in the sunitinib group, with the hazard ratio (HR) of 1.05 (95 % confidence interval [CI] 0.90–1.22) being within the acceptable boundaries of non-inferiority. Although pazopanib and sunitinib showed similar efficacy, safety and quality-of-life (QOL) profiles favored pazopanib. These findings were confirmed in the subsequent randomized, double-blind, crossover PISCES (PazopanIb versus Sunitinib patient preference Study) study, which compared QOL and patient preference in patients treated with pazopanib or sunitinib [9].

Based on these results, pazopanib has become one of the most frequently used VEGFR TKIs for metastatic RCC in Korea. However, the choice of a first-line TKI for an individual patient can be a clinical dilemma.

Factors that must be considered include the experiences of the treating oncologists, the activities of the TKIs, and the potential toxicities of these agents, especially for patients with symptoms or decreased performance status. Moreover, the efficacy and/or tolerability of pazopanib has been found to differ in Western and Asian populations. For example, subset analysis of the COMPARZ trial [10] found that, in Asian patients, median PFS was longer with sunitinib than with pazopanib (11.1 versus 8.4 months, HR 1.07, 95 % CI 0.81–1.42), although the difference was not statistically significant. In addition, Asian and non-Asian RCC patients experienced different adverse events: hematologic toxicities, hypertension, and hand-foot-syndrome were more frequently observed in Asian patients, whereas fatigue and gastrointestinal symptoms were more frequent in non-Asians, regardless of treatment arm. Patients in phase III clinical studies, including COMPARZ, were selected on the basis of a fairly preserved performance status and normal organ function. However, RCC is a highly aggressive disease, which often shows rapid progression and clinical decline; therefore, the clinical trial population may not be representative of all patients seen in real-world daily oncology practice. Based on these considerations, this multi-center retrospective studywas designed to evaluate the efficacy and safety of first-line pazopanib in Korean patients with RCC.

Methods

The medical records of 93 consecutive adults with histologically proven mRCC and predominant clear cell histology who were treated with pazopanib as first-line TKI therapy in 2012 were retrospectively reviewed. The decision to treat with pazopanib was solely at the discretion of the treating oncologist. Patients enrolled in clinical trials were excluded to ensure that the study population reflected daily clinical practice in our institutions. Patients were also excluded if they had: (1) received prior chemotherapy or anti-angiogenic therapy for advanced or metastatic disease, (2) 100% non-clear cell carcinoma,(3) another malignancy within 5 years, and (4) inappropriate laboratory findings or severe comorbid illness during treatment with the standard dose of pazopanib (800 mg/day). This study was approved by the Institutional Review Boards of Samsung Medical Center, Asan Medical Center, and Seoul National University Hospital. Written informed consent was provided by all patients prior to starting pazopanib treatment, according to institutional standards.

All patients were treated with 800 mg/day pazopanib, administered orally without interruption. Supportive care, including the administration of blood products and analgesics, was provided if judged appropriate by the treating physician. Before treatment with pazopanib, patients had a complete history taken and underwent complete blood counts and serum chemistries, chest x-rays, and computed tomography scans of all involved sites. Patients were assessed every 4 weeks because pazopanib therapy was repeated at this interval. Therapy was continued until objective disease progression per Response Criteria in Solid Tumors [11], unacceptable toxicity or deterioration of hepatic function, or patient refusal. Baseline characteristics and outcome data were collected using a uniform case report form. Clinical and laboratory parameters collected at the time of starting pazopanib treatment included, but were not restricted to, those described inthe Memorial Sloan Kettering Cancer Center (MSKCC) [2] and Heng [12] prognostic criteria: age, sex, Eastern Cooperative Oncology Group (ECOG) performance status, the presence of other histologic types than clear cell carcinoma, previous nephrectomy, previous cytokine therapy, neutrophil count, platelet count, hemoglobin, serum lactate dehydrogenase, corrected serum calcium, time between diagnosis and TKI therapy, and sites of metastases. Responses were evaluated every 8 weeks by chest and abdominopelvic computed tomography or by the same tests that were used to stage initial tumors. Adverse events were graded according to the National Cancer Institute criteria (CTCAE v4). Causes of death and discontinuation of therapy were evaluated by a structured review of medical records.

The primary endpoint was PFS, defined as the time between pazopanib initiation and the date of documented disease progression or death, whichever occurred first. Secondary endpoints included OS, response rate, and toxicity profile. OS was defined as the time from the first day of pazopanib administration to death from any cause. PFS and OS were calculated using the Kaplan–Meier method. The impact of baseline parameters on PFS and OS was assessed using a Cox proportional hazards model. Laboratory parameters and age were recorded as continuous variables and were evaluated as both continuous and categorical variables. The potential presence of interaction effects between baseline parameters was tested by defining product terms for the respective factors in a regression model. All P values were two-sided, with $P < 0.05$ indicating statistical significance. All statistical analyses were performed using the SPSS package (version 16.0) and R for Windows v2.11.1 software (R Core Team, Vienna, Austria; http://www.Rproject.org).

Results

Medical records were collected from 93 consecutive patients who were treated with first-line pazopanib at three tertiary Korean cancer centers between January and December 2012. Patient characteristics are given in Table 1.

Table 1 Baseline characteristics

	No. of patients	Percent
Age, years		
Median (range)	65 (19–84)	
Sex		
Male	72	77
Female	21	23
ECOG performance status		
0	4	4
1	78	84
2 or higher	11	12
Comorbid illness		
Any	52	
Diabetes	23	
Hypertension	42	
Obstructive lung disease	11	
Renal insufficiency	3	
Histology		
Clear cell carcinoma (100 %)	87	93
Mixed	6	7
Time from diagnosis to treatment, months		
Median (range)	14 (0–83)	
Prior therapy		
Nephrectomy	74	80
Cytokine immunotherapy	9	10
Radiotherapy	6	7
Laboratory findings (mean, SD)		
Hemoglobin, g/dL	12.6 (2.0)	
Corrected calcium, mg/dL	9.3 (0.7)	
Lactate dehydrogenase, U/L	372 (243)	
Number of metastatic site(s)		
Median (range)	2 (1–5)	
Sites of metastases		
Lung	66	
Lymph nodes	21	
Bone	18	
Liver	11	
Brain	17	
MSKCC risk		
Favorable	46	49
Intermediate	36	39
Poor	11	12
Heng score		
Favorable	40	43
Intermediate	38	40
Poor	15	17

Of the 93 patients, 72 (77 %) were male individuals and 21 (23 %) were female individuals. Nine (10 %) patients had previously been treated with cytokine therapy, the majority with high-dose interleukin-2. Eighty-two (88 %) patients had favorable or intermediate MSKCC risk scores, whereas 11 (12 %) had an ECOG performance status of 2 or higher. Approximately 60 % of the patients had two or more metastatic disease sites, mostly involving the lungs and lymph nodes. At the time of data collection, corresponding to a median follow-up of 21 months, 82 patients (88 %) had discontinued pazopanib treatment and 40 (43 %) had died.

The 93 patients received a total of 1,086 4-week cycles of pazopanib (median 12, range 1–34). In 32 cycles (0.03 %), involving 12 (13 %) of the 93 patients, doses were reduced by 25 %. The reasons for dose reduction were available for 11 patients, the most common being non-hematologic toxicities, including fatigue (4/11, 36 %), gastrointestinal discomfort (3/11, 27 %), and hypertension (2/11, 18 %). In addition, two (18 %) of these 11 patients required dose reductions for hematologic toxicities, both being grade 3 thrombocytopenia. The most common reason for therapy discontinuation was disease progression, Overall, first-line pazopanib was generally well tolerated, with hypertension, anemia, and oral mucositis being the most commonly observed toxicities (Table 2). Twelve (13 %) patients experienced transient and reversible elevation of liver function tests (LFTs); of these, one patient had early liver cirrhosis owing to hepatitis B virus infection and three were heavy consumers of alcohol, whereas the other eight had no underlying hepatic diseases. All 12 patients received ursodeoxycholic acid to normalize LFTs, but none requirement pazopanib dose modification or delay. Abnormal LFTs were all normalized within

3 months. Two patients died of causes for which we could not completely rule out a relationship to pazopanib. One patient died of a pulmonary thromboembolism during the middle of the second cycle of pazopanib treatment, with no clinical evidence of progression. The second patient, who had multiple lung and lymph node metastases, died of interstitial pneumonitis after 12 months of clinical response to pazopanib. Although the size of involved lymph nodes remained unchanged, the possibility of disease progression could not be completely excluded.

Of the 93 patients, two could not be evaluated for response to pazopanib because of the absence of measurable lesions or early discontinuation of therapy. Three (3 %) patients showed a complete response (CR) and 52 (56 %) had a partial response, making the objective response rate 59 % (95 % CI 45–65 %). In addition, 21 (23 %) patients had stable disease, making the disease control rate 82 %. Patients with poor MSKCC risk scores were significantly less likely to respond to pazopanibthan patients with favorable or intermediate risk scores (P = 0.03). Response rate was not significantly influenced by age, sex, number and site of metastases, or baseline laboratory parameters.

The median OS forthe 93 patients analyzed in the study was21.9 months (95 % CI 12.9–30.9 months, Fig. 1) and the median PFS was 12.2 months (95 % CI 7.1–17.4 months, Fig. 2). Median PFS was significantly shorter for patients with poor risk than for patients with favorable or intermediate MSKCC riskscores (2.4 months [95 % CI 2.0–2.8 months] vs. 12.5 months [95 % CI 8.3–16.7 months], $P < 0.0001$). Similarly, median OS was shorter for patientswith poor risk than for patient with favorable or intermediate MSKCC risk scores (7.2 months [95 % CI 1.5–12.9 months] vs. 26.5 months [95 % CI 18.9–34.1 months], $P < 0.001$; Fig. 3). This model suggested that mRCC patients with poor MSKCC risk scores had a 4-fold higher risk of death than

Table 2 Maximum grade toxicity recorded per patient (n = 93)

	Grade 1–2		Grade 3–4	
	N	%	N	%
Anemia	19	20	1	1
Neutropenia	2	2	0	
Thrombocytopenia	12	13	0	
Nausea	3	3	0	
Vomiting	2	2	0	
Anorexia	6	7	0	
Stomatitis	20	22	2	2
Diarrhea	15	16	3	3
Fatigue	9	10	1	1
Skin	11	12	0	
Hepatic	12	13	0	
Hypertension	22	24	0	

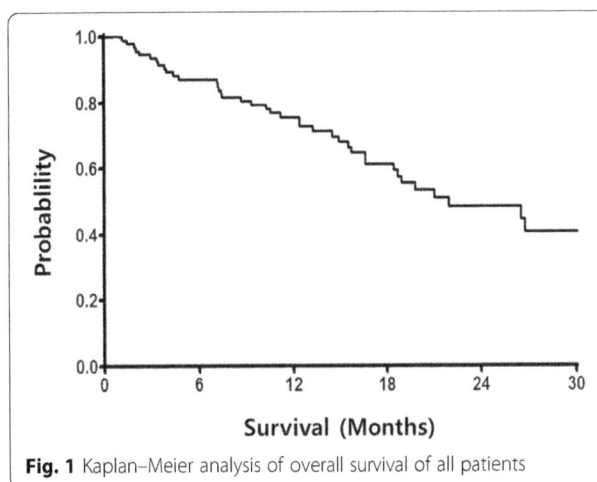

Fig. 1 Kaplan–Meier analysis of overall survival of all patients

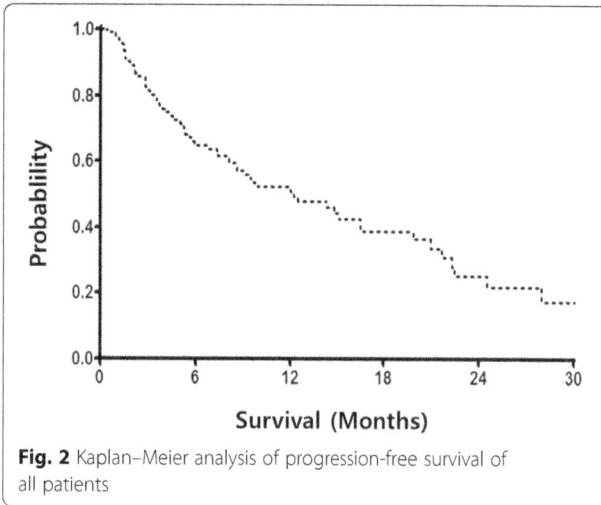

Fig. 2 Kaplan–Meier analysis of progression-free survival of all patients

patients with favorable or intermediate risk scores. We also tested whether OS was altered by interactions with poor MSKCC risk scores and other clinical characteristics by entering the first-level interaction term between these variables into separate multivariate models; however, the results were not significant.

For exploratory purposes, we compared OS according to the clinical response to pazopanib. OS was longer in responders (26.7 months) than in non-responders (18.6 months), although this difference was statistically insignificant ($P = 0.106$).In contrast, OS was significantly longer in patients who did than did not achieve clinical response or stable disease (26.5 months vs. 14.8 months, $P = 0.007$). After the failure of pazopanib treatment, 37 % of the patients received second-line therapy, mostly with everolimus ($n = 30$) or another VEGFR TKI ($n = 4$).

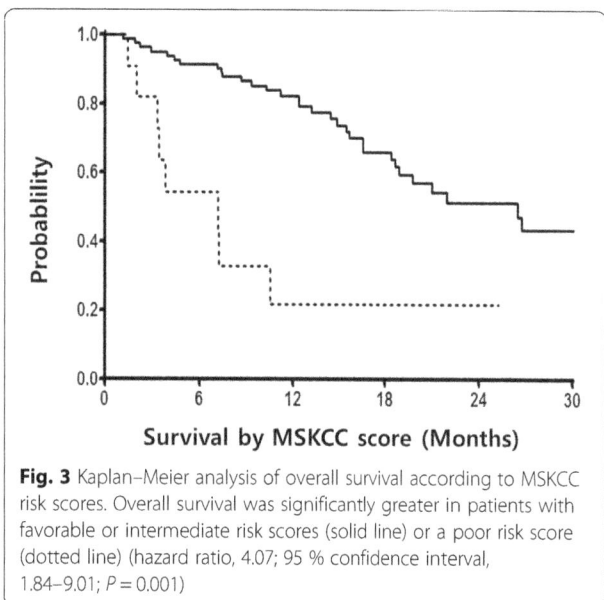

Fig. 3 Kaplan–Meier analysis of overall survival according to MSKCC risk scores. Overall survival was significantly greater in patients with favorable or intermediate risk scores (solid line) or a poor risk score (dotted line) (hazard ratio, 4.07; 95 % confidence interval, 1.84–9.01; $P = 0.001$)

Discussion

This retrospective study on a limited number of Korean RCC patients showed that first-line therapy with pazopanib was both well tolerated and effective, regardless of performance status or the number of metastases. Pazopanib achieved an objective response and stable disease in 59 and 23 % of patients, respectively. The estimated median PFS and OS were 12.2 months (95 % CI, 7.1–17.4 months) and 21.9 months (95 % CI, 12.9–30.9 months), respectively. These results compared favorably with the outcomes of large phase III trials [6, 8]. Although this study was retrospective in nature, its results indicate that Korean patients with metastatic RCC may derive clinically relevant benefits from pazopanib. Most adverse events were transient and self-limiting, and there were few severe non-hematologic toxicities, with grade 3 or 4 stomatitis or diarrhea occurring in only 2–3 % of patients.

VEGFR TKIs have been the mainstay of treatment of patients with clear cell mRCC. Because the main goal of treatment remains palliation, the choice of TKI is based not only on efficacy, but on the consideration of other parameters, include patient preference, relief of symptoms, and/or QOL. The phase III COMPARZ trial, a direct head-to-head comparison between sunitinib and pazopanib indicated that both TKIs are effective and feasible for the first-line treatment of patients with mRCC [8]. Although these two TKIs had similar efficacy, safety and QOL data favored pazopanib. Interestingly, subgroup analysis of patients in the COMPARZ trial showed marked geographic and/or ethnic differences in toxicity profiles and efficacy. In Asian patients, the median PFS was longer with sunitinib (11.1 months) than with pazopanib (8.4 months) [10], although the difference was not statistically significant (HR 1.07, 95 % CI 0.81–1.42). One possible explanation is that the incidence of adverse events differs according to ethnicity. The discontinuation rate owing to adverse events in the COMPARZ trial was 20 % for sunitinib and 24 % for pazopanib. Asian RCC patients experienced hematologic toxicities, hypertension, hand-foot syndrome, liver dysfunction, and proteinuria more frequently than non-Asian patients, whereas fatigue and gastrointestinal symptoms were observed less frequently in Asian patients, regardless of the treatment arm.

In contrast to the COMPARZ subgroup results [10], sunitinib is thought to be less well tolerated by Asian than Western RCC patients, leading to the widespread administration of reduced suboptimal doses of sunitinib to Asian patients [13]. Because of the clear-cut relationship between drug exposure and efficacy [14], maintaining adequate TKI doses is essential to optimize treatment outcomes in Asian RCC patients [15]. These ethnicity-based differences may be owing to chance, to differences in tumor biology between Asian and Western patients, or to a pharmacogenomic difference in drug metabolism leading to differences in drug exposure.

It is difficult to determine whether pazopanib or sunitinib is more effective in Asian patients with mRCC, even when including results from the analysis of Asian subpopulations in a sunitinib expanded access program [16]. Choice of a first-line TKI regimen for individual patients with mRCC requires careful considerations of eachpatient's disease status, symptoms, general condition, and preference. The results of the present study indicate that pazopanib is a reasonable option for Korean mRCC patients and that poor MSKCC risk score is a significant predictor of reduced survival. Studies are underway to identify possible molecular markers, as well as specific genotypic variations in different ethnicities, which may be linked to responsiveness or resistance to VEGFR TKIs.

The strength of the current study includes its multi-center nature and the enrollment of patients who were treated with pazopanib as routine clinical practice to avoid selection bias. The patients included in this study were those treatedat academic tertiary cancer centers, reflecting real-world experience with first-line pazopanib. This population may differ from those in clinical trials and may be more relevant to those seen by the clinicians in daily practice. That is, the results of this study may better reflect real-world outcomes that may not necessarily be seen in randomized controlled trials of selected patients.

This study also had several limitations, including its retrospective nature, which may have introduced selection bias and issues regarding missing data. However, selection bias can be minimized by evaluating a consecutive series of patients, as in the current study. Other limitations include the lack of central radiology review, the use of various imaging modalities, and different intervals between scans; however, these variations better reflect the real-world clinical experience of oncologists who administer targeted therapy. Finally, the lack of a comparative arm precludes our ability to determine whether pazopanib is superior, or at least equivalent, to other agents such as sunitinib.

Conclusions

The results obtained in the present study suggest that pazopanib is active and safe in the first-line treatment of Korean patients with mRCC. Better patient selection may improve clinical outcomes of mRCC patients in a first-line setting. Emerging clinical data and greater knowledge of the disease may further guide the development of individualized treatment regimens for patients with mRCC.

Abbreviations
mRCC, metastatic renal clear-cell carcinoma; OS, overall survival; PFS, progression-free survival; VEGFR, vascular endothelial growth factor receptor

Acknowledgments
The inclusion of co-authors reflects the fact that the work came from active collaboration between researchers and acknowledges input into team-based research.

Authors' contributions
MJK, J-LL, and S-HL analyzed and interpreted the data. MJK participated in revising the manuscript. SHP made substantial contributions to the conception and design of this study and was involved in drafting the manuscript. SJL and HYL participated in the study design and coordination and helped to draft the manuscript. All authors read and approved the final manuscript.

Competing interests
The authors declare that they have no competing interests.

Author details
[1]Division of Hematology–Oncology, Department of Medicine, Samsung Medical Center, Sungkyunkwan University School of Medicine, Seoul, Korea. [2]Department of Oncology, Asan Medical Center, University of Ulsan College of Medicine, Seoul, Korea. [3]Department of Internal Medicine, Seoul National University Hospital, Seoul, Korea. [4]Department of Medicine, Myongji Hospital, Goyang-si, Gyeonggi-do, Korea.

References
1. Siegel R, Ma J, Zou Z, Jemal A. Cancer statistics, 2014. CA Cancer J Clin. 2014;64:9–29.
2. Motzer RJ, Mazumdar M, Bacik J, Berg W, Amsterdam A, Ferrara J. Survival and prognostic stratification of 670 patients with advanced renal cell carcinoma. J Clin Oncol. 1999;17:2530–40.
3. Hutson TE. Targeted therapies for the treatment of metastatic renal cell carcinoma: clinical evidence. Oncologist. 2011;16 Suppl 2:14–22.
4. Motzer RJ, Hutson TE, Tomczak P, Michaelson MD, Bukowski RM, Rixe O, et al. Sunitinib versus interferon alfa in metastatic renal-cell carcinoma. N Engl J Med. 2007;356:115–24.
5. Escudier B, Eisen T, Stadler WM, Szczylik C, Oudard S, Siebels M, et al. TARGET Study Group. Sorafenib in advanced clear-cell renal-cell carcinoma. N Engl J Med. 2007;356:125–34.
6. Sternberg CN, Davis ID, Mardiak J, Szczylik C, Lee E, Wagstaff J, et al. Pazopanib in locally advanced or metastatic renal cell carcinoma: results of a randomized phase III trial. J Clin Oncol. 2010;28:1061–8.
7. Motzer RJ, Jonasch E, Agarwal N, Beard C, Bhayani S, Bolger GB, et al. National Compresive Cancer Networks. Kidney cancer, version 2.2014. J Natl Compr Canc Netw. 2014;12:175–82.
8. Motzer RJ, Hutson TE, Cella D, Reeves J, Hawkins R, Guo J, et al. Pazopanib versus sunitinib in metastatic renal-cell carcinoma. N Engl J Med. 2013;369: 722–31.
9. Escudier B, Porta C, Bono P, Powles T, Eisen T, Sternberg CN, et al. Randomized, controlled, double-blind, cross-over trial assessing treatment preference for pazopanib versus sunitinib in patients with metastatic renal cell carcinoma: PISCES Study. J Clin Oncol. 2014;32:1412–8.
10. Guo J, Jin J, Huang Y, Wang JW, Lim HY, Uemura H, et al. Comparison of PFS and safety for Asian compared to North American and European populations in the phase III trial of pazopanib versus sunitinib in patients with treatment-naive RCC (COMPARZ). J Clin Oncol. 2013;31(Suppl 6): Abstr 366.
11. Therasse P, Arbuck SG, Eisenhauer EA, Wanders J, Kaplan RS, Rubinstein L, et al. New guidelines to evaluate the response to treatment in solid tumors. European Organization for Research and Treatment of Cancer, National Cancer Institute of the United States, National Cancer Institute of Canada. J Natl Cancer Inst. 2000;92:205–16.
12. Heng DY, Xie W, Regan MM, Warren MA, Golshayan AR, Sahi C, et al. Prognostic factors for overall survival in patients with metastatic renal cell carcinoma treated with vascular endothelial growth factor-targeted agents: results from a large, multicenter study. J Clin Oncol. 2009;27:5794–9.

13. Yoo C, Kim JE, Lee JL, Ahn JH, Lee DH, Lee JS, et al. The efficacy and safety of sunitinib in Korean patients with advanced renal cell carcinoma: high incidence of toxicity leads to frequent dose reduction. Jpn J Clin Oncol. 2010;40:980–5.

14. Houk BE, Bello CL, Poland B, Rosen LS, Demetri GD, Motzer RJ. Relationship between exposure to sunitinib and efficacy and tolerability endpoints in patients with cancer: results of a pharmacokinetic/pharmacodynamic meta-analysis. Cancer Chemother Pharmacol. 2010;66: 357–71.

15. Kim HS, Hong MH, Kim K, Shin SJ, Ahn JB, Jeung HC, et al. Sunitinib for Asian patients with advanced renal cell carcinoma: a comparable efficacy with different toxicity profiles. Oncology. 2011;80:395–405.

16. Lee SH, Bang YJ, Mainwaring P, Nq C, Chang JW, Kwong P. Sunitinib in metastatic renal cell carcinoma: an ethnic Asian subpopulation analysis for safety and efficacy. Asia Pac J Clin Oncol. 2014;10:237–45.

29

Renal capsule metastasis from renal pelvic cancer

Yasuyuki Kobayashi[1]* (iD), Hiroki Arai[1], Masahito Honda[1], Takashi Matsumoto[2] and Kyotaro Yoshida[3]

Abstract

Background: Metastatic renal cancers are relatively common. Most are metastases to the renal parenchyma via a hematogenous route and are derived from lung, breast, and gastrointestinal cancer, malignant melanoma, and hematologic malignant cancer. However, little is known about renal capsule metastasis from other cancers.

Case presentation: We report a 71-year-old woman with breast cancer who was treated with endocrine therapy. She presented with gross hematuria and was diagnosed as having right renal pelvic cancer and renal cell cancer. She underwent right laparoscopic radical nephroureterectomy. Pathological findings revealed right pelvic cancer and renal capsule metastasis.

Conclusion: Renal capsule metastasis derived from renal pelvic cancer is very rare. When diagnosing renal capsule cancer, we believe that renal capsule metastasis should also be taken into consideration. Clinical and radiological differential diagnosis of renal capsule metastasis from renal cell cancer and primary renal capsule cancer is difficult. Assessment of the histopathological findings of the surgical specimens seems to be the only realistic approach to achieving the correct diagnosis.

Keywords: Breast cancer, Renal capsule metastasis, Renal cell cancer, Renal pelvic cancer, Urothelial carcinoma

Background

Metastatic renal cancer is relatively common and is mainly derived from lung, breast, and gastrointestinal cancer, malignant melanoma, and hematologic malignant cancer [1–4]. Almost all of the metastases are to the renal parenchyma, and to our best knowledge, there is no case report describing metastasis to the renal capsule. We report a rare case of renal capsule metastasis derived from renal pelvic cancer.

Case presentation

A 71-year-old woman was diagnosed as having breast cancer (left breast, invasive lobular carcinoma, T4cN3cM1, Stage IV) in September 2014 and was treated with endocrine therapy (exemestane 25 mg/day). Gross hematuria was pointed out in January 2015, and hematuria was detected by urinalysis. Her past history included hypertension and diabetes mellitus but no history of smoking. Urinary cytology was Class III (Papanicolaou classification) [5].

Blood tests showed a hemoglobin of 12.0 g/dL, serum creatinine of 0.87 mg/dL, lactate dehydrogenase of 251 U/L, aspartate aminotransferase of 18 U/L, and alanine aminotransferase of 6 U/L. Computed tomography (CT) showed a hypovascular mass 25 mm diameter in the right renal pelvis and a hypervascular mass of 22 mm in diameter in the upper pole of the right kidney. The hypervascular mass showed a contrast effect in the early phase. There were no signs of metastasis in the lung, liver, or abdominal lymph nodes. A retrograde pyelogram showed a filling defect in the right renal pelvis, and catheterized urine cytology was class III (Papanicolaou classification). No obvious findings were observed on radiographic imaging of the ureter.

We diagnosed her as having right renal pelvic cancer (cT3N0M0) and right renal cell cancer (cT1aN0M0). Because her metastatic breast cancer prognosis was expected to be relatively good, she thus underwent right laparoscopic radical nephroureterectomy via a retroperitoneal approach. As described below, we diagnosed right pelvic cancer and renal capsule metastasis.

Macroscopically, the renal pelvic tumor was 4 cm in diameter, yellowish white, and soft. It was located in the right renal pelvis and infiltrated into the parenchyma.

* Correspondence: ya_su_koba@yahoo.co.jp
[1]Departments of Urology, Kinki Central Hospital of Mutual Aid Association of Public Teachers, 3-1 Kurumazuka, Itami, Hyogo 664-8533, Japan
Full list of author information is available at the end of the article

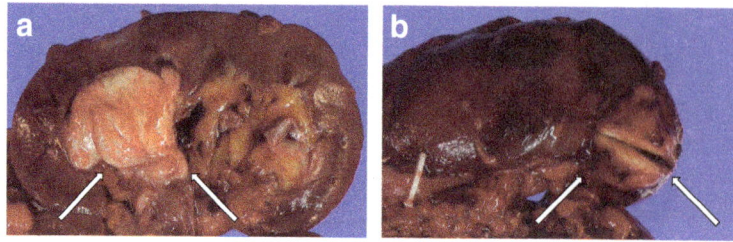

Fig. 1 Gross appearance of the right kidney. **a** Renal pelvic cancer occupying the renal pelvis and invading the renal parenchyma (arrows). **b** The renal capsule cancer coating the renal capsule was easily peeled off from the renal parenchyma (arrows)

The other renal tumor was 2.5 cm in diameter, well-circumscribed, yellowish white, and hard (Fig. 1). It was coated with renal capsular tissue and was easily decapsulated from the renal parenchyma. This tumor was considered to be a renal capsule tumor. The ureteral wall was thickened, but its mucosa was normal.

Microscopically, the renal pelvic tumor invaded the parenchyma but not the capsule beyond the parenchyma. The renal capsule tumor was circumscribed by the renal capsule and did not invade neighboring tissue. Both tumor cells were similar and had eosinophilic cytoplasm, round nuclei, and an alveolar pattern of growth, and they were concordant with urothelial carcinoma. Tumor cells of the ureter had eosinophilic cytoplasm, round nuclei, and a trabecular pattern of growth similar to those of the breast cancer cells.

Immunohistochemically, the cancer cells of the renal pelvis were similar to those of the renal capsule (Fig. 2), whereas the cancer cells of the ureter were similar to those of the breast cancer (Table 1). We concluded that the renal capsule cancer was derived from the renal pelvic cancer, and the ureter cancer was derived from the breast cancer.

We thus diagnosed right pelvic cancer (urothelial carcinoma, G2 > G3, pT3) and renal capsule metastasis. We explained the necessity of adjuvant chemotherapy for the metastatic renal pelvic cancer to the patient, but she rejected chemotherapy and continued only with endocrine therapy. She then developed bilateral pleural effusions, mediastinal lymph node metastasis, para-aortic lymph node metastasis, and liver metastasis. She underwent a thoracentesis in October 2015, and the pleural effusion cytology was class V (Papanicolaou classification), compatible with breast cancer. Endocrine therapy was changed to letrozole 2.5 mg, but she died of breast cancer progression in January 2016.

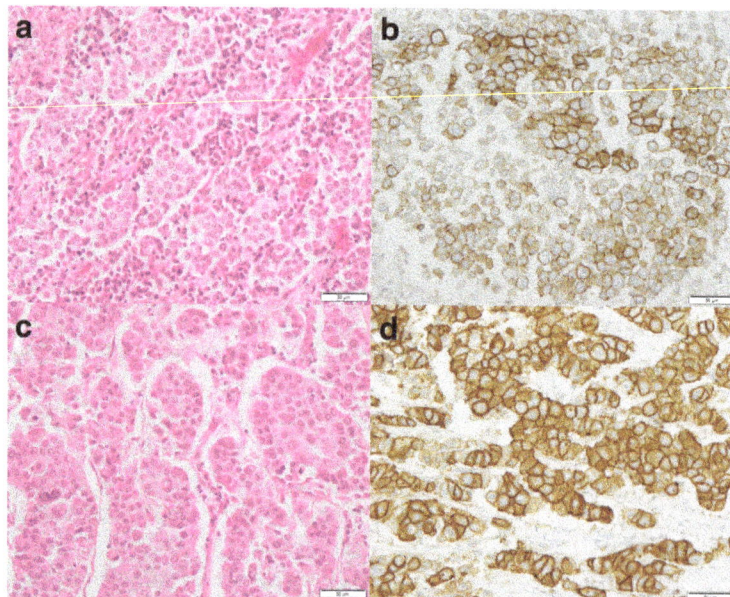

Fig. 2 Histopathologic examination of the renal pelvic cancer and renal capsule cancer. **a** Hematoxylin and eosin (H&E)-stained section of the pelvic cancer. **b** H&E-stained section of the renal capsule cancer. **c** HER2-stained section of the pelvic cancer showing positive staining. **d** HER2-stained section of the renal capsule cancer showing positive staining

Table 1 Immunohistochemical examination

	HER2	ER	CK7
Renal pelvic cancer	+	–	+
Renal capsule cancer	+	–	+
Ureter cancer	–	+	±
Breast cancer	–	+	±

HER human epidermal growth factor receptor 2, *ER* estrogen receptor, *CK* cytokeratin

Discussion

Metastatic renal cancer is relatively common, and autopsy studies indicate that 12% of patients who die of cancer have renal metastasis [2]. Mostly, the metastases are to the renal parenchyma, and few are to the renal capsule. Most renal metastases develop via a hematogenous route and are derived from lung, breast, and gastrointestinal carcinoma, malignant melanoma, and hematologic malignant cancer [1–4]. Renal metastasis is generally accompanied by systemic metastasis, and renal metastatic lesions are often small and multifocal [6].

The renal capsule is a fibrous membrane that surrounds the renal parenchyma and can be separated from the renal parenchyma [7]. Primary renal capsule cancer is relatively rare. It originates from renal capsule structures and is derived from mesenchymal components, and almost all renal capsule cancer is sarcoma such as leiomyosarcoma [8]. Because high-grade renal sarcoma often grows rapidly, it is difficult to distinguish from sarcomatoid RCC in the clinical presentation and radiographic findings. The clinical presentation of renal sarcoma is similar to that of rapidly growing RCC, i.e., a palpable mass, abdominal or flank pain, and hematuria. In patients with renal capsule cancer, renal sarcoma should also be considered [9]. Wide local excision with negative margins is desirable in the case of localized renal sarcoma because the most important prognostic factors for renal sarcoma are margin status and tumor grade [8]. Contrastingly, metastatic renal capsule cancer is very rare and has never been reported in detail.

The *HER2* gene is an oncogene that has a similar structure to the epidermal growth factor receptor gene. Overexpression of HER2 protein occurs in 20% of patients with breast cancer and 13.5% of patients with upper urinary tract urothelial carcinoma [10, 11]. In the present patient, we concluded that the renal capsule metastasis was derived from the HER2-positive renal pelvic cancer, and the ureteral metastasis was derived from the HER2-negative breast cancer.

Ureter metastasis derived from breast cancer was reported in 7.8% of patients with disseminated breast cancer in an autopsy series [12] and can cause ureteral obstruction and renal insufficiency. It occurs in long-standing hormonal-dependent breast cancer with bone metastasis. The prognosis after diagnosis is relatively poor [13]. However, 8 of 15 (53%) patients with ureter metastasis derived from breast cancer did not show any clinical findings of ureteral obstruction [14]. The present patient did not have right hydronephrosis at surgery.

During the preoperative assessment of this patient, we diagnosed her renal capsule cancer as renal cell cancer because it was solitary and showed a contrast effect in the early phase of CT. Based on the pathological findings, we concluded that the renal capsule cancer was derived from the renal pelvic cancer.

Conclusion

Renal capsule metastasis derived from renal pelvic cancer is very rare. When diagnosing renal capsule cancer, we believe that renal capsule metastasis should also be taken into consideration. Clinical and radiological differential diagnosis of renal capsule metastasis from renal cell cancer and primary renal capsule cancer is difficult. For this reason, assessment of the histopathological findings of the surgical specimens seems to be the only realistic approach to achieving the correct diagnosis.

Abbreviation
CT: Computed tomography

Acknowledgments
The authors thank the members of the ethics committee who reviewed the contents of the present study.

Funding
This research did not receive any specific grant from funding agencies in the public, commercial, or not-for-profit sectors.

Authors' contributions
YK drafted the manuscript and was responsible for critical revision of the manuscript. YK, HA, and MH performed the operation. YK and TM made substantial contributions to patient management. TM made substantial contributions to analysis and interpretation of data. YK and KY analyzed the patient data. YK was responsible for the conception and design of this study and interpretation of the data. All authors read and approved the final manuscript.

Competing interests
The authors declare that they have no competing interests.

Author details
[1]Departments of Urology, Kinki Central Hospital of Mutual Aid Association of Public Teachers, 3-1 Kurumazuka, Itami, Hyogo 664-8533, Japan. [2]Surgery, Kinki Central Hospital of Mutual Aid Association of Public Teachers, 3-1 Kurumazuka, Itami, Hyogo 664-8533, Japan. [3]Pathology, Kinki Central Hospital of Mutual Aid Association of Public Teachers, 3-1 Kurumazuka, Itami, Hyogo 664-8533, Japan.

References

1. Choyke PL, White EM, Zeman RK, Jaffe MH, Clark LR. Renal metastases: clinicopathologic and radiologic correlation. Radiology. 1987;162:359–63.
2. Pollack HM, Banner MP, Amendola MA. Other malignant neoplasms of the renal parenchyma. Semin Roentgenol. 1987;22:260–74.
3. Aron M, Nair M, Hemal AK. Renal metastasis from primary hepatocellular carcinoma. A case report and review of the literature. Urol Int. 2004;73:89–91.
4. Stage AC, Pollock RE, Matin SF. Bilateral metastatic renal synovial sarcoma. Urology. 2005;65:389.
5. Papanicolaou GN, Marshall VF. Urine sediment smears as a diagnostic procedure in cancers of the urinary tract. Science. 1945;101:51920.
6. Choyke PL, Glenn GM, Walther MM, Zbar B, Linehan WM. Hereditary renal cancers. Radiology. 2003;226:33–46.
7. Zhu G, Wu D, Wu K, Song W, Yang Z, Zhang Y, et al. The retroperitoneal laparoscopic renal capsulectomy for spontaneous renal subcapsular fluid collection: a case-series report and literature review. Medicine (Baltimore). 2016;95:e3751.
8. Wang X, Xu R, Yan L, Zhuang J, Wei B, Kang D, et al. Adult renal sarcoma: clinical features and survival in a series of patients treated at a high-volume institution. Urology. 2011;77:836–41.
9. Wein AJ, Kavoussi LR, Partin AW, Peters CA. Campbell-Walsh urology. 11th ed. Philadelphia: Elsevier; 2015. p. 1360–4.
10. Yaziji H, Goldstein LC, Barry TS, Werling R, Hwang H, Ellis GK, et al. HER-2 testing in breast cancer using parallel tissue-based methods. JAMA. 2004; 291:1972–7.
11. Sasaki Y, Sasaki T, Kawai T, Morikawa T, Matsusaka K, Kunita A, et al. HER2 protein overexpression and gene amplification in upper urinary tract urothelial carcinoma-an analysis of 171 patients. Int J Clin Exp Pathol. 2014;7:699–708.
12. Abrams HL, Spiro R, Goldstein N. Metastases in carcinoma; analysis of 1000 autopsied cases. Cancer. 1950;3:74–85.
13. Recloux P, Weiser M, Piccart M, Sculier JP. Ureteral obstruction in patients with breast cancer. Cancer. 1988;61:1904–7.
14. Geller SA, Lin C. Ureteral obstruction from metastatic breast carcinoma. Arch Pathol. 1975;99:476–8.

30

Neutrophil-lymphocyte ratio as a predictive biomarker for response to high dose interleukin-2 in patients with renal cell carcinoma

James A. Kuzman[1], David D. Stenehjem[1,2], Joseph Merriman[1], Archana M. Agarwal[3], Shiven B. Patel[1], Andrew W. Hahn[1], Anitha Alex[1], Dan Albertson[1], David M. Gill[1] and Neeraj Agarwal[1*]

Abstract

Background: Immunotherapy with high-dose interleukin-2 (HD-IL2) results in long-term survival in some metastatic renal cell carcinoma (mRCC) patients but has significant acute toxicities. Biomarkers predicting response to therapy are needed to better select patients most likely to benefit. NLR (absolute neutrophil count (ANC)/absolute lymphocyte count (ALC)) is a prognostic and predicative biomarker in various malignancies. The goal was to determine whether NLR can predict response to HD-IL2 in this setting.

Methods: Patients with clear cell mRCC treated with HD-IL2 were identified from an institutional database from 2003–2012. Baseline variables for the assessment of IMDC risk criteria, and neutrophil and lymphocyte count, were collected. Best response criteria were based on RECIST 1.0. Wilcoxon rank-sum test was used to evaluate the association of continuous baseline variables with disease control. NLR was stratified by ≤4 or >4. Progression free survival (PFS) and overall survival (OS) were estimated with the Kaplan-Meier method and Cox proportional hazard models assessed associations of NLR with survival.

Results: In 71 eligible patients, median NLR in those with an objective response ($n = 14$, 20%) was 2.3 vs 3.4 in those without ($n = 57$, 80%, $p = 0.02$). NLR ≤4 was associated with improved progression free and overall survival. After adjustment for IMDC risk criteria, NLR remained a significant predictor of OS (ANC/ALC ≤4 vs >4, HR 0.41, 95% CI 1.09-5.46, $p = 0.03$; ANC/ALC continuous variable per unit change in NLR, HR 1.08, 95% CI 1.01-1.14, $p = 0.03$).

Conclusions: In this discovery set, NLR predicts overall survival in patients treated with HD-IL2 in mRCC, and may allow better patient selection in this setting. Data needs validation in an independent cohort.

Keywords: Renal cell carcinoma, Neutrophil lymphocyte ratio, High dose interleukin-2

Background

The landscape of metastatic renal cell carcinoma (mRCC) has significantly improved in the last decade as the biology is better understood and novel treatments are developed. Targeting various signal transduction molecules has been shown to be effective in improving progression free and overall survival. Despite these developments, the prognosis remains relatively poor, and most die of their disease within a few years of onset of metastatic disease. High dose interleukin-2 (HD-IL2) is an approved therapy for select patients with mRCC. It was one of the first immunotherapy agents used that resulted in a durable response in a small population of patients. However, the therapy is associated with many acute and rare chronic toxicities and requires experienced management of these acute toxicities in a critical care setting. Clearly a subset of patients derives benefit

* Correspondence: neeraj.agarwal@hci.utah.edu
[1]University of Utah Huntsman Cancer Institute, Salt Lake City, UT, USA
Full list of author information is available at the end of the article

from HD-IL2, but at the current time there are no predicative markers to help identify these patients.

Prognostic models have been used for about a decade to help stratify patients with mRCC into different risk categories [1, 2]. However, currently there is not a single biomarker, which is used in the clinic to predict response to therapy in patients with mRCC. Current prognostic models include interval from diagnosis to treatment, Karnofsky performance status, serum LDH, corrected serum calcium, and serum hemoglobin. Later absolute neutrophil count greater than upper limit of normal was found to be an independent adverse prognostic factor [2]. Recently addition of NLR has been proposed to be used to help risk stratify patients with metastatic prostate cancer [3].

Neutrophil-lymphocyte ratio has been shown to be a prognostic marker for a wide variety of malignancies including renal cell carcinoma. It was also previously shown that increase in absolute lymphocyte number correlated with objective response in patients undergoing therapy with interleukin-2. Given that NLR is a crude measure of immune function it may be useful in predicting response with immune related treatments such as checkpoint inhibition or HD-IL2.

This study investigates the role of using NLR as a predicative marker of response to HD-IL2 in patients with mRCC. We hypothesized that lower NLR would be associated with better OR, PFS, and OS in patients treated with HD-IL2.

Methods
Study cohort
All sequential patients with clear cell mRCC treated with HD-IL2 at the University of Utah Huntsman Cancer Institute from 2003–2013 were identified. Any patient with clear cell mRCC with good performance status, and intact organ function was offered treatment with HDIL-2, regardless of the prognostic risk category. These are also the selection criteria currently recommended by the National Comprehensive Cancer Network (NCCN) guidelines for treatment with HDIL-2 [4]. Patients were excluded if date of last follow-up or death was not available or date of HD-IL2 administration was not recorded. Patient age, gender, Karnofsky performance status, and absolute neutrophil and lymphocyte values were collected prior to HD-IL2 therapy. Clear cell histology was confirmed by pathology reports and number and sites of metastasis prior to HD-IL2 was recorded. Demographics, as well as clinical and laboratory were collected. The Institutional Review Board of the University of Utah approved the study design, and informed consent was obtained from all patients.

HD-IL2 treatment protocol
One course of HD-IL2 consisted of two cycles – cycle administered over 5–6 days, followed by one week off,

followed by cycle two over 5–6 days. HD-IL2 dosing comprised the standard regimen of 600,000 IU/kg IV every 8 h for a total of 14 planned doses per cycle. Restaging scans were done approximately 8 weeks after the first course. Thereafter, restaging scans were done every 12 weeks.

HD-IL2 response criteria
Best response criteria were based on RECIST 1.0. A PR was defined as a >30% decrease in target lesion size. Progressive disease was a >20% increase in target lesion size or new lesion. CR indicated no imaging evidence of disease. Patients not meeting criteria for PR or progressive disease (PD) were considered to have stable disease (SD). Patients without appropriate follow-up between radiographic imaging and treatment, who were lost to follow-up or died before determining response were classified as not evaluable (NE) and grouped with PD for statistical analysis.

NLR ratio
The absolute neutrophil and lymphocyte values immediately prior to initiating HD-IL2 and within 30 days were used to calculate the NLR ratio. The 75% quartile of NLR values was used to stratify outcomes. The NLR was also assessed as a continuous variable.

Objective
The primary objective was progression free survival (PFS) and overall survival (OS) stratified by NLR patients with mRCC treated with HD-IL2.

Statistical analysis
Descriptive statistics were used to summarize patient and treatment characteristics. Kaplan-Meier method with log-rank tests were used to assess PFS and OS by HD-IL2 response. PFS was defined as the time from first HD-IL2 initiation to disease progression, death, or last follow-up. OS was defined as the time from first HD-IL2 administration to death or last follow-up. In the PFS analysis, censoring occurred at the time of treatment discontinuation if treatment was discontinued for any other reason than progression or death. In both the PFS and OS analysis, censoring occurred at the time of last follow-up in those who had not progressed or were still alive at the end of the designated study period. Cox proportional-hazards models were created with IMDC prognostic risk criteria, gender, and NLR ratio both as a continuous variable and with a cut off of at the 75% quartile for PFS and OS. Significance was set at less than 0.05 for the analysis.

Results
In 71 eligible patients ANC and ALC values were obtained and 53 (75%) of the patients were male with a

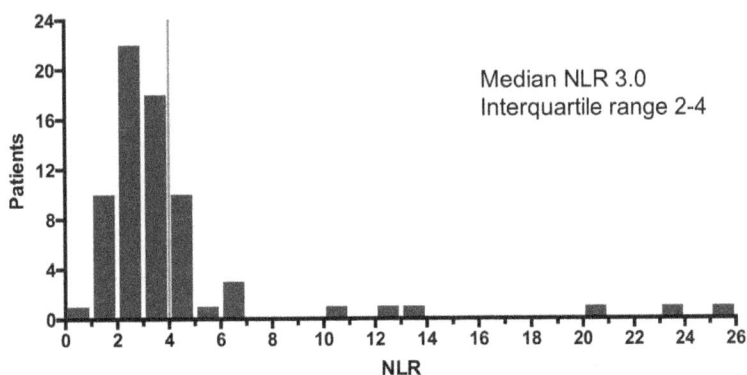

Fig. 1 Histogram of the NLR at initiation of HD-IL2

median age at diagnosis of metastatic disease of 55 years. IMDC criteria was favorable for 9 (13%), intermediate for 49 (69%), and poor for 13 (18%) patients (Table 1). The median NLR was three and the 75% quartile was 4 (Fig. 1). There was a trend for better objective response rate in patients with NLR < 4 though this was not significant (24% vs 10%, p = 0.32). There was also a trend for higher complete response rate in patients with NLR <4 vs ≥4 with CR rates of 18% vs 0% (p = 0.086), respectively (Tables 1 and 2). NLR ≤4 (versus NLR >4) was associated with significant improvement in both progression free and overall

survival (Figs. 2a and 1b). Median PFS was improved by 4.7 months (8.0 vs. 3.3, p = 0.024), and median OS was improved by 28.4 months (40.9 vs 12.5, p = 0.0003). The role of NLR to predict survival outcomes after adjustment for IMDC risk criteria was also investigated. NLR was significant predictor of PFS in univariate analysis and OS by univariate and OS for multivariate analysis after correction for IMDC criteria and sex (Table 3).

Discussion

This study shows that NLR could be used to help predict response to HD-IL2. HD-IL2 is a very effective treatment for a small population of patients with mRCC. Given its several acute but rare chronic toxicities, a predictive biomarker in this setting is expected to optimize selection of patients, who are most likely to derive benefit from therapy. Low NLR has been associated with a better prognosis for many different types of malignancies. This is the first report to suggest that low NLR may be "predictive" of improved survival outcomes to HD-IL2 in the setting of mRCC.

It is clear that inflammation and immune response play a pivotal role in neoplastic progression [5]. Indeed novel treatment strategies targeting the immune system, such as immune check point inhibitors, have been shown to

Table 1 Demographics and disease characteristics between NLR ≤4 vs NLR >

	NLR ≤ 4 n = 51	NLR > 4 n = 20	P-value
Age			
Years of age, median (IQR)	55 (49–58)	55 (49–59)	0.9[a]
Sex			
Males, n (%)	42 (82%)	11 (55%)	*0.021*[b]
Prior Therapy, n (%)			
Nephrectomy	51 (100%)	20 (100%)	-
Previous systemic treatment	7 (14%)	6 (30%)	0.12[b]
Number of metastatic disease sites, n (%)			
1	11 (22%)	6 (30%)	0.40[c]
2	15 (29%)	2 (40%)	
3	12 (24%)	5 (25%)	
≥ 4	13 (26%)	7 (35%)	
IMDC risk factors, n (%)			
Favorable	7 (14%)	2 (10%)	*0.013*[c]
Intermediate	39 (76%)	10 (50%)	
Poor	5 (10%)	8 (40%)	

[a]Wilcoxon Rank Sum
[b]Chi-Square
[c]Fisher's Exact
Italicized values are less than 0.05

Table 2 Best Reponses to HD-IL2 between NLR ≤4 vs NLR >4

	NLR ≤ 4 n = 51	NLR > 4 n = 20	P-value
Best response			
CR	9 (18%)	0 (0%)	0.086[a]
PR	3 (6%)	2 (10%)	
SD	18 (35%)	5 (25%)	
PD/NE	21 (41%)	13 (65%)	
Objective response	12 (24%)	2 (10%)	0.32[a]
Clinical benefit	30 (59%)	7 (35%)	0.11[b]

[a]Fisher's Exact
[b]Chi-Square

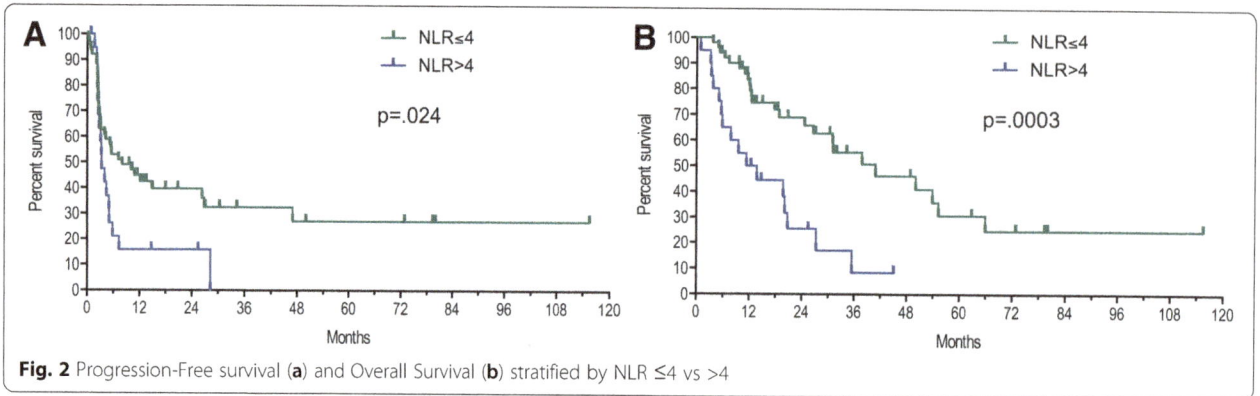

Fig. 2 Progression-Free survival (**a**) and Overall Survival (**b**) stratified by NLR ≤4 vs >4

improve outcomes and are approved for multiple malignancies. One of simplest estimations of the balance of inflammation and immune response is neutrophil/lymphocyte ratio [6, 7].

NLR has been reported to be a predictive and prognostic factor for localized renal cell carcinoma [8, 9]. In a large meta-analysis of 15 cohorts including 3357 patients, NLR predicted poorer OS (hazard ratio = 1.82, 95% CI 1.51-2.19) [10]. Additionally, high preoperative NLR was associated with larger tumor size, higher nuclear grade, histologic tumor necrosis, and sarcomatoid differentiation [8]. Recently, on treatment neutropenia was shown to be an independent biomarker of favorable outcome in mRCC, independent of treatment type [11]. NLR was also recently shown to predict response to ipilimimab in melanoma patients. In a recent report, lower NLR ratio predicted improved overall survival in patients with metastatic melanoma [12].

Unlike recently developed immunotherapeutic agents, the mechanism of action of HD-IL2 is not fully understood. Interleukin-2 is a recombinant protein that has a wide range of effects on the immune system, including promoting proliferation and differentiation of CD4(+) T cell into specific effector T cell subsets, of CD8(+) T cells into effector T cells, and in to memory cells, but also expansion of immunosuppressive CD4(+)FOXP3 T regulatory cells in certain situations [13].

Historically, HD-IL2 therapy has generally been shown to have an objective response rate of approximately 10-20%, including complete responses in ~10% of patients. More recently, in a large cohort of patients with mRCC ($n = 391$) treated with HDIL-2, a clinical benefit with HD-IL2 was seen in ~50% of patients. In addition to ~20% patients who experienced objective responses (CR in 9% and PR in 10%), an additional 32% experienced SD as the best response to treatment. The survival outcomes were

Table 3 Univariate and Multivariate analysis results for PFS and OS

Variable	Univariate		Multivariate Model 1		Multivariate Model 2	
	PFS HR (95% CI), P-value	OS HR (95% CI), P-value	PFS HR (95% CI), P-value	OS HR (95% CI), P-value	PFS HR (95% CI), P-value	OS HR (95% CI), P-value
Sex						
Male vs Female	0.49 (0.27-0.93), p = .031	0.35 (0.17-0.71), p = .005	0.64 (0.33-1.28), p = .20	0.67 (1.09-5.46), p = .33	0.56 (0.30-1.08), p = .08	0.45 (0.22-0.93), p = .03
IMDC Criteria						
Favorable	ref	ref	ref	ref	ref	ref
Intermediate	2.20 (0.93-6.50), p = .08	4.13 (1.23-25.62), p = .02	2.02 (0.83-6.06), p = .13	4.02 (1.16-25.33), p = .03	1.91 (0.78-5.73), p = .17	3.42 (1.00-21.48), p = 0.05
Poor	4.46 (1.56-14.65), p = .005	10.43 (2.65-69.34), p = .0004	3.38 (1.12-11.55), p = .03	7.00 (1.68-47.83), p = .006	3.23 (1.03-11.30), p = .04	5.41 (1.20-38.24), p = .03
NLR						
≤ 4 vs >4	0.51 (0.28-0.95), p = .034	0.31 (0.16-0.61), p = .001	0.68 (0.35-1.39), p = .28	0.41 (1.09-5.46), p = .03	NA	NA
Continuous (per unit change in NLR	1.05 (0.99-1.10), p = .08	1.10 (1.04-1.15), p = .002	NA	NA	1.03 (0.97-1.09), p = .30	1.08 (1.01-1.14), p = .03

CI, 95% confidence interval

HR hazard ratio, NA not applicable, NLR neutrophil to lymphocyte ratio, OS overall survival, PFS progression-free survival

Italicized p-values are less than 0.05

similar in those experiencing PR and SD, and were significantly superior to those who did not experience objective responses or SD [14]. Although the use of HDIL-2 declined after the approval of targeted therapies starting in 2005, in the recent years with the resurgence of cancer immunotherapy in general, the use of HDIL-2 has stabilized and may have picked up [15]. Identification of predictive biomarkers in this setting is expected to further allow more patients to experience benefits of HDIL-2 while limiting toxicities and cost in others. No other therapy in the mRCC setting has been shown to be associated with durable long-term response, albeit in a small proportion of patients, in a consistently reproducible fashion. Absolute number of peripheral blood lymphocytes have been correlated with objective response in patients treated with IL-2, interferon alpha, and histamine. There was no difference in baseline levels of lymphocytes of responding versus non-responding patients [16]. This further supports that NLR probably acts as a better marker to predict response in patients with mRCC treated with HD-IL2.

One of the main limitations of this study is the retrospective nature of the study and the relatively small sample size.

Conclusion
In conclusion, these hypotheses generating data provides initial evidence that low NLR may predict improved survival outcomes in mRCC, and help better selection of patients for HD-IL2 therapy. Low NLR was associated with significantly improved PFS and OS with a trend for improved objective responses with HD-IL2. Data need further validation in a larger and an independent cohort.

Abbreviations
ALC: Absolute lymphocyte count; ANC: Absolute neutrophil count; CI: Confidence interval; HD-IL2: High-dose interleukin-2; HR: Hazard ratio; mRCC: Metastatic renal cell carcinoma; NE: No effect; NLR: Neutrophil to lymphocyte ratio; OS: Overall survival; PD: Progressive disease; PFS: Progression free survival; SD: Stable disease

Acknowledgements
No further individuals contributed to this manuscript.

Funding
This study was supported in whole or in part by funding from the Cancer Clinical Investigator Team Leadership Award awarded by the National Cancer Institute through a supplement to P30CA042014.

Authors' contribution
JAK and DDS contributed equally to the preparation of this manuscript. JAK, DDS, and NA developed the hypothesis behind this research. JM, SBP, NA, and AWH compiled the database used for this research. DDS performed all statistical analyses. JAK, DMG, DDS, and NA wrote the original manuscript. AMA performed pathology over reads. JAK, DDS, AMA, AWH, AA, DA, DMG, and NA made revisions to the final manuscript. All authors read and approved the final manuscript.

Competing interests
The authors declare that they have no competing interests.

Author details
[1]University of Utah Huntsman Cancer Institute, Salt Lake City, UT, USA. [2]Department of Pharmacotherapy, College of Pharmacy, University of Utah, Salt Lake City, UT, USA. [3]Department of Pathology and ARUP Laboratories, University of Utah, Salt Lake City, UT, USA.

References
1. Heng DY, Xie W, Regan MM, et al. Prognostic factors for overall survival in patients with metastatic renal cell carcinoma treated with vascular endothelial growth factor–targeted agents: results from a large, multicenter study. J Clin Oncol. 2009;27:5794–9.
2. Mekhail TM, Abou-Jawde RM, BouMerhi G, et al. Validation and extension of the Memorial Sloan-Kettering prognostic factors model for survival in patients with previously untreated metastatic renal cell carcinoma. J Clin Oncol. 2005;23:832–41.
3. Templeton AJ, Pezaro C, Omlin A, et al. Simple prognostic score for metastatic castration-resistant prostate cancer with incorporation of neutrophil-to-lymphocyte ratio. Cancer. 2014;120:3346–52.
4. Motzer RJ, Jonasch E, Agarwal N, et al. Kidney cancer, version 3.2015. J Natl Compr Canc Netw. 2015;13:151–9.
5. Hanahan D, Weinberg RA. Hallmarks of cancer: the next generation. Cell. 2011;144:646–74.
6. Guthrie GJ, Charles KA, Roxburgh CS, et al. The systemic inflammation-based neutrophil–lymphocyte ratio: experience in patients with cancer. Crit Rev Oncol Hematol. 2013;88:218–30.
7. Zahorec R. Ratio of neutrophil to lymphocyte counts–rapid and simple parameter of systemic inflammation and stress in critically ill. Bratisl Lek Listy. 2000;102:5–14.
8. Viers BR, Boorjian SA, Frank I, et al. Pretreatment neutrophil-to-lymphocyte ratio is associated with advanced pathologic tumor stage and increased cancer-specific mortality among patients with urothelial carcinoma of the bladder undergoing radical cystectomy. Eur Urol. 2014;66:1157–64.
9. de Martino M, Pantuck AJ, Hofbauer S, et al. Prognostic impact of preoperative neutrophil-to-lymphocyte ratio in localized nonclear cell renal cell carcinoma. J Urol. 2013;190:1999–2004.
10. Hu K, Lou L, Ye J, et al. Prognostic role of the neutrophil–lymphocyte ratio in renal cell carcinoma: a meta-analysis. BMJ Open. 2015;5:e006404.
11. Soerensen AV, Geertsen PF, Christensen IJ, et al. A five-factor biomarker profile obtained week 4–12 of treatment for improved prognostication in metastatic renal cell carcinoma: Results from DARENCA study 2. Acta Oncologica. 2016;55(3):341–8.
12. Ferrucci P, Gandini S, Battaglia A, et al. Baseline neutrophil-to-lymphocyte ratio is associated with outcome of ipilimumab-treated metastatic melanoma patients. Br J Cancer. 2015;112:1904–10.
13. Boyman O, Sprent J. The role of interleukin-2 during homeostasis and activation of the immune system. Nat Rev Immunol. 2012;12:180–90.
14. Stenehjem DD, Toole M, Merriman J, et al. Extension of overall survival beyond objective responses in patients with metastatic renal cell carcinoma treated with high-dose interleukin-2. Cancer Immunol Immunother. 2016;65:941–9.
15. Allard CB, Gelpi-Hammerschmidt F, Harshman LC, et al. Contemporary trends in high-dose interleukin-2 use for metastatic renal cell carcinoma in the United States. Urol Oncol. 2015;33:496.e11–6.
16. Donskov F, Bennedsgaard K, von der Maase H, et al. Intratumoural and peripheral blood lymphocyte subsets in patients with metastatic renal cell carcinoma undergoing interleukin-2 based immunotherapy: association to objective response and survival. Br J Cancer. 2002;87:194–201.

31

Spontaneous regression of adrenal metastasis from renal cell carcinoma after sunitinib withdrawal

Ti-Yuan Yang[1,2], Wun-Rong Lin[1,2]* and Allen W. Chiu[1,2,3]

Abstract

Background: The spontaneous regression of metastatic renal cell carcinoma is a rare phenomenon, with an estimated incidence of < 1%. We report a case of post-nephrectomy renal cell carcinoma adrenal metastasis, followed by the spontaneous regression of the metastasis after withdrawal of sunitinib.

Case presentation: The patient was a 55-year-old male with clear cell type renal cell carcinoma who previously underwent a left laparoscopic radical nephrectomy. After 51 months of follow up, a recurrence in the left renal fossa was observed and subsequently excised. Four months after excision, an abdominal Computerized tomography (CT) identified an adrenal metastasis of 1.6 cm. The patient was treated with sunitinib. However, the treatment was discontinued because of gastrointestinal side effects and fatigue. Eleven months after the discontinuation of sunitinib treatment, a progression in the adrenal metastasis growth (5.7 cm) was observed, whereas 16 months after the discontinuation, a regression of the adrenal metastasis growth (3.4 cm) was observed. During subsequent follow-ups, a gradual reduction in the size of the adrenal metastasis (1.8 cm) was observed. After 44 months from the discontinuation of sunitinib treatment, the patient was still alive and followed up in the outpatient department.

Conclusions: Sunitinib is a multi-targeted inhibitor of vascular endothelial growth factor (VEGF) receptors. This compound reduces tumor angiogenesis and has been approved worldwide for the treatment of advanced renal cell carcinoma. To our knowledge, this is the fourth case of the spontaneous regression of metastatic renal cell carcinoma after the discontinuation of sunitinib treatment.

Background

Approximately 21% of patients with renal cell carcinoma present with a metastatic disease at diagnosis, and 23% of patients who undergo radical nephrectomy for clinically localized disease develop metastasis/local recurrence during a 5-year follow-up [1]. The spontaneous regression of metastatic renal cell carcinoma is a rare but well-known phenomenon, with an estimated incidence of < 1% [2]. Several case reports have described the spontaneous regression of metastatic renal cell carcinoma. Such an occurrence has been associated with multiple different events that might influence the immune system, including primary tumor surgical debulking, radiation or embolization of the primary tumor, palliative hormonal treatment with tamoxifen, surgical abortion, and discontinuation of sunitinib treatment [3–6]. However, the exact mechanism remains unclear. We report a case of a post-nephrectomy adrenal metastasis of a renal cell carcinoma followed by the spontaneous regression of the metastasis after a short-term sunitinib treatment. To our knowledge, this is the fourth case of the spontaneous regression of metastatic renal cell carcinoma after withdrawal of sunitinib.

Case presentation

A 55-year-old man presented with chronic testicular pain. An ultrasonography of the abdomen detected left renal tumor. The patient had a history of hypertension and left renal urolithiasis. CT showed a heterogeneous

* Correspondence: vincent751051@gmail.com
[1]Department of Urology, Mackay Memorial Hospital, Taipei, Taiwan
[2]Department of Medicine, Mackay Medical College, Taipei, Taiwan
Full list of author information is available at the end of the article

left upper pole renal tumor (5.3 cm in diameter). A laparoscopic radical nephrectomy was performed in May 2008. Left adrenalectomy and lymph node dissection were not performed because the CT scan showed no adrenal gland invasion or lymphadenopathy. The histological evaluation of the tissue revealed a clear cell renal cell carcinoma and negative surgical margins (pathological stage, T2N0M0). Three years after nephrectomy, following a cerebrovascular accident, the Eastern Cooperative Oncology Group score changed from 0 to 2. No tumor recurrence (CT scan was performed every 6 months) was found until 51 months later. A CT scan detected two nodules in the renal fossa (1.8 and 0.9 cm, respectively). Retroperitoneal exploration confirmed recurrent clear cell carcinoma with microscopically positive surgical margins. Lymph node dissection was not performed because of severe adhesion around the aorta. Lymph nodes that could be detected by palpation were not identified during the surgery. Four months after excision, an abdominal CT showed a nodule (1.6 cm) over the right adrenal gland. At that time, tumor target therapy was not covered by the national health insurance in Taiwan. Therefore, because of economic reasons, the patient could not afford the treatment until 2013. A repeat CT evaluation confirmed the disease progression of the adrenal metastasis (2.1 cm). The patient was treated with sunitinib (37.5 mg/d) for 4 weeks, but the treatment was discontinued because of gastrointestinal side effects and fatigue. After 3 months, a CT scan showed the progression of the adrenal metastasis (3.8 cm) and no lower lung lesion. A chest X-ray revealed the absence of lung metastasis. The patient refused to undergo hormonal survey, biopsy, and adrenalectomy. Eleven months after sunitinib treatment, a CT scan showed an obvious growth of the adrenal metastasis (5.7 cm) (Fig. 1a), whereas 16 months after the treatment, a regression of the metastasis (3.4 cm) was observed (Fig. 1b). Twenty-two months after sunitinib treatment, a CT scan demonstrated a gradual reduction in the size of the adrenal metastasis (1.8 cm) (Fig. 1c). The patient was still alive and followed up at the outpatient department 44 months after the discontinuation of sunitinib treatment.

Discussion and conclusions

The spontaneous regression of cancer is defined as the partial or complete disappearance of a tumor without any treatment or with a treatment considered inadequate to exert a significant influence on the progression of cancer [7]. The spontaneous regression of metastatic renal cell carcinoma following nephrectomy was first described by Bumpus in 1928 [8]. It is a rare phenomenon, which is estimated to represent < 1% of renal cell carcinoma cases [9]. The regression of metastatic sites has been reported to occur at the lungs and at other visceral

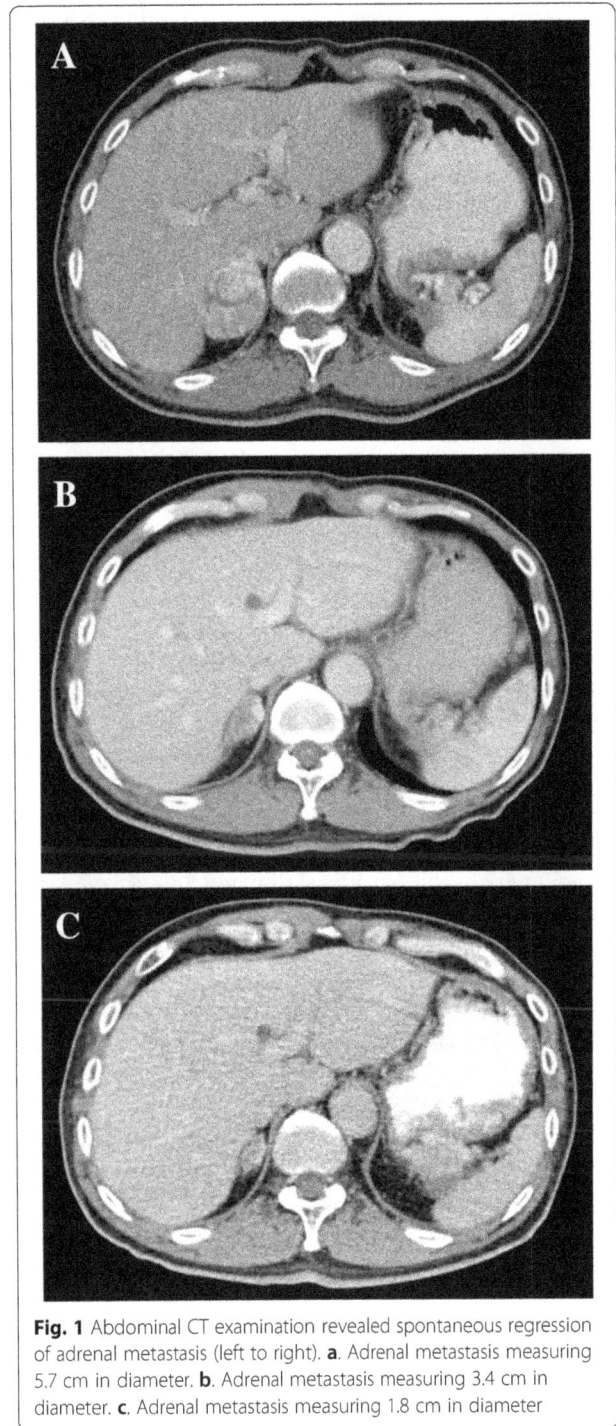

Fig. 1 Abdominal CT examination revealed spontaneous regression of adrenal metastasis (left to right). **a**. Adrenal metastasis measuring 5.7 cm in diameter. **b**. Adrenal metastasis measuring 3.4 cm in diameter. **c**. Adrenal metastasis measuring 1.8 cm in diameter

organs including liver, bones, brain, choroid, pancreas, and adrenal glands [10]. The mechanism of the spontaneous regression of renal cell carcinoma remains unclear. Humoral, immunological, and vascular factors, such as autoinfraction, have been previously proposed to be possible pathophysiologic mechanisms [11]. Nephrectomy is not necessary and accounts for < 50% of the documented cases [12]. Because the oncologic benefits of lymph node dissection in the management of renal cell carcinoma remain controversial [13], we routinely performed nephrectomy and renal fossa recurrent tumor resection without lymph node dissection.

Sunitinib is a multi-targeted inhibitor of vascular endothelial growth factor (VEGF) receptors. The mechanism of action includes the reduction of tumor angiogenesis, which makes it an approved treatment for advanced renal cell carcinoma worldwide [14]. It has been shown that response rates are comparable among groups treated with 50 mg/d of sunitinib for 4 weeks followed by 2 weeks off treatment or with 37.5 mg/d of sunitinib on a continuous daily dosing treatment [15]. A study performed on 1059 patients treated with sunitinib for metastatic renal cell carcinoma has shown that 398 (38%) patients had an objective response and 12 (1.1%) had a complete response. The median time to tumor response was 10.6 weeks [16]. Our report describes the case of a patient who experienced metastasis progression after discontinuation of sunitinib treatment because of adverse effects on day 28 and spontaneous regression 16 months later. To our knowledge, there are only three other reports that have described a similar phenomenon. Rothermundt et al. reported a 63-year-old female patient who had a right renal tumor with the invasion of the right renal vein and the vena cava, bilateral adrenal metastasis, multiple lung metastases, and bone metastasis [17]. The patient was treated with 50 mg of sunitinib 4 weeks on and 2 weeks of. A decrease in the size of all involved tumor sites was observed at the beginning of treatment. After 10 months, because an obvious disease was detected on CT, sunitinib treatment was discontinued. A CT scan performed for trial purposes after 1 month revealed disease regression in all tumor locations. Yanagihara et al. were the second to report a case of the regression of metastatic renal cancer after the discontinuation of sunitinib treatment [18]. The authors reported the case of a 61-year-old female patient with a left renal tumor along with multiple bone and liver metastases. Left radical nephrectomy revealed disease progression in each metastatic site. The patient was treated with sunitinib, but the treatment was discontinued on day 11 because of thrombocytopenia and digestive symptoms. Disease regression was

detected after 18 months. Teo et al. reported the case of a 65-year-old male patient [6] with lung metastasis, which was detected by CT scan 7 years after a right radical nephrectomy was performed for right renal cell carcinoma. Sunitinib was started for the metastasis. A partial response was achieved 9 months after starting the treatment; however, the treatment was discontinued because of disease progression after 6 months, which was followed by the regression of lung metastasis. The patient remains clinically well with a follow up of 44 months since the discontinuation of sunitinib treatment. A summary of the published cases of the discontinuation of sunitinib treatment is listed in Table 1. Data from three published cases and those from our patient showed that the interval of sunitinib treatment varied from 11 days to 15 months. The interval between spontaneous regression and the last sunitinib dose varied from 1 to 18 months. Two cases discontinued sunitinib treatment because of disease progression and two discontinued it because of the side effects of the drug.

The mechanisms of spontaneous regression after an incomplete use of the multiple kinase inhibitor sunitinib remain unclear. Rothermundt et al. drew an analogy with the antiandrogen withdrawal syndrome of prostate cancer. Gene mutations of the androgen receptor might be a possible mechanism of antiandrogen withdrawal syndrome, which cause the antiandrogens to act as partial agonists. A withdrawal of these antiandrogens can promote disease regression [19].

Another possible mechanism is the immunomodulatory effect of sunitinib. Sunitinib improved the type-1 T-cell cytokine response in patients with metastatic renal cell carcinoma while reducing the T-regulatory cell function [20]. Furthermore, sunitinib has been shown to inhibit the proliferation and function of human peripheral T cells and to prevent T-cell-mediated immune response in mice [21]. In the present report, sunitinib treatment, or its discontinuation, might have modified the immune response.

The phenomenon of spontaneous regression after the discontinuation of sunitinib treatment may be masked by further treatment. The disease regression might have been missed or attributed to other second line therapies if our patient had not refused the suggestion of a right

Table 1 Summary of published sunitinib withdrawal phenomenon cases

Ref, year	Age/sex	Location	Dose and length of sunitinib treatment	Reason for discontinuing sunitinib treatment	Interval between spontaneous regression and sunitinib
Rothermundt, 2009 [17]	63/F	bilateral adrenal glands, lung and bone	sunitinib 50 mg 4 weeks on and 2 weeks off, 10 months	disease progression	1 month
Yanagihara, 2011 [18]	61/F	bone and liver	sunitinib 50 mg per day, 11 days	thrombocytopenia and digestive symptoms	18 months
Teo, 2013 [6]	65/M	lung	50 mg/d, 4 weeks on and 2 weeks off for 6 months and 37.5 mg per day for 9 months	disease progression	No mention

adrenalectomy. Thus, the number of patients with spontaneous regression associated with the discontinuation of sunitinib treatment may be underestimated, and this case report is a reminder of that for urologists.

Because recurrence has been reported after spontaneous regression [5], we will closely follow up our patient.

Acknowledgements
The authors are grateful to the operating room staff and ward staff of Mackay Memorial Hospital who participated in the management of this patient.

Funding
There are no sources of funding to be declared for this study.

Authors' contributions
WRL did the clinical evaluation of the patient, came to a diagnosis and operated on the patient. TYY and AWC participated literature review and wrote the manuscript. All authors read and approved the final manuscript to be published. All authors agreed to be accountable for all aspects of the work.

Competing interests
The authors declare that they have no competing interests.

Author details
1Department of Urology, Mackay Memorial Hospital, Taipei, Taiwan.
2Department of Medicine, Mackay Medical College, Taipei, Taiwan. 3School of Medicine, National Yang-Ming University, Taipei, Taiwan.

References
1. Dabestani S, Thorstenson A, Lindblad P, Harmenberg U, Ljungberg B, Lundstam S. Renal cell carcinoma recurrences and metastases in primary non-metastatic patients: a population-based study. World J Urol. 2016;34(8): 1081–6.
2. Nakajima T, Suzuki M, Ando S, Iida T, Araki A, Fujisawa T, Kimura H. Spontaneous regression of bone metastasis from renal cell carcinoma; a case report. BMC Cancer. 2006;6:11.
3. Lekanidi K, Vlachou PA, Morgan B, Vasanthan S. Spontaneous regression of metastatic renal cell carcinoma: case report. J Med Case Rep. 2007;1:89.
4. Mangel L, Bíró K, Battyáni I, Göcze P, Tornóczky T, Kálmán E. A case study on the potential angiogenic effect of human chorionic gonadotropin hormone in rapid progression and spontaneous regression of metastatic renal cell carcinoma during pregnancy and after surgical abortion. BMC Cancer. 2015; 15:1013.
5. de Riese W, Goldenberg K, Allhoff E, Stief C, Schlick R, Liedke S, Jonas U. Metastatic renal cell carcinoma (RCC): spontaneous regression, long-term survival and late recurrence. Int Urol Nephrol. 1991;23(1):13–25.
6. Teo M, Downey FP, McDermott RS. Beyond the maths of biology: long-term spontaneous tumoral regression after sunitinib withdrawal. Clin Genitourin Cancer. 2013;11(2):198–200.
7. Cole WH, Everson TC. Spontaneous regression of cancer: preliminary report. Ann Surg. 1956;144(3):366–83.
8. Bumpus HCJ. The apparent disappearance of pulmonary metastasis in a case of hypernephroma following nephrectomy. J Urol. 1928;20:185.
9. Kim H, Park BK, Kim CK. Spontaneous regression of pulmonary and adrenal metastases following percutaneous radiofrequency ablation of a recurrent renal cell carcinoma. Korean J Radiol. 2008;9(5):470–2.
10. Janiszewska AD, Poletajew S, Wasiutynski A. Spontaneous regression of renal cell carcinoma. Contemp Oncol (Pozn). 2013;17(2):123–7.
11. Kobayashi K, Sato T, Sunaoshi K, Takahashi A, Tamakawa M. Spontaneous regression of primary renal cell carcinoma with inferior vena caval tumor thrombus. J Urol. 2002;167(1):242–3.
12. Lokich J. Spontaneous regression of metastatic renal cancer. Case report and literature review. Am J Clin Oncol. 1997;20(4):416–8.
13. Gershman B, Thompson RH, Boorjian SA, Larcher A, Capitanio U, Montorsi F, Carenzi C, Bertini R, Briganti A, Lohse CM, et al. Radical nephrectomy with or without lymph node dissection for high-risk non-metastatic renal cell carcinoma: a multi-institutional analysis. J Urol. 2017;199:1143–8.
14. Motzer RJ, Hutson TE, Tomczak P, Michaelson MD, Bukowski RM, Rixe O, Oudard S, Negrier S, Szczylik C, Kim ST, et al. Sunitinib versus interferon alfa in metastatic renal-cell carcinoma. N Engl J Med. 2007;356(2):115–24.
15. Motzer RJ, Hutson TE, Olsen MR, Hudes GR, Burke JM, Edenfield WJ, Wilding G, Agarwal N, Thompson JA, Cella D, et al. Randomized phase II trial of sunitinib on an intermittent versus continuous dosing schedule as first-line therapy for advanced renal cell carcinoma. J Clin Oncol. 2012;30(12):1371–7.
16. Molina AM, Lin X, Korytowsky B, Matczak E, Lechuga MJ, Wiltshire R, Motzer RJ. Sunitinib objective response in metastatic renal cell carcinoma: analysis of 1059 patients treated on clinical trials. Eur J Cancer. 2014;50(2):351–8.
17. Rothermundt CA, Omlin A, Gillessen S. Sunitinib withdrawal phenomenon' or spontaneous regression in renal cell cancer. Ann Oncol. 2009;20(6):1144–6.
18. Yanagihara Y, Tanji N, Nishida T. Spontaneous regression of metastatic renal cancer after short-term treatment with sunitinib. Int J Urol. 2011;18(3):258–9.
19. Miyamoto H, Rahman MM, Chang C. Molecular basis for the antiandrogen withdrawal syndrome. J Cell Biochem. 2004;91(1):3–12.
20. Finke JH, Rini B, Ireland J, Rayman P, Richmond A, Golshayan A, Wood L, Elson P, Garcia J, Dreicer R, et al. Sunitinib reverses type-1 immune suppression and decreases T-regulatory cells in renal cell carcinoma patients. Clin Cancer Res. 2008;14(20):6674–82.
21. Gu Y, Zhao W, Meng F, Qu B, Zhu X, Sun Y, Shu Y, Xu Q. Sunitinib impairs the proliferation and function of human peripheral T cell and prevents T-cell-mediated immune response in mice. Clin Immunol. 2010;135(1):55–62.

32

SDH-deficient renal cell carcinoma –clinical, pathologic and genetic correlates

Ravi Kumar[1*] ⓘ, Michael Bonert[2], Asghar Naqvi[2], Kevin Zbuk[3] and Anil Kapoor[4]

Abstract

Background: Succinate dehydrogenase (SDH)- deficient renal cell carcinoma (RCC) is a newly identified rare subtype of RCC, having only gained acceptance from the World Health Organization in 2016. To the best of our knowledge, there are only 55 reported cases worldwide. Here, we report a new case of SDH-deficient RCC.

Case presentation: A 49-year-old male patient was incidentally found to have a large right renal mass. He had no personal or family history of paragangliomas (PGL), pheochromocytomas (PC), or gastrointestinal stromal tumors (GIST). The neoplasm was unilateral and unifocal. He underwent an open partial nephrectomy. Detailed pathological analysis was conducted to confirm the diagnosis. Genetic testing revealed a pathogenic mutation in the *SDHB* gene. He has been followed for 24 months now and has remained well without any evidence of local or distant recurrence. In this report we describe our experience with this diagnosis and review the relevant clinical, pathological, and genetic features.

Conclusions: Without the identification of SDHB deficiency, this patient's personal and familial predisposition to PC, PGL, GIST and metachronous RCCs may have gone undetected despite his RCC diagnosis. When faced with an eosinophilic RCC, pathologists should routinely search for vacuoles or flocculent cytoplasmic inclusions. When these are present, or in cases of difficult eosinophilic renal tumors, staining for SDHB is recommended. For tumours without adverse pathologic features (i.e. high nuclear grade, coagulative necrosis, or sarcomatoid differentiation) excision alone may be a reasonable option, with the addition of regular surveillance for PC and PGLs in those found to harbor germline SDH mutations.

Keywords: Succinate dehydrogenase-deficient renal cell carcinoma, Kidney cancer

Background

Succinate dehydrogenase (SDH)- deficient renal cell carcinoma (RCC) was first identified in 2004 [1]. In 2013, it was integrated into the International Society of Urological Pathology (ISUP) Vancouver classification and in 2016 it was accepted by the WHO organization as a unique subtype of RCC [2].

Succinate dehydrogenase is an enzyme complex consisting of four subunits (SDHA, SDHB, SDHC, and SDHD) that is required for energy metabolism in cells. The majority of patients with SDH-deficient RCC have germline mutations in SDH, with the most commonly mutated gene being *SDHB*, followed by *SDHC, SDHD,* and *SDHA* respectively [3, 4]. Since its first description there have been two cohort studies that have helped identify further clinical and pathological features of this tumour [3, 5]. SDH-deficient RCC is estimated to make up between 0.05 to 0.2% of all renal carcinomas. In patients with a SDHB mutation, the lifetime risk of developing a renal tumour has been estimated at 14% [6]. Patients have developed renal tumours as early as 14 years old, with the mean age estimated around 37 years [3]. SDH-deficient RCC affects both genders, with a slight male predominance. Patients harbouring such mutations are also predisposed to the development of paragangliomas, pheochromocytomas, and gastrointestinal stromal tumors [3, 5]. Given the nascency of SDH-deficient RCC, there are currently no diagnostic or therapeutic guidelines in place to guide management.

* Correspondence: rkuma015@uottawa.ca
[1]Division of Urology, Department of Surgery, The Ottawa Hospital, University of Ottawa, Ottawa, Canada
Full list of author information is available at the end of the article

Here, we report our experience with a new case of SDH-deficient RCC and review the current literature for this rare RCC variant.

Case

A 49-year-old male presented to the urology clinic after incidental detection of a renal mass. He was asymptomatic, without any hematuria, flank pain, constitutional symptoms, or prior urological history. His past medical history was remarkable for morbid obesity, hypertension, atrial fibrillation, asthma, osteoarthritis, and gastro-esophageal reflux disease. His only prior surgery was a pannulectomy. He reported no relevant family history. Physical examination was unremarkable, except for an obese abdomen and a large ventral hernia. Patient weighed 400 lbs., having previously weighed 500 lbs. His bloodwork showed a hemoglobin of 131 g/L, creatinine of 96 umol/L, and eGFR of 80 ml/min/1.73m^2.

A CT scan of the abdomen was done as part of a workup for abdominal pain. This revealed a large exophytic heterogeneous mass measuring $9.1 \times 9.1 \times 10.5$ cm in the lower pole of the left kidney (Fig. 1). There was no lymphadenopathy, regional invasion, or distant metastases seen. Bilaterally there were renal cysts without hydronephrosis or hydroureter. A pre-operative CT scan of the chest and bone scan were both negative for metastatic disease. A renogram showed that the large left renal mass was poorly functioning and that there was significant tubular dysfunction affecting both kidneys symmetrically. The function was estimated as 43% on the left and 57% on the right. Review of CT with urology and radiology was suggestive of T2A, N0, M0 renal cell carcinoma. Because of the high likelihood of RCC diagnosis, pre-operative biopsy was offered to the patient, but felt to be unnecessary.

Four months after presentation, he underwent an uncomplicated open left partial nephrectomy. He recovered expectantly post-operatively. The tumor was confined to the kidney with negative surgical margins; pathological stage was pT2a, Nx, Mx.

Since the patient's surgery, he has been seen in follow up every 6 months with CT imaging. To date, he has remained without evidence of any local or distant tumour recurrence.

Pathologic correlate

Gross examination revealed a firm-to-rubbery 10 cm tumor located in the lower pole of the left kidney. The tumor was tan brown with areas of hemorrhage and a pale yellow scarred area measuring 3.2 cm.

Microscopic examination showed a solid renal tumor. The cells were intermediate to large in size with partially vacuolated eosinophilic cytoplasms. The nuclei were round (non-resinoid) and without prominent nucleoli or apparent perinuclear halos. The tumor was classified as ISUP nucleolar grade 1 of 4. (Fig. 2). There was no necrosis, sarcomatoid change or increased number of mitotic figures. The tumor cells stained positive for PAX8, AE1/AE3, CAM 5.2, p504S, and EMA. The tumor cells were negative for SDHB, CD117, CK7, CK20, CD10, vimentin, RCC, S100, HMB-45, Melan-A, myogenin, SMA, calretinin, inhibin, DOG1, E-cadherin, and CD56 (Fig. 3).

Genetic testing and counselling

The absence of SDHB staining by immunohistochemistry confirmed SDH -deficient RCC. Most individuals with SDH -deficient RCC have underlying germline mutations in one of the SDH genes. The patient subsequently underwent genetic counselling and germline mutation analysis of the SDH genes was carried out. This revealed a pathogenic mutation in the *SDHB* gene.

Since there is an increased risk of paragangliomas and pheochromocytomas in SDHB mutation carriers, surveillance for these neoplasms was carried out. A baseline CT scan of the neck/chest/abdomen/pelvis, utilized as the patient's body habitus precluded MRI scanning, revealed no significant abnormalities aside from post-operative changes post partial nephrectomy. Similarly, baseline 24-h urinary collection for metanephrines and catecholamines was within normal limits. He will continue to undergo annual

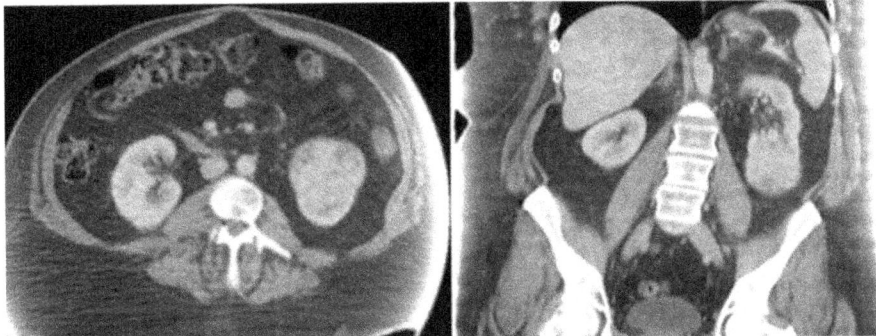

Fig. 1 Abdominal computed tomography imaging of the patient shows a large exophytic heterogeneous mass in the lower pole of the left kidney

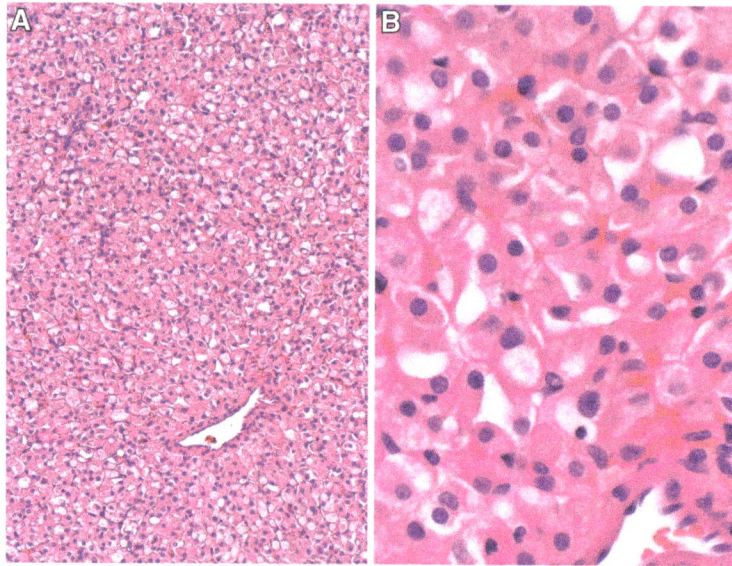

Fig. 2 H&E stain. (**a**) 100x original magnification and (**b**) 400x original magnification micrographs showing abundant eosinophilic cytoplasm that is partially vacuolated. The nuclei are round and low grade without no prominent nucleoli or perinuclear halos

or biennial biochemical and radiographic surveillance for PC and PGL. Additionally, genetic testing has been offered to family members, who are at risk of inheriting the *SDHB* mutation.

Discussion and conclusions

Succinate dehydrogenase is required for energy metabolism in cells. It is a part of the Krebs tricarboxylic acid cycle and the mitochondrial electron transport chain. It is composed of four subunits: SDHA, SDHB, SDHC, and SDHD. Anchored by SDHC and SDHD, the catalytic subunits SDHA and SDHB convert succinate to fumarate and pass it on to the next enzyme in the cycle, fumarate hydroxylase (FH) [7]. Mutations in FH are known to underlie the development of Hereditary Leiomyomatosis and Renal Cell Carcinomas (HLRCCs), a hereditary syndrome of RCC [8]. Mutations in SDH had been implicated in familial and sporadic pheochromocytomas and paragangliomas, but not in the development of RCC until recently.

Given the common mitochondrial location of SDH and FH, the possibility of mutations in SDH underlying the pathogenesis of RCCs was explored by Vanharanta et al. in 2004 [1]. By examining a database of patients with symptomatic paragangliomas, they identified 2 members form the same family who had mutations in SDH as well as RCCs (24 and 26 years old respectively). Similarly, in a database of early onset RCC patients they identified a 22-year-old patient with an SDH mutation, who had a RCC and whose mother had a cardiac paraganglioma. These findings suggested a connection between SDH mutations, pheochromocytomas/paragangliomas, and RCCs [1].

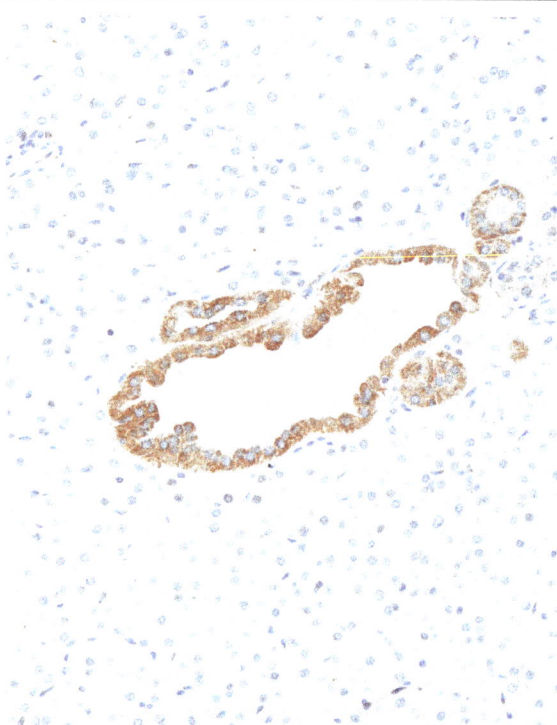

Fig. 3 Micrograph showing a section of tumor stained with an SDHB immunostain. The tumour characteristically has lost staining; however, staining is preserved in an entrapped benign tubular structure (200x original magnification)

Since its first description there have been additional larger studies exploring characteristics of patients with SDH deficient tumours. One of the larger cohorts was the Gill series which included 27 patients with SDH-deficient RCC [3]. From these studies clinical and pathological features were able to be identified.

The mean age of patients was about 37 years, with a slight male predominance of 1.7:1. Approximately 15% of patients had a personal history of gastrointestinal stromal tumours (GISTs), 15% a personal history of paragangliomas (PGLs), 22% had a family history for RCC, 26% had a family history positive for PGLs, and 4% had a positive family history of GISTs [3]. Our patient was a 49-year-old male who did not have a personal or family history of RCC, GISTs, pheochromocytomas, or PGLs.

Pathologically, the colour of SDH-deficient RCC tumours range from tan to red. The majority are well-circumscribed solid lesions with cystic changes being common. The average size of the tumor is about 55 mm. Microscopically, SDH-deficient RCC have solid architecture, eosinophilic cells with clear (flocculent) cytoplasmic inclusions, round nuclei with mildly granular chromatin pattern, and solid architecture. The most characteristic feature is the vacuoles or flocculent cytoplasmic inclusions; however, it may not be prominent in all areas of the tumour. Typically they are low ISUP nucleolar grade but may be sarcomatoid [3]. Our patient's morphologic findings were largely in keeping the typical findings described for SDH-deficient RCC.

Immunohistochemically, SDH-deficient RCCs are generally positive for PAX8 and EMA, and negative for CK7, CK20, AE1/AE3, and CD117. Immunohistochemical loss of SDHB is a diagnostic requirement. In SDHB-, SDHC- and SDHD-deficient RCCs, tumour cells are negative for SDHB but positive for SDHA. In contrast tumor cells are negative for both SDHA and SDHB in SDHA-deficient RCC [4]. Neuroendocrine markers and epithelial markers are also generally negative. Gill et al. reported that all patients with SDH-deficient RCC who underwent germline mutation testing were found to harbour a pathogenic mutation in one of the SDH subunits. Our patient's tumour was negative for SDHB and matched the expected immuno-profile. Subsequent germline mutation analysis confirmed a mutation in SDHB, the most commonly mutated gene in SDH deficient RCC.

The main differential diagnosis to consider are other renal tumours with eosinophilic cytoplasms such as renal oncocytoma and chromophobe RCC [9]. A full list of differential diagnoses to consider and defining features for each are summarized in Table 1.

Table 1 Differential diagnosis of eosinophilic renal cell carcinoma and associated characteristic features

	Macroscopic features	Microscopic features	Immunohistochemistry
Renal Oncocytoma	Classically mahogany brown, well-circumscribed lesion with a central scar	Small solid nests of cells within myxoid or hyalinized stroma. Densely eosinophilic cytoplasm. Nuclei are uniform and round. Prominent nucleoli, typically lacking binucleanation.	Cytokeratin 7: isolated scattered cell staining.
Chromophobe RCC	Usually solitary well-circumscribed grey-beige colored lesion	Solid growth pattern with thin fibrovascular septa. Abundant cytoplasm with prominent cell borders. Nuclei with preserved chromatin and irregular, winkled nuclear membrane.	Cytokeratin 7; usually diffuse staining
Clear cell RCC, eosinophilic variant	Generally golden/yellow color with extensive hemorrhage and necrosis.	Clear cells, although the cytoplasm may be eosinophilic in higher grade tumours. Nested growth pattern. Rich sinusoidal vasculature, often called "chicken wire-like" vasculature.	Positive for CD10, CA-9, EMA, vimentin, and RCC antigen. Negative for CK7 and high-molecular weight keratin. SDHB signal may be weak due to the abundant clear cytoplasm.
TF3 translocation RCC	Yellow-tan with areas of hemorrhage and necrosis	Papillary architecture lined by clear and eosinophilic cells with abundant psammoma bodies. Clear to pale pink fluffy cytoplasm.	Positive for TFE3
SDH-deficient RCC	Tan to red well-circumscribed solid lesions with cystic changes common.	Eosinophilic cells with clear (flocculent) cytoplasmic inclusions, round nuclei with mildly granular chromatin pattern, and solid architecture.	Loss of SDHB is a diagnostic requirement Positive for PAX8 and EMA Negative for CK7, CK20, AE1/AE3, and CD117
Other:	Hybrid oncocytic/chromophobe tumour, tubulocystic carcinoma, papillary RCC, Follicular thyroid-like carcinoma, hereditary leiomyomatosis-associated RCC, acquired cystic kidney disease-associated RCC, epitheloid angiomyolipoma, unclassified RCC, Rhabdoid RCC, MiTF translocation carcinomas		

In the Gill series, the follow up ranged from 0 to 368 months with a mean of 55 months [2]. During that time 9 out of the 27 patients (33%) developed metastatic disease. Two of them occurred after prolonged follow-up (5.5 and 30 years). Four died of metastatic disease at a mean of 18 months after presentation, all of whom had ISUP nuclear grade of 3 or 4 and 3 of whom had coagulative necrosis. Based on this, targeted therapy against vascular endothelial growth factor, mammalian target of rapamycin, and tyrosine kinase have been considered for patients with adverse prognostic factors such as high nuclear grade, coagulative necrosis, or sarcomatoid differentiation. Patients with low-grade tumors showing typical histologic features and an ISUP nuclear grade 2 were usually cured by excision alone. For our patient, a nephron-sparing surgery in the form of left partial nephrectomy was chosen. He had negative margins and no adverse prognostic indicators on pathology. Given these findings no adjuvant treatments were recommended.

Our case illustrates the importance of being familiar with SDH-deficient RCC. The patient described had no personal or family history of RCC, PGL/PC or GIST. The neoplasm was unilateral and unifocal. Finally, the age of onset was not particularly early. Without the identification of SDHB deficiency, this patient's predisposition to PC/PGL and metachronous RCCs may have gone undetected despite his RCC diagnosis. The identification of an SDH mutation in such cases additionally allows for predictive genetic testing for at risk family members, and subsequent surveillance for RCC and PC/PGL if they harbor the familial mutation. Therefore, when faced with an eosinophilic RCC, pathologists should routinely look for vacuoles or flocculent cytoplasmic inclusions. SDHB immunostaining is useful in eosinophilic renal tumours, especially if the tumor cells are negative for CD117 or there is vacuoles or flocculent cytoplasmic inclusions.

In summary, SDH-deficient renal cell carcinoma is the newest sub-type of RCC that shows distinctive clinical and pathologic features. The tumor can be recognized primarily on the basis of morphology alone, and confirmed with immunohistochemistry. For tumours without adverse pathologic features, excision alone may be a reasonable option, with the addition of regular surveillance for PC and PGLs in those found to harbor germline SDH mutations.

Abbreviations
FH: Fumarate hydroxylase; GIST: Gastrointestinal stromal tumors; HLRCCs: Hereditary Leiomyomatosis and Renal Cell Carcinomas; HOCT: Hybrid oncocytic/chromophobe tumour; ISUP: International Society of Urological Pathology; PC: Pheochromocytomas; PGL: Paragangliomas; RCC: Renal cell carcinoma; SDH: Succinate dehydrogenase; WHO: World Health Organization

Acknowledgements
Dr. Andrew Evans (University Health Network) kindly took the image of the SDHB immunostain and we would like the thank him for this contribution to the manuscript.

Authors' contributions
RK and AK designed and drafted the manuscript. MB, AN, and KZ revised the manuscript. MB and AN contributed the figures. All authors read and approved the final manuscript. All authors are accountable for all aspects of the work.

Consent for publication
Written informed consent was obtained from the patient for publication of this Case Report and any accompanying images.

Competing interests
The authors declare that they have no competing interests.

Author details
[1]Division of Urology, Department of Surgery, The Ottawa Hospital, University of Ottawa, Ottawa, Canada. [2]Division of Pathology, Department of Pathology and Molecular Medicine, McMaster University, Hamilton, ON, Canada. [3]Division of Medical Oncology, Department of Oncology, Juravinski Cancer Centre, McMaster University, Hamilton, ON, Canada. [4]Division of Urology, Department of Surgery, Juravinski Cancer Centre, McMaster University, Hamilton, ON, Canada.

References
1. Vanharanta S, Buchta M, McWhinney SR, et al. Early-onset renal cell carcinoma as a novel extraparaganglial component of SDHB-associated heritable paraganglioma. Am J Hum Genet. 2004;74:153–9.
2. Srigley JR, Delahunt B, Eble JN, Egevad L, Epstein JI, Grignon D, Hes O, Moch H, Montironi R, Tickoo SK, Zhou M. The International Society of Urological Pathology (ISUP) Vancouver classification of renal neoplasia. Am J Surg Pathol. 2013;37(10):1469–89.
3. Gill AJ, Hes O, Papathomas T, et al. Succinate dehydrogenase (SDH) – deficient renal carcinoma: a morphologically distinct entity. Am J Surg Pathol. 2014;38:1588–602.
4. Yakirevich E, Ali SM, Mega A, et al. A novel SDHA-deficient RCC revealed by comprehensive genomic profiling. Am J Surg Pathol. 2015;39(6):858–63.
5. Williamson SR, Eble JN, Amin MB, et al. Succinate dehrdrogenase-deficient renal cell carcinoma: detailed characterization of 11 tumors defining a unique subtype of renal cell carcinoma. Mod Pathol. 2015;28:80–94.
6. Ricketts CJ, Shuch B, Vocke CD, et al. Succinate dehydrogenase-deficient kidney cancer (SDH-RCC): an aggressive example of the Warburg effect in cancer. J Urol. 2012;188:2063–71.
7. Eng C, Kiuru M, Fernandez MJ, Aaltonen LA. A role for mitochondrial enzymes in inherited neoplasia and beyond. Nat Rev Cancer. 2003;3:193–202.
8. Tomlinson IPMT, Alam NA, Rowan AJ, et al. Germline mutations in the fumarate hydratase gene predispose to dominantly inherited uterine fibroids, skin leiomyomata and renal cell cancer. Nat Genet. 2002;30:406–10.
9. Kryvenko ON, Jorda M, Argani P, Epstein JI. Diagnostic approach to eosinophilic renal neoplasms. Arch Pathol Lab Med. 2014;138(11):1531–41.

Permissions

List of Contributors

Jeanette E Eckel-Passow
Division of Biomedical Statistics and Informatics, Mayo Clinic, Rochester, MN, USA

Daniel J Serie and Alexander S Parker
Department of Health Sciences Research, Mayo Clinic, 4500 San Pablo Road, Jacksonville, FL 32224, USA

Brian M Bot
Statistical Genetics, Sage Bionetworks, Seattle, WA, USA

Richard W Joseph
Department of Hematology and Oncology, Mayo Clinic, Jacksonville, FL, USA

John C Cheville
Laboratory Medicine and Pathology, Mayo Clinic, Rochester, MN, USA

Difu Fan, Leming Song, Donghua Xie, Min Hu, Zuofeng Peng, Tairong Liu, Chuance Du, Lunfeng Zhu, Lei Yao, Jianrong Huang, Zhongsheng Yang, Shulin Guo, Wen Qin and Jiuqing Zhong
Department of Urology, The Affiliated Ganzhou City People's Hospital of Nanchang University, Ganzhou, Jiangxi 341000, China

Xiaohui Liao
Dermatology Institute of Gan County, Jiangxi 341100, China

Zhangqun Ye
Department of Urology, Tongji Hospital, Tongji Medical College, Huazhong University of Science and Technology, Wuhan, Hubei 430030, China

Bishoy A Gayed, Ganesh Raj, Arthur I Sagalowsky and Yair Lotan
Department of Urology, University of Texas Southwestern Medical Center, Dallas, Texas, USA

Jessica Gillen
Department Internal Medicine, University of Texas Southwestern Medical Center, Dallas, Texas, USA

Alana Christie, Xian-Jin Xie and Jingsheng Yan
Department of Clinical Science, University of Texas Southwestern Medical Center, Dallas, Texas, USA

Samuel Peña-Llopis
Department of Developmental Biology, University of Texas Southwestern Medical Center, Dallas, Texas, USA

Jose A Karam
Department of Urology, MD Anderson Cancer Center, Houston, Texas, USA

Vitaly Margulis
Department of Urology, University of Texas Southwestern Medical Center, Dallas, Texas, USA
Department of Urology, UT Southwestern Medical Center at Dallas, 5323 Harry Hines Blvd., Dallas 75390-9110, Texas, USA

James Brugarolas
Department Internal Medicine, University of Texas Southwestern Medical Center, Dallas, Texas, USA
Department of Developmental Biology, University of Texas Southwestern Medical Center, Dallas, Texas, USA

XiaWa Mao, Gang Xu, HuiFeng Wu and JiaQuan Xiao
Department of Urology, The Second Affiliated Hospital of Zhejiang University School of Medicine, Hangzhou, P.R. China

Linfeng Xu, Rong Yang, Weidong Gan, Xiancheng Chen, Xuefeng Qiu, Kai Fu, Jin Huang, Guancheng Zhu and Hongqian Guo
Department of Urology, The Affiliated Drum Tower Hospital of Medical College of Nanjing University, Zhongshan Road 321, Nanjing, Jiangsu Province 210008, China

Akinori Sato, Takako Asano, Makoto Isono, Keiichi Ito and Tomohiko Asano
Department of Urology, National Defense Medical College, 3-2 Namiki, Tokorozawa, Saitama 359-8513, Japan

Yimin Wang, Shanwen Chen, Wei Wang and Baiye Jin
Department of Urology, the First Affiliated Hospital of Medical College, Zhejiang University, No. 79 Qing Chun Road, 310003 Hangzhou, China

Jianyong Liu
Sidney kimmel Comprehensive Cancer Center, Johns Hopkins University School of Medicine, 21128 Baltimore, USA

Teele Kuusk, Fausto Biancari, Vito D'Andrea, Aare Mehik and Markku H. Vaarala
Department of Surgery and Medical Research Center Oulu, Oulu University Hospital and University of Oulu, 90029 OYS Oulu, Finland

Brian Lane and Conrad Tobert
Division of Urology, Michigan State University, Grand Rapids, Michigan, USA

Steven Campbell
Department of Urology, Glickman Urological and Kidney Institute, Cleveland Clinic, Cleveland, Ohio, USA

Uri Rimon
Sheba Medical Center, Tel-Hashomer, Sackler School of Medicine, Tel-Aviv University, Tel-Aviv, Israel

Takuya Koie, Chikara Ohyama, Takahiro Yoneyama, Hayato Yamamoto, Atsushi Imai, Shingo Hatakeyama, Yasuhiro Hashimoto, Tohru Yoneyama, Yuki Tobisawa and Kazuyuki Mori
Department of Urology, Hirosaki University Graduate School of Medicine, 5 Zaifucho, Hirosaki 036-8562, Japan

Yi-Ting Lin
Department of Urology, St. Joseph's Hospital, 74, Sinsheng Road, Huwei County, Yunlin Hsien 632, Taiwan
Research Institute of Biotechnology, Hungkuang University, 34 Chung-Chie Road, Shalu County, Taichung City 43302, Taiwan

Charng-Cherng Chyau and Robert Y Peng
Research Institute of Biotechnology, Hungkuang University, 34 Chung-Chie Road, Shalu County, Taichung City 43302, Taiwan

Chia-Chun Huang
Department of Radiation Oncology, Changhua Christian Hospital, No.135 Nan Shiau Street, Changhua 500, Taiwan

Kuan-Chou Chen
Department of Urology, Taipei Medical University-Shuang Ho Hospital, Taipei Medical University, 250, Wu-Xin St, Xin-Yi District 110 Taipei, Taiwan

Department of Urology, School of Medicine, Taipei Medical University, 250, Wu-Xin St, Xin-Yi District 110 Taipei, Taiwan

Kyu-Hyun Han, Ji-Jing Yan, Jae-Ghi Lee and Eun Mi Lee
Transplantation Research Institute, Seoul National University College of Medicine, Seoul, Republic of Korea

Ki Won Kim
Nephrology clinic, Center for Clinical Specialty, National Cancer Center, Seoul, Republic of Korea

Miyeon Han and Eun Jin Cho
Department of Internal Medicine, Seoul National University College of Medicine, Seoul, Republic of Korea

Seong Sik Kang, Hye Jin Lim and Tai Yeon Koo
Transplantation Center, Seoul National University Hospital, 101 Daehak-ro, Jongno-gu, Seoul 110-744, Republic of Korea

Curie Ahn
Transplantation Research Institute, Seoul National University College of Medicine, Seoul, Republic of Korea
Department of Internal Medicine, Seoul National University College of Medicine, Seoul, Republic of Korea
Transplantation Center, Seoul National University Hospital, 101 Daehak-ro, Jongno-gu, Seoul 110-744, Republic of Korea

Jaeseok Yang
Transplantation Research Institute, Seoul National University College of Medicine, Seoul, Republic of Korea
Transplantation Center, Seoul National University Hospital, 101 Daehak-ro, Jongno-gu, Seoul 110-744, Republic of Korea

Hui Zhang, Xinyu Ren, Di Yang and Ruie Feng
Department of Pathology, Peking Union Medical College Hospital, Chinese Academy of Medical Sciences and Peking Union Medical College, 1 Shuaifu Yuan, Beijing 100730, PR China

Wen Zhang
Department of Rheumatology, Peking Union Medical College Hospital, Chinese Academy of Medical Sciences and Peking Union Medical College, Beijing 100730, PR China

Cezary Szczylik
Department of Oncology, Military Institute of Medicine, Warsaw, Poland

Pawel Sobczuk
Department of Oncology, Military Institute of Medicine, Warsaw, Poland
The Second Faculty of Medicine with the English Division and the Physiotherapy Division, Medical University of Warsaw, Warsaw, Poland

Fei Lian
Emory University School of Medicine, Atlanta, GA, USA

Anna M Czarnecka
Department of Oncology, Military Institute of Medicine, Warsaw, Poland
Department of Oncology, Military Institute of Medicine, Laboratory of Molecular Oncology, Szaserow 128, 04-141 Warsaw, Poland

Peng Jiang, Chaojun Wang and Liping Xie
Department of Urology, The First Affiliated Hospital, School of Medicine, Zhejiang University, Qingchun Road 79, Hangzhou 310003, Zhejiang Province, China

Jun Li
Department of Pathology, The First Affiliated Hospital, School of Medicine, Zhejiang University, Hangzhou, Zhejiang Province, China

Jianjian Xiang
Department of Ultrasonography, The First Affiliated Hospital, School of Medicine, Zhejiang University, Hangzhou, Zhejiang Province, China

Honghan Gong, Lei Gao, Xi-Jian Dai, Fuqing Zhou, Ning Zhang, Xianjun Zeng, Jian Jiang and Laichang He
Department of Radiology, the First Affiliated Hospital of Nanchang University, 17 Yongwai Zheng Street, Donghu District, Nanchang, Jiangxi 330006, China

Go Noguchi, Sohgo Tsutsumi, Masato Yasui, Susumu Umemoto and Takeshi Kishida
Department of Urology, Kanagawa Cancer Center, 2-3-2, Nakao, Asahi-ku, Yokohama, Kanagawa 2418515, Japan

Shinji Ohtake, Noboru Nakaigawa and Masahiro Yao
Department of Urology, Yokohama City University Graduate School of Medicine, Yokohama, Japan

Abdelmoneim E. M. Kheir
Department of Paediatrics and Child Health, Faculty of Medicine, University of Khartoum and Soba University Hospital, Khartoum, Sudan

Aziza M. Elnaeema
Paediatric Surgeon and Paediatric Urologist, Soba University Hospital, Ahfad University for Women, Omdurman, Sudan

Sara M. A. Gafer
Department of Paediatrics, Soba University Hospital, Khartoum, Sudan

Sawsan A. Mohammed
Department of Histopathology, Soba University Hospital, Khartoum, Sudan

Mustafa E. Bahar
Department of Radiology, Soba University Hospital, Khartoum, Sudan

Joo Yong Lee, Won Sik Ham and Young Deuk Choi
Department of Urology, Severance Hospital, Urological Science Institute, Yonsei University College of Medicine, Seoul, South Korea

Seong Uk Jeh
Department of Urology, Gyeongsang National University Hospital, Gyeongsang National University School of Medicine, Jinju, South Korea

Man Deuk Kim
Department of Radiology, Severance Hospital, Research Institute of Radiological Science, Yonsei University College of Medicine, Seoul, South Korea

Dong Hyuk Kang
Department of Urology, Inha University School of Medicine, Incheon, South Korea

Jong Kyou Kwon
Department of Urology, Severance Check-Up, Yonsei University Health System, Seoul, South Korea

Kang Su Cho
Department of Urology, Gangnam Severance Hospital, Urological Science Institute, Yonsei University College of Medicine, 211 Eonju-ro, Gangnam-gu, Seoul 06273, South Korea

Simon Ouellet, Alexander Nguyen and Robert Sabbagh
Department of Surgery, Division of Urology, Université de Sherbrooke, Centre Hospitalier Universitaire de Sherbrooke (CHUS), 3001 12e avenue Nord, Sherbrooke, QC J1H 5N4, Canada

Audrey Binette
Department of Obstetrics and Gynaecology, Université de Sherbrooke, Centre Hospitalier Universitaire de Sherbrooke (CHUS), 3001 12e avenue Nord, Sherbrooke, Canada

Perrine Garde-Granger
Department of Pathology, Université de Sherbrooke, Centre Hospitalier Universitaire de Sherbrooke (CHUS), 3001 12e avenue Nord, Sherbrooke, Canada

Victor C. Kok
Division of Medical Oncology, Cancer Center of Kuang Tien General Hospital, 117 Shatien Rd, Taichung 43303, Taiwan
Department of Biomedical Informatics, Asia University, Taichung 41354, Taiwan

Jung-Tsung Kuo
Division of Biostatistics, Institute of Public Health, School of Medicine, National Yang-Ming University, Taipei 11221, Taiwan

William Keith Ballentine III and Majid Mirzazadeh
Department of Urology, Wake Forest Baptist Health, Medical Center Blvd, Winston-Salem, NC 27157, USA

Fernandino Vilson
Wake Forest School of Medicine, Winston-Salem, NC 27157, USA

Raymond B Dyer
Department of Radiology, Wake Forest Baptist Health, Winston-Salem, NC 27157, USA

Kentaro Mizuno, Akihiro Nakane, Hidenori Nishio, Yoshinobu Moritoki, Hideyuki Kamisawa, Satoshi Kurokawa, Taiki Kato, Ryosuke Ando, Tetsuji Maruyama and Takahiro Yasui
Department of Nephro-urology, Nagoya City University Graduate School of Medical Sciences, Nagoya, Japan

Yutaro Hayashi
Department of Pediatric urology, Nagoya City University Graduate School of Medical Sciences, 1 Kawasumi, Mizuho-cho, Mizuho-ku, Nagoya, Japan

Alissar El Chediak, Deborah Mukherji, Sally Temraz and Ali Shamseddine
Department of Internal Medicine, Division of Hematology/Oncology, American University of Beirut - Medical Center, Riad El Solh, Beirut 110 72020, Lebanon

Samer Nassif, Sara Sinno and Rami Mahfouz
Department of Pathology and Laboratory Medicine, American University of Beirut - Medical Center, Beirut, Lebanon

Jeanette E. Eckel-Passow
Division of Biomedical Statistics and Informatics, Mayo Clinic, Rochester, MN, USA

Daniel J. Serie and Alexander S. Parker
Department of Health Sciences Research, Mayo Clinic, 4500 San Pablo Road, Jacksonville, FL 32224, USA

John C. Cheville
Laboratory Medicine and Pathology, Mayo Clinic, Rochester, MN, USA

Thai H. Ho
Division of Hematology and Medical Oncology, Mayo Clinic, Scottsdale, AZ, USA

Payal Kapur
Department of Pathology, University of Texas Southwestern Medical Center, Dallas, TX, USA

James Brugarolas
Kidney Cancer Program, Simmons Comprehensive Cancer Center, University of Texas Southwestern Medical Center, Dallas, TX, USA
Division of Hematology-Oncology, University of Texas Southwestern Medical Center, Dallas, TX, USA

R. Houston Thompson, Bradley C. Leibovich and Eugene D. Kwon
Department of Urology, Mayo Clinic, Rochester, MN, USA

Richard W. Joseph
Division of Hematology/Oncology, Mayo Clinic, Jacksonville, FL, USA

Xiangming Cheng, Gutian Zhang and Xiaogong Li
Department of Urology, Nanjing Drum Tower Hospital, the Affiliated Hospital of Nanjing University Medical School, No. 321 Zhongshan Road, Nanjing 210008, Jiangsu Province, China

Takashi Karashima, Takahira Kuno, Hirofumi Satake, Satoshi Fukata, Chiaki Kawada, Ichiro Yamasaki, Taro Shuin and Keiji Inoue
Department of Urology, Kochi University, Kochi Medical School, Kohasu, Oko, Nankoku, Kochi 783-8505, Japan

Naoto Kuroda
Department of Diagnostic Pathology, Kochi Red Cross Hospital, Kochi-Shi, Kochi 780-0062, Japan

Masakazu Chikazawa
Department of Urology, Izumino Hospital, Kochi-Shi, Kochi 781-0011, Japan

Makoto Hiroi
Laboratory of Diagnostic Pathology, Kochi Medical School Hospital, Kohasu, Oko, Nankoku, Kochi 783-8505, Japan

Weijin Fu, Zhanbin Yang, Zhibin Xie and Haibiao Yan
Department of Urology, The First Affiliated Hospital of GuangXi Medical University, 6 Shuangyong Road, Nanning 530021, GuangXi Zhuang Autonomous Region, People's Republic of China

Se Hoon Park, Su Jin Lee and Ho Yeong Lim
Division of Hematology–Oncology, Department of Medicine, Samsung Medical Center, Sungkyunkwan University School of Medicine, Seoul, Korea

Jae-Lyun Lee
Department of Oncology, Asan Medical Center, University of Ulsan College of Medicine, Seoul, Korea

Se-Hoon Lee
Department of Internal Medicine, Seoul National University Hospital, Seoul, Korea

Moon Jin Kim
Department of Medicine, Myongji Hospital, Goyang-si, Gyeonggi-do, Korea

Yasuyuki Kobayashi, Hiroki Arai and Masahito Honda
Departments of Urology, Kinki Central Hospital of Mutual Aid Association of Public Teachers, 3-1 Kurumazuka, Itami, Hyogo 664-8533, Japan

Takashi Matsumoto
Surgery, Kinki Central Hospital of Mutual Aid Association of Public Teachers, 3-1 Kurumazuka, Itami, Hyogo 664-8533, Japan

Kyotaro Yoshida
Pathology, Kinki Central Hospital of Mutual Aid Association of Public Teachers, 3-1 Kurumazuka, Itami, Hyogo 664-8533, Japan

James A. Kuzman, Joseph Merriman, Shiven B. Patel, Andrew W. Hahn, Anitha Alex, Dan Albertson, David M. Gill and Neeraj Agarwal
University of Utah Huntsman Cancer Institute, Salt Lake City, UT, USA

David D. Stenehjem
University of Utah Huntsman Cancer Institute, Salt Lake City, UT, USA
Department of Pharmacotherapy, College of Pharmacy, University of Utah, Salt Lake City, UT, USA

Archana M. Agarwal
Department of Pathology and ARUP Laboratories, University of Utah, Salt Lake City, UT, USA

Ti-Yuan Yang and Wun-Rong Lin
Department of Urology, Mackay Memorial Hospital, Taipei, Taiwan
Department of Medicine, Mackay Medical College, Taipei, Taiwan

Allen W. Chiu
Department of Urology, Mackay Memorial Hospital, Taipei, Taiwan
Department of Medicine, Mackay Medical College, Taipei, Taiwan
School of Medicine, National Yang-Ming University, Taipei, Taiwan

Ravi Kumar
Division of Urology, Department of Surgery, The Ottawa Hospital, University of Ottawa, Ottawa, Canada

Michael Bonert and Asghar Naqvi
Division of Pathology, Department of Pathology and Molecular Medicine, McMaster University, Hamilton, ON, Canada

Kevin Zbuk
Division of Medical Oncology, Department of Oncology, Juravinski Cancer Centre, McMaster University, Hamilton, ON, Canada

Anil Kapoor
Division of Urology, Department of Surgery, Juravinski Cancer Centre, McMaster University, Hamilton, ON, Canada

Index